THE
EVERYTHING
LOW-FODMAP DIET
COOKBOOK

Dear Reader,

I understand what it's like to endure irritable bowel syndrome (IBS) because I once suffered on a daily basis. Ever since I was a child my family remembers my not feeling well after most meals, but we never knew why. Like many others, my symptoms became worse in my early thirties after a series of stressful events. Doctors were unable to help me, and no one knew how to take care of my awfully bloated abdomen or my need to sprint to the bathroom. One day I finally reached the point when I had had enough of my symptoms and I began researching a better way to treat my gut and my body, without the use of drugs.

Nutrition, wellness, and healthy food are just a few of my favorite things and when I started writing my blog *www.FODMAPLife.com* and pouring my passion into my posts, I realized I could help others to feel better too. I began studying to become a Certified Nutritionist Consultant (CNC) with the Natural Healing Institute. I received training in the Low-FODMAP Diet Training Program™ and I now use my training and education to teach people about the low-FODMAP diet, nutrition, and mind-body wellness.

With this book I hope to inspire you to cook delicious, flavorful dishes, and learn a few wellness tips on how to be better to your gut, body, and mind. You'll find more inspiration, advice, and recipes on *www.FODMAPLife.com* as well as *www.BonCalme.com* and don't forget to connect with others on all my FODMAP Life social media channels.

Be good to yourself and your gut!

Colleen Francioli, CNC

T0057230

Welcome to the EVERYTHING® Series!

These handy, accessible books give you all you need to tackle a difficult project, gain a new hobby, comprehend a fascinating topic, prepare for an exam, or even brush up on something you learned back in school but have since forgotten.

You can choose to read an Everything® book from cover to cover or just pick out the information you want from our four useful boxes: e-questions, e-facts, e-alerts, and e-ssentials.

We give you everything you need to know on the subject, but throw in a lot of fun stuff along the way, too.

We now have more than 400 Everything® books in print, spanning such wide-ranging categories as weddings, pregnancy, cooking, music instruction, foreign language, crafts, pets, New Age, and so much more. When you're done reading them all, you can finally say you know Everything®!

QUESTION

Answers to common questions

FACT

Important snippets of information

ALERT

Urgent warnings

ESSENTIAL

Quick handy tips

PUBLISHER Karen Cooper

MANAGING EDITOR, EVERYTHING® SERIES Lisa Laing

COPY CHIEF Casey Ebert

ASSISTANT PRODUCTION EDITOR Jo-Anne Duhamel

ACQUISITIONS EDITOR Hillary Thompson

SENIOR DEVELOPMENT EDITOR Brett Palana-Shanahan

EVERYTHING® SERIES COVER DESIGNER Erin Alexander

Visit the entire Everything® series at *www.everything.com*

THE
EVERYTHING®
LOW-FODMAP DIET
COOKBOOK

Colleen Francioli, CNC

Adams Media
New York London Toronto Sydney New Delhi

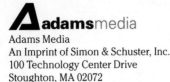

Adams Media
An Imprint of Simon & Schuster, Inc.
100 Technology Center Drive
Stoughton, MA 02072

Copyright © 2016 by Simon & Schuster, Inc.

All rights reserved, including the right to reproduce this book or portions thereof in any form whatsoever. For information address Adams Media Subsidiary Rights Department, 1230 Avenue of the Americas, New York, NY 10020.

An Everything® Series Book.
Everything® and everything.com® are registered trademarks of Simon & Schuster, Inc.

ADAMS MEDIA and colophon are trademarks of Simon and Schuster.

For information about special discounts for bulk purchases, please contact Simon & Schuster Special Sales at 1-866-506-1949 or business@simonandschuster.com.

The Simon & Schuster Speakers Bureau can bring authors to your live event. For more information or to book an event contact the Simon & Schuster Speakers Bureau at 1-866-248-3049 or visit our website at www.simonspeakers.com.

Nutritional statistics by Nicole Cormier, RD, LDN.

Manufactured in the United States of America

4 2021

Library of Congress Cataloging-in-Publication Data has been applied for.

ISBN 978-1-4405-9529-5
ISBN 978-1-4405-9530-1 (ebook)

This book is intended as general information only, and should not be used to diagnose or treat any health condition. In light of the complex, individual, and specific nature of health problems, this book is not intended to replace professional medical advice. The ideas, procedures, and suggestions in this book are intended to supplement, not replace, the advice of a trained medical professional. Consult your physician before adopting any of the suggestions in this book, as well as about any condition that may require diagnosis or medical attention. The author and publisher disclaim any liability arising directly or indirectly from the use of this book.

Always follow safety and commonsense cooking protocol while using kitchen utensils, operating ovens and stoves, and handling uncooked food. If children are assisting in the preparation of any recipe, they should always be supervised by an adult.

Many of the designations used by manufacturers and sellers to distinguish their products are claimed as trademarks. Where those designations appear in this book and Simon & Schuster, Inc., was aware of a trademark claim, the designations have been printed with initial capital letters.

Contains material adapted from *The Everything® Guide to the Low-FODMAP Diet* by Barbara Bolen and Kathleen Bradley, copyright © 2014 by Simon & Schuster, Inc., ISBN 13: 978-1-4405-8173-1.

Colleen Francioli would like to dedicate this book to her mother, Rita, who was loving, caring, and selfless and helped so many people to feel better. She would also like to dedicate the book to all the fans and friends of FODMAP Life, for their honesty, kindness, and support.

The author would like to thank her mentors Patsy Catos, MS, RD, LD, and Barbara Bolen, PhD, for their partnership on past projects and for answering a few questions along the way. Many thanks also to Kathleen Bradley, CPC.

Contents

Introduction **9**

01 What Is the Low-FODMAP Diet? / 11

Who Developed the Diet? **12**

Why Go on the Low-FODMAP Diet? **13**

Working with Your Doctor **16**

What Are FODMAPs? **17**

A Breakdown of FODMAP Groups **19**

The Elimination and Challenge Phases **23**

How to Read Labels **25**

Understanding Servings **26**

Wheat and Gluten **28**

Make Ahead **30**

Eating Out **31**

Wellness Tips **33**

02 Breakfast / 37

03 Appetizers / 63

04 Soups and Salads / 77

05 Vegetables and Sides / 105

06 Sandwiches / 121

07 Poultry, Pork, and Beef / 127

08 Fish and Shellfish / 155

09 Vegan and Vegetarian Main Dishes / 171

10   Snacks and Main Dishes for Kids / 193

11   Cookies and Bars / 213

12   Desserts / 229

13   Condiments, Sauces, and Dressings / 245

14   Snacks / 265

15   Drinks / 271

16   From Scratch / 281

Appendix A: Sample Menu Plans and Snack Suggestions **288**

Appendix B: Low- and High-FODMAP Foods List **292**

Appendix C: Sources **308**

Appendix D: Additional Resources **311**

Standard U.S./Metric Measurement Conversions **312**

Index **313**

Introduction

NOT MANY PEOPLE LIKE to talk about irritable bowel syndrome (IBS) because it is so personal and oftentimes utterly embarrassing. Some people dread the thought of talking to friends and family or even their doctors about the IBS symptoms they endure, such as gas, bloating, distension, constipation (IBS-C), diarrhea (IBS-D), alternating constipation and diarrhea (IBS-M), and abdominal pain.

After all, it's not easy to look a doctor in the face and describe your bowel habits, color, and consistency of stool! You absolutely can't tell your boss why you were late (again). Your friends or family wonder why you were late or didn't show up (again), and having to return to the table after an almost-missed rendezvous with the toilet is "gut-wrenching" all on its own, never mind the episode that just took place in the bathroom. And sometimes you never know when it's truly "safe" to leave home or if you'll find a bathroom in time.

There is still no known cure for IBS, and receiving a diagnosis can take months or even years. Doctors cannot do much to help bring about symptom relief, and some prescribed medications can make matters worse.

If you have IBS, your wardrobe has evolved to pants with elastic bands, or long shirts and skirts, billowy dresses and sweaters. You try to hide under your clothes; meanwhile, wearing larger clothes doesn't make you happier and neither does the pain and pressure you feel in your gut and abdomen.

While some people enjoy eating, the thought of eating may bring about some level of fear for you—are you going to feel sick afterward? Will this food or combination of foods keep you from having a bowel movement for a long time or will it catapult you into the nearest bathroom?

Living with IBS can make it hard to lead a normal life, but don't worry, it's not "all in your head." You are not alone. IBS affects over 58 million (1 in 7) Americans and in developed countries, it may affect up to 1 in 5 adults. The cause of IBS is still unknown. Some experts believe symptoms of IBS are brought on by a disruption to the interaction between the brain, nervous system, and the gut, and that food, stress, and/or a person's environment can act as "triggers" for symptoms.

Mild or debilitating IBS symptoms can be chronic or episodic, meaning they can come and go or last for weeks or even years. In a survey of 1,597 patients with IBS, 50 percent said they suffered from IBS symptoms for more than 10 years and 16 percent suffered for 21–30 years. With regard to the frequency of IBS, 57 percent said they experienced it daily, 25 percent said weekly, and 14 percent said monthly.

If all of this rings true to you, the low-FODMAP diet may be the answer you have been looking for. The low-FODMAP diet is an evidence-based dietary treatment plan that provides an effective approach for functional gut symptoms.

If you've heard about the low-FODMAP diet, you might have heard "FODMAP" pronounced several ways and wondered what it's all about. FODMAP is an acronym that stands for certain short-chain carbohydrates found in foods that produce undesirable feelings, pain, and discomfort within the digestive system. FODMAPs aren't necessarily a bad thing, as they are present in many healthy, natural foods. They can just become problematic for people with IBS. With proper guidance, dieters learn how to relieve symptoms by restricting all foods high in FODMAPs for a short period of time and then reintroducing them to see what foods they should exclude from their diet, the foods they should limit, and the foods they can enjoy. The low-FODMAP diet helps take the guesswork out of wondering which ingredient(s) in a meal or which foods over the course of a day caused you to become bloated, distended, or constipated—or made you run for the bathroom.

This book provides a short basic guide on FODMAPs to help get you acquainted and confident with the diet and also includes meal plans, snack ideas, and additional health resources. The recipes steal the show, as they are flavorful and fun; some have been inspired by different cultures; most are very easy to make; and some are popular favorites re-created to be low-FODMAP. After you try a few recipes in this book and get more acquainted with low-FODMAP foods and ingredients, your confidence will be boosted, your creative juices will be flowing, and hopefully you too will be inspired to create your own low-FODMAP dishes.

For more information and tips around the science and dietary approach of the diet check out *The Everything® Guide to the Low-FODMAP Diet.*

CHAPTER 1

What Is the Low-FODMAP Diet?

The low-FODMAP diet is an elimination diet designed to help people who endure symptoms of irritable bowel syndrome (IBS) and other digestive issues. This plan is a dietary approach to IBS, and it can help you identify common foods you eat regularly that may actually be triggering issues in your body. The diet is based on food components known as FODMAPs (fermentable, oligosaccharides, disaccharides, monosaccharides, and polyols)—components that contribute to digestive symptoms in patients with IBS. Ultimately, this diet will help you identify and eliminate the types of FODMAPs that are causing your problems, and get you to a place where you can enjoy a wide range of foods without experiencing symptoms.

Who Developed the Diet?

Witnessing her patients with celiac disease and difficult-to-treat symptoms led nutritionist Dr. Sue Shepherd to study the role of fructose and fructans in gut symptoms and develop the fructose malabsorption diet. Then after some research and looking at the role of other poorly absorbed, short-chain carbohydrates in patients with IBS and other FGIDs (functional gastrointestinal disorders), Dr. Peter Gibson at Monash University in Australia collaborated with Dr. Shepherd in 1999 to create a more restrictive diet called the low-FODMAP diet. They developed the acronym FODMAP when labeling the food components that contribute to digestive symptoms in patients with IBS. These components consist of short-chain carbohydrates (saccharides) and sugar alcohols (polyols). Dr. Shepherd and Dr. Gibson created the Elimination and Challenge Phases of this diet as a way for IBS patients to understand which foods trigger symptoms. In the beginning of the diet, you will avoid all foods that are high in FODMAPs, and then you will systematically identify which specific FODMAPs are causing your problems.

FACT

Many people are living in pain right now and are unaware their discomfort could be due to consuming onions, garlic, wheat, apples, lactose, sugar-free candy, or other foods high in FODMAPs. Pain and symptoms can include constipation, diarrhea, abdominal pain and distension, lower back pain, lack of sleep, stress, sexual dysfunction, missed work days, and an overall disinterest in social activities.

Prior to the development of the FODMAP concept, a dietary approach was rarely used as first-line therapy for management of IBS and other FGIDs. Although FODMAPs are naturally present in food and the human diet, FODMAP restriction has been found to improve symptom control in people with IBS and other FGIDs. Today, Dr. Gibson, along with Dr. Jacqueline Barrett, Dr. Jane Muir, and a team of researchers are helping to further develop the diet by continuing to test a wide variety of foods for high-FODMAP content and classify which particular FODMAP each food contains.

ALERT

There are several sources online with lists for low-FODMAP and high-FODMAP foods. The best list to follow is that of Monash University. You can download a printable *Low-FODMAP Grocery List* (*www.FODMAPLife .com*) with foods and servings as reported by Monash University, and also download the *Monash FODMAP App* at (*www.med.monash.edu.au/cecs/ gastro/fodmap/iphone-app.html*). If you're using the app, be sure to read this blog post from Monash University first: *http://fodmapmonash .blogspot.com/2015/02/talking-about-traffic-light-system.html.*

Why Go on the Low-FODMAP Diet?

The low-FODMAP diet was designed to offer patients with conditions such as IBS, other functional gastrointestinal disorders (FGIDs) such as SIBO (small intestinal bacterial overgrowth), GERD (gastroesophageal reflux disease), celiac disease, or a gluten intolerance a way of eating that does not aggravate symptoms. It does not necessarily "cure" the underlying problem, but it has been shown to be effective in reducing abdominal pain, bloating, flatulence, constipation, and diarrhea. There is also emerging evidence that the diet may be helpful for people who don't have one of these illnesses, yet experience these same symptoms on a regular basis.

If you have been suffering from intestinal pain or discomfort and think you may be suffering from one of these conditions—but do not yet have a formal diagnosis—it would be helpful to learn more about them so you know the right questions to ask your doctor at your next appointment. Remember, before you begin the low-FODMAP diet, it is essential that you discuss the diet with your doctor. Your doctor is in the best position to ascertain whether the diet is safe for you.

ALERT

If you are experiencing chronic digestive difficulties, it is essential that you speak with your doctor. Many other health problems have symptoms that are quite similar to IBS. It is important to ensure that you have an accurate diagnosis so that you will be assured that you are getting optimal treatment before you start to follow a low-FODMAP diet.

IBS

Doctors have a set of diagnostic criteria, called the Rome III criteria, for making a firm diagnosis of IBS. The Rome criteria require that a person experiences abdominal pain or discomfort along with a marked change in bowel habit for at least six months. In addition, symptoms must have occurred on at least three days of at least three months. At least two of the following must apply:

- Pain is relieved by a bowel movement.
- The onset of pain symptoms is associated with a change in the frequency of bowel movements.
- The onset of pain symptoms is related to a change in the way stool appears.

In the real world, doctors tend to give the diagnosis to anyone who has chronic digestive symptoms without any identifiable reason, regardless of whether or not the symptoms meet the Rome III criteria.

ESSENTIAL

Many people who have IBS report a wide variety of other symptoms that seem to go along with their IBS. Some of these symptoms are also gastrointestinal, such as nausea and heartburn. Other symptoms include dizziness, fatigue, head, back, and overall muscle pain, heart palpitations, and urinary problems.

The diagnosis of IBS is based on symptom report and is made after ruling out other disorders. Typically, your doctor will conduct a comprehensive physical exam, order blood work, and ask you for a stool sample to look for the presence of rectal bleeding. Depending on your symptom picture, the doctor may recommend that you undergo further testing, such as a colonoscopy or endoscopy. These tests are not essential for a diagnosis of IBS, but rather are used to rule out other reasons behind your symptoms. The Rome III criteria were designed to come up with a definitive diagnosis of IBS so as to prevent having patients undergo unnecessary diagnostic procedures.

Food Allergy and Intolerance

A food allergy is an immune system reaction to a particular food that is not harmful to most people. When a person has a food allergy, eating even a small amount of the offending food will prompt the immune system to release chemicals that cause a variety of symptoms. You are probably familiar with typical allergy symptoms—hives, itching, and lip swelling—in addition to the more serious symptoms of difficulty breathing and swelling of the throat. Food allergies can also create gastrointestinal symptoms such as vomiting, diarrhea, and/or abdominal pain. The most common food allergens include eggs, fish and shellfish, milk, peanuts, soy, tree nuts, and wheat.

In an allergic reaction, the body produces antibodies when it encounters what it perceives as an invader. These antibodies are known as immunoglobulin E, or IgE. The IgE reaction triggers the release of histamine and other chemicals, causing allergy symptoms. IgE release can be identified through the use of allergy tests, thus helping to confirm a diagnosis of a food allergy.

A food intolerance, also known as a food sensitivity, is when a person has a negative reaction to a food without it being an allergy. An allergy involves a clear reaction on the part of the immune system (with an IgE response), while a food intolerance is a reaction on the part of the gastrointestinal system (although there may still be some immune system involvement). Therefore, symptoms of a food intolerance are often gastrointestinal in nature.

Celiac Disease

Celiac disease is an autoimmune condition in which the body's immune system reacts to the presence of gluten. Gluten is a protein found in products containing barley, rye, and wheat. When a person with celiac disease eats something containing gluten, the immune system attacks and damages the villi lining the small intestine. The damage to the villi prevents the body from being able to absorb important nutrients. This can result in serious health problems and a wide variety of symptoms. Celiac disease is diagnosed according to initial blood screening, followed by an endoscopy with a biopsy of the lining of the small intestine.

The gastrointestinal symptoms of celiac disease are very similar to those of IBS—abdominal pain, bloating, and diarrhea. Research indicates that IBS patients are at a significantly higher risk for celiac disease. Therefore, if you have IBS, it is essential that you be screened for celiac disease. If you are subsequently diagnosed with celiac disease, you must follow a strict gluten-free diet for the rest of your life.

FACT

Due to a growing recognition of the high number of IBS patients who react poorly to gluten, researchers have come up with the term "non-celiac gluten sensitivity (NCGS)" as a diagnosis for such patients. NCGS is theorized to be a subset of IBS.

Gluten Intolerance

Gluten intolerance is a condition in which a person reacts negatively to foods containing gluten, but who does not have celiac disease. When a person has a gluten intolerance, their immune system does not attack the villi, so there is no concern about damage to the small intestine. Unlike a person with celiac disease, a person with gluten intolerance can eat gluten without the concern of permanent damage, but may suffer the consequence of undesirable symptoms.

The symptoms of gluten intolerance may be gastrointestinal in nature, with symptoms such as abdominal pain, constipation, and diarrhea. There is also the theory that a gluten intolerance may cause other symptoms throughout the body—symptoms such as brain fog, fatigue, headaches, and joint pain. Like other intolerances, a gluten intolerance is typically identified through the use of an elimination diet and challenge test.

Working with Your Doctor

A medical diagnosis is needed for IBS, but sometimes it can take a long time to be properly diagnosed. Take an active part in your own health by asking for tests. Make an appointment with a gastroenterologist if you frequently experience symptoms of IBS and ask to be tested for lactose intolerance, fructose intolerance, and sorbitol intolerance. Ask your doctor to rule out small intestinal bacterial overgrowth (SIBO) and also test for celiac disease.

If you have IBS, SIBO, IBD (inflammatory bowel disease)—not during a flare—GERD, celiac disease, gluten sensitivity, or chronic stress, consider following the low-FODMAP diet along with your doctor's recommendations. When you have IBS, most clinical doctors can only help in suggesting medications or running tests. Consider working with your doctor and a nutritionist or registered dietitian who has been trained in the low-FODMAP approach. They can help you to carefully navigate the diet and take into consideration your past and current health status and any special dietary needs you may have. Some of the best partners in health to work with are those who will take a holistic approach, helping you to heal both your body and mind.

QUESTION

Will the diet work for me?
While medical approaches exist for IBS, the low-FODMAP dietary approach has been touted to help over 75 percent of people who follow the diet carefully and with their doctor's guidance.

The low-FODMAP diet is fascinating because it has helped people feel better overnight or over a couple of months, oftentimes following years of pain and misdiagnoses from doctors. In order to fully reap the benefits of what the low-FODMAP diet can offer your body, it is also wise to consider some form of stress relief every day. Your lifestyle can also affect the way food is broken down in your body, resulting in adverse physical and emotional responses.

What Are FODMAPs?

The acronym FODMAP stands for:
    Fermentable
    oligosaccharides (fructans and galacto-oligosaccharides, GOS)
    Disaccharides (lactose)
    Monosaccharides (excess fructose)

and

Polyols (sugar alcohols)

FODMAPs are short-chain carbohydrates (sugars and fibers) that are poorly absorbed in the small intestine and are then rapidly fermented by bacteria in the gut. The bacteria then produces hydrogen, carbon dioxide, and methane gases that contribute to symptoms—otherwise known as unpleasant times for people with IBS! In the small and large intestine, an osmotic effect draws more fluid and gas into the bowel, which is why people with IBS complain of bloating and distension. From the distended bowel comes symptoms of diarrhea or constipation, or both, as well as lower back pain and abdominal pain and pressure.

FACT

Internationally, more women than men report having IBS. All age groups are affected by IBS, including children and the elderly, but most report symptoms occurring in their late twenties or early thirties.

Some other medical conditions may have symptoms similar to those of IBS, including:

- Celiac disease
- Diverticulitis
- Endometriosis
- Fibromyalgia
- Gallstones
- Inflammatory bowel disease (IBD)
- Pancreatic conditions
- Parasitic infestation
- Thyroid disease
- Tumors of the digestive system

Due to this long list of other possible causes for IBS-like symptoms, patients run more of a chance of being incorrectly diagnosed. Receiving an accurate diagnosis may take time, and that is why it's vital to get as many opinions as possible.

ESSENTIAL

People without IBS can also experience issues with malabsorption of FODMAPs but they may not react to FODMAPs due to their own motility (the speed at which their bowel muscles move); they may not be as hypersensitive to all the inner workings of the gut; their bodies may have a different response to stress, anxiety, or trauma; or they might have an overall healthy balance of bacteria.

When you have IBS, sometimes it can take days or weeks for symptoms to ease up. Symptoms may ease up just slightly or almost completely and then return. Everyone's gut, body chemistry, environment, and stress level is different. So from one person to the next, food can have varying effects. This is why the low-FODMAP diet is so effective—it can be individualized to your particular sensitivities. The trial and error of the low-FODMAP diet is what helps you determine what's best for you and only you.

A Breakdown of FODMAP Groups

The following sections describe the different FODMAP groups, explain how they can impact your body, and reveal what foods they are found in.

Fermentation

Fermentation is a process that triggers the release of gases in the digestive system. It is a result of your gut's bacteria interacting with the carbohydrates you have consumed. The fermented carbohydrates can contribute to bloating, burping, or flatulence.

oligosaccharides and Fructans

oligosaccharides and fructans are carbohydrates that are poorly digested in humans, as the body does not have the proper enzymes to break them down. Since they are not able to be fully digested, gut bacteria perform the job of fermentation in the large intestine. oligosaccharides include:

- Fructo-oligosaccharides (FOS)—fructans found in wheat, rye, onions, and garlic
- Galacto-oligosaccharides (GOS)—legumes/pulses

Fructans are seen as the most common FODMAP to cause symptoms of IBS and they are found in several different types of foods, both natural and processed. Wheat is only a problem ingredient when consumed as a wheat-based carbohydrate food such as cereal, bread, or pasta. This is not a gluten-free diet; if you do not have celiac disease, non-celiac gluten sensitivity, or certain autoimmune conditions, you can have oats and small amounts of wheat, barley, and rye.

FACT

Although garlic and onions are considered to be high-FODMAP foods, you can still benefit from their flavor in cooking. FODMAPs are water soluble but they are not soluble in oil, so you can sauté garlic and onion in oil for a few minutes at the start of a recipe, then discard them. This allows for a flavor-infused oil without the concerns about the FODMAPs found in the actual garlic and onions.

Disaccharides

Lactose is a disaccharide—the "D" in FODMAP. Lactose is found in milk, soft cheese, and yogurts. As you probably know, many people are lactose intolerant, a digestive problem also known as lactose malabsorption. Problems with lactose occur in individuals who lack enough of the enzyme lactase. Lactase is an enzyme essential for the digestion of lactose. Lactase breaks lactose down into two monosaccharides, glucose and galactose, so that they can be absorbed into the bloodstream by the small intestine. When there is a deficiency in lactase, lactose is not absorbed and is fermented by gut bacteria, resulting in symptoms.

Dairy products differ in the amount of lactose that they contain. Therefore, certain dairy products are allowed as part of a low-FODMAP diet. Milk is very high in lactose so it is avoided on the diet. Soft cheeses are allowed but only up to 2 ounces. Harder cheeses, such as pecorino-style, are allowed on the diet because of their lower lactose content (0.1–1 percent).

Monosaccharides

Fructose is a monosaccharide—the "M" in FODMAP. Fructose is the sugar found in many fruits, honey, and high-fructose corn syrup (HFCS). Fructose malabsorption is experienced by approximately one-third of all humans, with higher rates seen in those with an FGID or with Crohn's disease.

Fructose malabsorption is the result of fructose not being absorbed well at the level of the small intestine. In order for fructose to pass through the lining of the small intestine, it requires the presence of a transporter called GLUT-5. In some people, there is a lessened amount of this transporter, resulting in malabsorption.

Luckily, the extent of the malabsorption is strongly affected by the presence of glucose. When glucose is present, another transporter, known as GLUT-2, is activated, which facilitates the absorption of fructose. Therefore, foods that contain equal parts of fructose/glucose or have more glucose than fructose can be eaten in moderation without causing symptoms.

This factor plays strongly in the consideration of foods that are allowed in the low-FODMAP diet. For example, you might be surprised to see that sugar is allowed in the diet. This is because sugar has an equal amount of fructose and glucose. If you have IBS, foods can be a problem if they contain more than 0.2 grams fructose in excess of glucose per serving.

Just remember, if you have fructose malabsorption, you do not need to avoid fructose completely; as long as there is more glucose than fructose in a food, you can eat moderate amounts.

QUESTION

When is the best time to consume fruit?
Firm, less-ripe fruit tend to contain more fructose than other foods. Try to consume fruit a half hour before eating anything else. Since fruit breaks down in about a half hour, it can ferment if sitting on top of other slower-to-digest foods already in the digestive tract.

Aside from smaller servings or even whole servings of fruit and vegetables with excess fructose, high-fructose corn syrup (HFCS) may cause long-term harm. HFCS is an unnatural, industrial food product that you may want to consider steering clear of. HFCS is found in so many processed foods, it's overwhelming just trying to avoid it! Here is a short list of where you may find HFCS: beverages, sodas, breads, candy, cake, cereals, barbecue sauce, cookies, cough syrups, dairy, ice cream, ketchup, marinades, relish, salad dressings, and more.

And Polyols

Polyols—the "P" in FODMAP—are sugar alcohols with scientific names that typically end in "-ol." Polyols are used as artificial sweeteners and found naturally in some fruit and vegetables such as cauliflower, mushrooms, Asian pears, blackberries, and more. Polyol types include:

- Isomalt
- Maltitol
- Mannitol
- Polydextrose
- Sorbitol
- Xylitol

Polyol malabsorption is a quite common condition, present in more than half of all humans. In addition to contributing to excessive intestinal gas and bloating, polyols are also strong contributors to diarrhea due to their laxative effect. As you follow the low-FODMAP diet, you will become very good at reading ingredient labels and looking for the presence of polyol artificial sweeteners. Watch out for anything listed as "sugar-free" or having sugar alcohols (these ingredients often end in *ol*). These polyols can cause symptoms for people with digestive disorders if they contain more than 0.5 grams total polyols per serving.

ESSENTIAL

A hydrogen breath test can detect malabsorption of fructose, lactose, and polyols. Gastroenterologists administer hydrogen breath tests. It can sometimes take weeks to get an appointment, so consider booking a test as soon as you are able and before starting the low-FODMAP diet.

The Elimination and Challenge Phases

There is an Elimination Phase and a Challenge Phase to this diet. You will follow the Elimination Phase by strictly negating all high-FODMAP foods for two to six weeks. Most people who try the low-FODMAP diet see significant improvement in their symptoms by the four-week mark, but you may find that you feel better even sooner. However, don't despair if it takes longer for you to see improvement—everyone's body is unique and will be affected differently by the diet.

It will also depend on how you are feeling and how quickly your body responds to the absence of problem foods. If you are feeling significantly better one week into the Elimination Phase, you might be able to start the Challenge Phase after two weeks.

During the Elimination Phase be sure to use a food and symptom diary. You can create your own symptom diary using the following template, or download a copy at BonCalme.com: *www.boncalme.com/ booksresources-low-fodmap-digestive-disorder-books/food-symptom-diary.* This valuable resource will help you and your doctor and nutritionist to pinpoint your triggers.

DAILY SYMPTOM DIARY			
Date	**Foods Eaten**	**Other Factors**	**Symptoms**
Breakfast			
Snack			
Lunch			
Snack			
Dinner			
Dessert/Snack			

During the Challenge Phase (or reintroduction phase) you will detect personal triggers by reintroducing one FODMAP category at a time, one food at a time.

After the Challenge Phase, FODMAPs that do not trigger symptoms can be a part of your regular diet again, and some foods may still be limited but far better tolerated. It is important to finish the Challenge Phase so you can enjoy a varied diet full of different essential nutrients from the vitamins and minerals found in fruit, vegetables, legumes, nuts, seeds, healthy fats, and protein. Your body needs these foods in order to fight free radicals looking to do cellular damage. A diet that is not healthy or balanced can lead to type 2 diabetes, obesity, heart disease, osteoporosis, IBS, depression, sleep disorders, and stress.

As an example, if you follow the diet correctly, after the Challenge Phase you may find that polyols do not cause an issue for your gut. If you were to stay on the diet for a long time or even lifelong, you would miss out on the health benefits of foods such as cauliflower, mushrooms, snow peas, apples, apricots, Asian pears, blackberries, nectarines, peaches, pears, plums, prunes, and watermelon, which are all high in polyols, but are possibly okay for you whole or in specific servings.

ALERT

For some people in the long term, a certain level of FODMAP restriction may be necessary to regulate symptoms. It is never suggested to follow the low-FODMAP diet for life. After abstaining from FODMAPs it is highly suggested that a person tries a rechallenge phase again, but under the supervision of a dietitian.

Elimination Phase Overview

The Elimination Phase of the diet typically lasts two to six weeks. Without argument, this is certainly the strictest phase of the diet. Many foods that you typically eat will now be off-limits. But don't worry; although you will have to change the way you eat, you will still be able to eat lots of delicious foods! Also, you'll find that there are many substitutes you can use so you can still enjoy your favorite recipes.

In theory, the longer you can adhere to the Elimination Phase, the better. That being said, you can make the decision with the help of your physician or your nutritionist. It will also depend on how you are feeling and how quickly your body responds to the absence of problem foods.

A full list of high-FODMAP foods is found in Appendix B. These foods are not allowed at all during the Elimination Phase. However, if you've already undergone breath testing and know you don't have a problem with lactose, fructose, and/or polyols, you can include these tolerated foods right from the start. Although the lists of "no" and "yes" foods may seem a little overwhelming at first, with practice you'll find that it becomes almost second nature to know which foods are on the allowed and restricted lists.

Challenge Phase Overview

In this next phase, you will be reintroducing your body to the foods that you love. You will do this by working your way through the various FODMAP types, group by group. You will gain a better awareness of which foods contain which FODMAPs and which foods your body is able to tolerate. After you complete the diet, you will then be able to eat more of your favorite foods with confidence.

The first step of the Challenge Phase is to start to reintroduce foods back into your diet. You will be introducing foods into your diet one FODMAP group at a time. Before you begin, you will need to figure out the order you would like to follow. You will spend approximately 1 week on each FODMAP type starting with the smallest dose on a Monday. You can decide which order you would like to follow as you challenge yourself with each type of FODMAP. Your starting options include fructose, lactose, or polyols (sorbitol and mannitol). Fructans and GOS should be saved for last, as they are not absorbed by anyone.

If you do not experience a return of your digestive symptoms after introducing a new food, you can conclude that your body can tolerate that food and other foods from that FODMAP group. Make note of this in your symptom diary. If your symptoms return in response to a reintroduced food, go back to your Elimination Phase food until you feel better. If you experience a severe reaction to the small Monday dose, it is okay to conclude that you have a sensitivity to this FODMAP.

To learn more about both phases of the diet, please refer to *The Everything® Guide to the Low-FODMAP Diet* by Dr. Barbara Bolen and Kathleen Bradley, CPC.

How to Read Labels

Properly reading food labels will help ensure success with the low-FODMAP diet. Food labels list ingredients in descending order of weight with the highest amounts listed first. FODMAPs can be an issue only when consumed regularly and in significant amounts. If a high-FODMAP food is listed on an ingredient list but is present in small amounts (such as less than 5 percent), it most likely will be "suitable" to consume.

When first starting the diet, it will take some time to learn how to read labels. Rest assured that with each trip to the grocery store, your confidence will improve and time spent researching will decrease. You can improve your experience of shopping by downloading the low-FODMAP Grocery List and making notes before your trip, such as the one found here: *www .boncalme.com/the-fodmap-diet/grocery-list*. Or, use a low-FODMAP app such as Monash University's to quickly look up any foods and servings for which you are uncertain, and get acquainted with the high-FODMAP foods list at *http://fodmaplife.com/fodmap-foods-to-avoid*. Both low- and high-FOD-MAP food lists are included in this book for your reference in Appendix B.

Choose more whole foods such as low-FODMAP fruit, vegetables, nuts, grains, and seeds, as well as lean proteins and lactose-free products. Choose organic, non-GMO foods whenever possible as well as grass-fed meat and eggs. Choose sunflower or safflower oils over the vegetable oils you might be more familiar with.

ESSENTIAL

Steer clear of breads, cereals, biscuits, pastas, and other products that have labels listing wheat or rye as a main ingredient, where they appear anywhere from first to third on the ingredient list. If a FOD-MAP is listed near the bottom of an ingredient list, the product may be suitable to consume.

Understanding Servings

Paying attention to serving amounts on the low-FODMAP diet is another way to successfully manage the diet. "Everything in moderation" is how the saying goes, and being mindful of servings and how much you consume is key to the low-FODMAP diet. Not overloading the gut with too many FODMAPs in one sitting or day is how people start to feel relief.

Many people following the Elimination Phase believe they need to stay away from FODMAPs completely, or else they have failed the diet. This isn't always true. It depends on which FODMAP food you consume, how much you've consumed in one sitting or over the course of a day (overall load of FODMAPs), and if the serving was high or moderate in FODMAPs. As an example, any serving of apples, dried apples, or applesauce is very high in FODMAPs. Most contain excess fructose and the polyol sorbitol—so the *overall load* of FODMAPs becomes very high. Apples should be avoided completely during the Elimination Phase, unless you know you do not malabsorb fructose. Whether or not you have taken a hydrogen breath test, you could still play it safe and consume zero high-FODMAPs, as sometimes tests are not always accurate. Wouldn't it be nice if there were a one-size-fits-all approach to alleviating IBS?

Another example of a food loved by so many is avocados. As long as you do not consume more than ⅛ of a whole avocado, you're still in the clear and should continue following the diet. However, a ¼ serving of a whole avocado contains a moderate amount of the polyol sorbitol and a ½ serving contains a high amount. Intake should be avoided if you know you malabsorb sorbitol, or if you accidentally consumed a ¼ or ½ serving and are experiencing symptoms. When you know that a food is moderate in FODMAPs, you do not have to avoid the food completely if you know you do not have malabsorption issues with a particular FODMAP. A hydrogen breath test can determine if you suffer from malabsorption of fructose, lactose, or polyols. So if through a hydrogen breath test you have found that you do not malabsorb polyols, you should still be able to enjoy a ¼ serving of a whole avocado—moderate in the polyol sorbitol.

ESSENTIAL

A good rule of thumb for the low-FODMAP diet is to remember that when any one type of food is marked as moderate, it means it comes with a limit and may or may not trigger symptoms (IBS symptoms are always very individualized). When this is the case, stick to one low-FODMAP serving once per day (as in the example of the avocado in this section). If you feel you really need to try the food, you can always try the moderate low-FODMAP serving as long as you know you do not malabsorb the FODMAP it contains, but always keep a food and symptom diary handy in case you need to record any symptoms.

If you've gone completely off course and have consumed far too many FODMAPs at a party or social event, don't beat yourself up. It's important to remember that we are all human; accidents happen, and the best approach is to start the diet over. Become your own patient advocate. Pay attention to servings, learn as much as you can about the diet, and use the lists for low-FODMAP foods and high-FODMAP foods.

Foods that are low-FODMAP but might still be troublesome include:

- **All meats and animal proteins** (unless they are processed with high-FODMAP ingredients) are low-FODMAP; however, fatty meats take a much longer time to digest and could cause constipation or diarrhea. As an example, fruit takes about a half hour to digest while fatty meat can take days. It's wise to choose lean meats on the low-FODMAP diet because it will mean easier digestion and a more peaceful gut.
- **Broccoli and kale** are cruciferous vegetables and may cause gas due to their content of raffinose, an indigestible sugar. Beans (oligos—GOS and fructans) have more raffinose.
- **Eggs** that have been boiled can cause symptoms in people who do not have the right enzymes (protease) to break down the egg, otherwise known as egg intolerance. Try soft-boiling or poaching eggs instead.
- **Potatoes, corn, and other starchy vegetables** can produce gas in the large intestine.
- **Oatmeal, oatmeal cookies, and other oat products** (including oat bran) can all result in excessive gas because of their high soluble-fiber content. Quick-cooking oats are okay on the diet at a ¼-cup serving.

Wheat and Gluten

The low-FODMAP diet is not a gluten-free diet, but a diet that negates foods high in wheat or fructans, which fall under the "O" in FODMAPs, oligosaccharides. Foods containing wheat will also contain gluten. Wheat contains fructans but gluten does not. The diet can be confusing sometimes because several gluten-free products work on the low-FODMAP diet, so let's discuss gluten and celiac disease.

People with celiac disease and different forms of gluten sensitivity (non-celiac gluten sensitivity or autoimmune disease—refer to Gluten Intolerance section in this chapter for more information) need to avoid gluten and they must use caution when abiding by the low-FODMAP diet because not all low-FODMAP foods are free of gluten. For example, ½ cup cooked wheat pasta is low in FODMAPs (fructans) and has a small amount of wheat but it also has gluten and is off-limits for those avoiding gluten. Oats are gluten-free and allowed on the diet; however, someone with celiac disease or a gluten sensitivity is more apt to buy gluten-free oats to not run the risk of the oats being cross-contaminated with wheat during processing. Thankfully gluten-free products made at 100 percent gluten-free facilities are more widely available today than they've ever been before.

The part of gluten that is most harmful is the gliadin protein, which is a component of gluten and found in a wide variety of foods and ingredients. If people with celiac disease ingest foods with gluten, they could endure serious intestinal damage and become hospitalized. Exposure to gluten in celiac disease results in inflammation of the small intestine when any gluten is ingested. Symptoms include severe unexplained diarrhea, hypo-proteinemia, low blood count (anemia), and metabolic and electrolyte disturbances, malabsorption, bloating, gas, fatigue, and osteoporosis.

Of all the FODMAPs, fructans (found in wheat) are the greatest contributor to IBS. As humans, we are not made to have enzymes to break down fructans and GOS (galacto-oligosaccharides). Wheat, barley, and rye (which have gluten) as well as onions and garlic contain fructans, which account for most of the foods or ingredients within the Western diet.

FACT

More doctors are prescribing gluten-free diets to patients with autoimmune diseases to help combat inflammation and oxidative stress. However, there is still a lack of evidence-based information about dietary treatments for autoimmune diseases. In people with autoimmune disease a gluten-free diet may help promote a healthy immune balance.

So on the low-FODMAP diet, you are essentially avoiding these FODMAPs and negating a specific kind of carbohydrate in the wheat—you are *not* negating the gluten protein gliadin as people with celiac disease and gluten sensitivity need to.

A food that contains gluten but is low in FODMAPs is spelt sourdough bread—it is suitable on the diet at 2 slices per serving. Oats are often cross-contaminated with gluten, so many health experts agree it is safer for people with celiac disease to avoid oats; otherwise the packaging needs a guarantee for a lack of contamination by wheat, rye, or barley. Please refer to the Low-FODMAPs food list in Appendix B to see which other foods have wheat but are low in FODMAPs (again please abide by serving sizes).

Make Ahead

If you've never been much of a planner, now is the time. If you're used to buying your meals instead of making your own, now is the time to cook! Since you can't throw just anything together on the low-FODMAP diet and restaurant menus are limited, planning ahead will help keep you on track.

Making certain foods in bulk and also planning your meals ahead of time by choosing a specific day each week to do so (consider Sunday evenings) will give you peace of mind. You will have an easier time staying on track and feel satisfied and not excessively hungry. Also, when you are making a dish that includes any ingredients such as buckwheat, rice, rice pasta, or other gluten-free pastas, quinoa, stock, pasta sauce, or meat, make extra to use in other recipes included in this book. As an example, additional quinoa made for dinner could be used for breakfast, lunch, or even baking.

Please refer to Appendix A for sample meal plans and snack ideas. Here are some items you can make ahead and how you can use them:

- **Cooked meat or chicken:** use in soups, casseroles, sandwiches, pizzas, stir-fries, and more. Make shredded chicken ahead of time for Chicken Pizza Quesadilla (see recipe in Chapter 10). It can be stored in the refrigerator 3–4 days or frozen 2–6 months.
- **Marinara sauce, tomato sauce:** can be used with pasta, as a dipping sauce, for pizza, appetizers, or for Victor's Chicken Parmesan (see recipe in Chapter 7). It can be stored in the refrigerator 5 days or frozen 1–3 months.
- **Buckwheat:** use to make your own buckwheat flour, or use in soups, salads, casseroles, and baking. Try Buckwheat Thumbprint Cookies in Chapter 11 or make ahead for Pork Chops with Carrots and Toasted Buckwheat in Chapter 7. When you buy buckwheat, it is best to store it in

the refrigerator or freezer. Cooked buckwheat can be stored in the refrigerator 3–5 days or frozen up to 1 month.

- **Rice:** use in soups, reheat and use in stir-fries, wraps, casseroles, and more. Cooked rice can be stored in the refrigerator 4–6 days or frozen up to 6 months.
- **Rice pasta:** use in pasta dishes, soups, and casseroles. Cooked pasta can be stored in the refrigerator 7 days or frozen up to 6–8 months.
- **Quinoa:** use in soups, salads, casseroles, appetizers, and baking. Make ahead for Turkey Quinoa Meatballs with Mozzarella in Chapter 7 or Latin Quinoa-Stuffed Peppers in Chapter 9. Cooked quinoa can be stored in the refrigerator 2–4 days or frozen up to 1 month.
- **Stock:** Chicken and vegetable stock is great to have on hand to make a quick soup, to liven up rice or quinoa, to use with risotto recipes, or for Lemon and Mozzarella Polenta Pizza in Chapter 9. Take a look at Easy Onion- and Garlic-Free Chicken Stock in Chapter 4. Store homemade stock in an airtight container in the refrigerator 5–7 days.
- **Vegetables and fruit:** once you return from the grocery store, wash, peel, and chop up vegetables and fruit and place in airtight containers.

For more refrigerator- and freezer-safe time limits, visit *www.foodsafety.gov.*

Eating Out

Eating out doesn't have to be a stress-inducing event, especially if you have the chance to choose the restaurant. If the choice in restaurant is not yours to make, ask for grilled meat or fish, steamed vegetables, a baked potato, or a salad. Hold the salad dressing, as most are high in FODMAPs, and ask for olive oil instead and add lemon with a dash of salt and pepper. One tablespoon of balsamic vinegar is low in FODMAPs, but anything more is moderate to high. Keep your Low-FODMAP Grocery List and Monash University app handy so you can quickly look up foods if need be.

If the menu doesn't seem to include anything low-FODMAP, straight off the bat, explain to your server due to your dietary requirements, you can only eat foods free of gluten, dairy, onions, and garlic. That should help narrow down selections. Don't ever be afraid to ask which ingredients are included in a dish. Hopefully your server and the kitchen staff will do all they can to accommodate you.

Here is a list of cuisines that might have more low-FODMAP options:

- **American:** make-your-own omelets; chef salad, Cobb salad (watch serving of avocado and hold creamy dressing, ask for olive oil and lemon juice and use up to 1 tablespoon balsamic vinegar as well); egg, tuna, or chicken salad (as long as not made with onions); burger in a lettuce wrap or ask for a burger no bun, on top of a salad; potato skins; shrimp cocktail; fresh fruit; plain French fries or potatoes (skip if you are gluten-free); decaf tea.
- **Chinese:** steamed vegetables with chicken; egg drop soup made without garlic powder; chicken/beef with broccoli (as long as no garlic is present); mixed seafood with vegetables; chow fun and mei fun, which are usually made with rice noodles (skip if you are gluten-free as the sauce is usually made with soy); those who are gluten-free should stick to steamed shrimp and vegetables or beef unless the restaurant uses cornstarch instead of flour for white sauces. Chicken is okay at most Chinese restaurants but just know that some lower-end Chinese restaurants may make their "chicken" using chicken and texturized vegetable protein, which is definitely not gluten-free.
- **Greek:** Greek salad (hold onions, use olive oil for dressing); chicken stuffed with feta and spinach; broiled fish; meat or fish kabobs (hold onions); some Greek restaurants offer gluten-free pita bread.
- **Italian:** garden salad, Caprese salad, antipasto salad (no artichokes, onions, croutons, dried fruit etc.); low-FODMAP cheese board with rice crackers; gluten-free pizza, gluten-free pasta, hold the sauce; again make sure all do not contain high FODMAPs.
- **Japanese:** sashimi; seaweed; cooked fish; ask for gluten-free soy sauce (tamari) and avoid tempura as it has wheat.
- **Mexican:** corn tacos with fish or meat, cheese and lettuce; hold the salsa as it's usually made with onions and garlic; hold the beans; hold the guacamole; hold the hot sauce if you find it irritates your gut.
- **Steak houses:** choose lean meat, fish, or both (surf 'n' turf) that have not been marinated in high FODMAPs; potatoes, side dishes, or salads with no added high FODMAPS (examples: regular mashed potatoes instead

of garlic mashed potatoes; green salad, hold the dressing and use olive oil; steamed spinach instead of creamed spinach; no fried appetizers).

- **Thai and Vietnamese:** these restaurants have some of the best choices when eating out, such as rice noodles, rice, summer rolls, grilled meats and fish; Vietnamese: pho (without onions or chili sauce); bún cha (without FODMAPs); bánh xèo (as long as not pan-fried in flour). Thai: tom kah soups without high FODMAPs.

More restaurants are starting to offer gluten-free bread, buns, cookies, crackers, pancakes, pasta, wraps, and more. Ask if they have those options or look for "gluten-free" or "GF" printed on the menu.

Wellness Tips

The following are some tips on how you can make better choices in food and how you can improve your body and mind.

For Preventing Gas

You can try to prevent gas by NOT doing the following:

- **Chewing gum, drinking out of a straw, eating too fast, or sucking on candies:** all can cause you to swallow a lot of air, causing gas.
- **Drinking coffee:** coffee is a diuretic and has a stimulating effect on the intestines and can increase diarrhea, dehydrating the body.
- **Drinking smoothies:** often they are made with several and large servings of fruit, which is one big FODMAP bomb.

For Digestion

The following list includes foods that may aid in digestion or help when you have an IBS attack. Please keep in mind again that everyone is different, so not all foods or methods of relieving IBS symptoms work for everyone.

- **Cinnamon** is used in Ayurvedic medicine to balance digestion in order to help restore the stomach to a balanced state. Sprinkle it on lactose-free yogurt, lactose-free kefir, in gluten-free oats, or use it after you eat to aid in digestion by adding a teaspoon to decaf green tea. If you have diabetes, sprinkle cinnamon on high-carb foods to lower the impact on your blood sugar levels.

- **Flaxseeds** can prevent excessive gas and fend off constipation. Grind them before using in baking, cereals, salads, and smoothies.
- **Kombucha** contains probiotics that can bring balance to the flora of your digestive tract. The good bacteria can help improve digestion and ease symptoms. Look for ingredients such as "water, sugar, tea, culture." Be mindful of additional sweeteners, which could not only be high FODMAPs but also indicate that the Kombucha was sweetened *after* the fermentation process. Start out slow; try ¼ cup of Kombucha per day to start.
- **Lemon water** (warmed) first thing in the morning helps flush out toxins and aids in digestion to help the production of digestive juices and the production of bile. It can also help increase your body's alkaline levels.
- **Ginger** can help activate your digestive juices and also soothe the stomach.
- **Peppermint** "relaxes the muscles that allow painful digestive gas to pass," according to the University of Maryland's Medical Center. Try enteric coated peppermint capsules, peppermint leaves, and organic peppermints (not made with sugar alcohols).
- **Pineapple** (fresh, raw) contains bromelain, an enzyme that aids in digestion and helps prevent inflammation and swelling.
- **Sauerkraut and other fermented foods** contain beneficial bacteria that make them easier to digest. As you age, you produce less digestive enzymes and juices, which fermented foods can help produce acetylcholine, a neurotransmitter that helps movement within the bowel. Acetylcholine can help reduce constipation and increase the release of digestive juices and enzymes from the stomach, the pancreas, and the gallbladder.
- **Probiotics:** there is still a lack of conclusive evidence that probiotics can help improve gut health. Taking probiotics for the short term might be best. Talk to your doctor.
- **Fiber supplements:** you have been told for years that fiber is important for digestion but it's not for everyone, and not for everyone with IBS either. Fiber can actually increase gas production and bloating. If you were to try a fiber supplement, talk to your doctor about trying a nonfermentable fiber such as Citrucel.

For Relaxing

Issues in your gut can affect your energy level, weight, mood, or may lead to premature aging, chronic disease, or allergies. When you have IBS, a healthy diet is imperative, but so is taking care of the mind and body.

Signals from an upset gut can be sent to the brain just as the brain can send signals to the gut. Gastrointestinal upset can be the cause or product of anxiety, stress, or depression. That is why there is a strong link between the brain and the gut. Many in the field of health and science believe the nerves in our gut, which are actually controlled by our "second brain" (located within the gut), influence negative emotions, stress, or anxiety. The brain can influence our perception of what is happening in the gut as well as the activity or "tuning" of the enteric nervous system (ENS) "gut brain." Some research suggests that people with functional gastrointestinal disorders (FGIDs) identify pain more profoundly than people without FGIDs because their brains cannot decode pain signals from the GI tract. And any stress in someone with IBS can make it seem as though pain experienced is worse than it actually is. Also, psychological and physical stress as well as antibiotics and diet can create a loss of the balance in gut microbiota (microflora), also known as intestinal dysbiosis. IBS, inflammatory bowel disease (IBD), rheumatoid arthritis, and ankylosing spondylitis have all been linked to alterations in gut microbiota. Probiotics and prebiotics may help alleviate symptoms associated with these inflammatory diseases but the long-term effects are unknown. Consult with your doctor or nutritionist before trying any therapies.

Reducing Stress

Here are a few tips to help calm the mind and relieve stress:

- **Meditating** once per day for 15–30 minutes or a few times per day at 5-minute intervals can help relax the mind and the gut, allowing for better digestion and bowel movements.
- **Eating slowly** is beneficial for a few reasons. Eating too much food can trigger IBS symptoms, but by eating slowly, you're giving your gut a chance to tell your brain that it's full, helping you to not overeat. Eating slowly helps you to chew your food better, which improves digestion, giving the digestive system less work to do. And finally, eating slowly

keeps you more aware of the present and less inclined to take part in stress eating. Take 7–10 long slow breaths every time before you start to eat and notice the change in the way you eat, and the way you feel during and after your meal.

- **Eating without distraction** helps you to slow down and become more aware of your surroundings and your food. You may find that eating without your phone in hand, or a computer or TV in your face will improve your enjoyment of food—it may smell and taste better!
- **Cooking for yourself** and making food ahead of time to have low-FODMAP foods on hand will fuel your body and save money, time, headaches and unneeded stress.
- **Getting creative** is a wonderful way to relax your body and mind, and be in the present. Creativity can come from cooking, writing, taking a class to learn something new, dancing, photography, gardening, volunteering, painting, playing an instrument, and playing with kids, among other ideas.
- **Gentle exercising** may help you to release gas or pain and it's also good to calm the nervous system and get blood flowing through your body, and to keep your joints lubricated. Even if you lead a very busy life, a short walk or even cleaning the house can do wonders. Other types of gentle and mindful exercising are yoga, Pilates, qigong, tai chi, stretching, swimming, golfing, light aerobics, or an easy bike ride.
- **Being good to yourself** is one of the best gifts you can give. If negative talk is part of your everyday life, you need to start saying nicer things to yourself. Become your own health advocate and learn as much about the low-FODMAP diet as you can. Use your food and symptom diary every day. Become more connected to healthy foods and cooking for yourself. Every day send positive energy to your gut. Remind yourself why you are awesome. Life is full of ups and downs. There will always be hard times—so have a plan in place for when disaster strikes so you can keep your gut, body, and mind as healthy and calm as possible. Eat well, meditate, exercise, and be grateful for all the positives in your life, and all the negatives that made you stronger.

CHAPTER 2

Breakfast

Autumn Breakfast
Chia Bowl
38

Cinnamon Spice
Granola
38

Green Dragon
Smoothie Bowl
39

Tomato Spinach
Frittata Muffins
40

Flourless Banana
Cinnamon Pancakes
41

Flourless Vegan
Banana Peanut
Butter Pancakes
41

Vegan Buckwheat
Crepes
42

Ham and Cheese
Crepes
43

Pumpkin Spice
Crepes
44

Coconut Cacao
Hazelnut
Smoothie Bowl
45

Raspberry Banana
Mint Chia Pudding
45

Passionfruit
Smoothie Bowl
46

Jubilant Muesli Mix
47

Cream of Muesli
48

Eggs Baked in
Heirloom Tomatoes
49

Shakshuka for Two
50

Pesto Eggs
Rice Bowl
51

Raspberry Lemon
Oatmeal Bars
51

Quinoa, Egg,
Ham, and Cheese
Breakfast Muffins
52

Mexican Egg Brunch
53

Eggs with Spinach
and Chickpeas
54

Delicioso
Breakfast Tacos
55

Tomato and Leek
Frittata
56

Cranberry Almond
Granola
57

Overnight Peanut
Butter Pumpkin
Spice Oats
58

Overnight Banana
Chocolate Oats
59

Overnight Carrot
Cake Oats and
Walnuts
59

Amaranth Breakfast
60

Savory Sourdough
Strata
61

Autumn Breakfast Chia Bowl

When the cool of autumn starts to roll in, warm up with this healthy and hearty breakfast bowl.

INGREDIENTS | SERVES 2

3 cups water
¼ teaspoon salt
1 cup gluten-free steel-cut oats
½ cup lactose-free milk
3 tablespoons chia seeds
1 tablespoon halved macadamia nuts
1 tablespoon sliced almonds
½ teaspoon ground cinnamon
1 tablespoon no-sugar-added dried cranberries

1. In a medium saucepan, bring water and salt to a boil, then add oats. Add milk and stir.

2. Add chia seeds, macadamia nuts, almonds, cinnamon, and cranberries and stir again.

3. Cover and cook 15–20 minutes, stirring occasionally until chia seeds become soft and gel-like. Serve immediately.

Per Serving Calories: 328 | Fat: 16g | Protein: 11g | Sodium: 325mg | Fiber: 7g | Carbohydrates: 38g | Sugar: 6g

Cinnamon Spice Granola

This granola tastes great in a Pumpkin Parfait (see recipe in Chapter 10) mixed in with lactose-free yogurt.

INGREDIENTS | SERVES 8

2 cups quick-cooking oats
1 cup walnut pieces
1 teaspoon ground cinnamon
½ teaspoon ground nutmeg
¼ teaspoon ground cloves
3 tablespoons light brown sugar
¼ cup maple syrup
¼ cup safflower oil

1. Preheat oven to 350°F.

2. Combine all ingredients in a large bowl.

3. Spread mixture in an even layer on a baking sheet and bake 20 minutes; stir once halfway through baking.

4. Allow to cool before serving.

Per Serving Calories: 280 | Fat: 17g | Protein: 5g | Sodium: 4mg | Fiber: 3g | Carbohydrates: 28g | Sugar: 12g

Are Oats High in FODMAPs?

Stick with a ¼ serving (dry) of quick-cooking oats. Due to their high fiber content, larger servings of oats may cause intestinal gas for people with IBS.

Green Dragon Smoothie Bowl

Beautifully hued and healthy dragon fruit garnishes this delicious mix of fruit, vegetables, seeds, and nuts.

INGREDIENTS | SERVES 1

½ cup unsweetened almond milk

1 small (6-ounce) tub lactose-free vanilla yogurt

1 tablespoon suitable protein powder

1 teaspoon unsweetened cocoa powder

⅛ teaspoon Himalayan salt

1 cup baby spinach

½ frozen medium banana

1 large slice or 2 small slices dragon fruit

5 almonds

2 tablespoons shredded unsweetened coconut

½ tablespoon chia seeds

1. Pour almond milk and yogurt into a blender and then add protein powder, cocoa powder, salt, spinach, banana, and 1 cup ice. Blend to process. Mixture should be thick and icy; add more ice if needed. Pour into a shallow bowl.

2. Top with dragon fruit, almonds, coconut, and chia seeds. Enjoy!

Per Serving   Calories: 473 | Fat: 14g | Protein: 38g | Sodium: 763mg | Fiber: 8g | Carbohydrates: 55g | Sugar: 40g

Which Protein Powders Are Suitable on the Low-FODMAP Diet?

When choosing protein powder for smoothies, it's again very important to pay close attention to labels. Steer clear of polyols such as xylitol and other sugar alcohols; FOS (fructo-oligosaccharides) such as fructose, high-fructose corn syrup, inulin, agave, honey, artificial sweeteners; and whey protein concentrate that is not lactose-free. Pea protein, gums, and pectins might also cause symptoms.

Tomato Spinach Frittata Muffins

Easy to make and fun to bake! Enjoy frittatas in a new way with these muffins.

INGREDIENTS | SERVES 12

2 cups finely chopped spinach

1½ cups halved cherry tomatoes

1 scallion, finely chopped, green part only

½ cup crumbled feta cheese

10 large eggs

2 tablespoons lactose-free milk

1 teaspoon dried oregano

⅛ teaspoon salt

¼ teaspoon freshly ground black pepper

1. Preheat oven to 375°F. Grease a 12-cup muffin pan with cooking spray.

2. Fill muffin cups with chopped spinach, tomatoes, scallion, and feta.

3. In a medium bowl, whisk together eggs, milk, oregano, salt, and pepper. Pour egg mixture evenly into each muffin cup.

4. Bake 15–20 minutes or until eggs are completely set.

Per Serving   Calories: 82 | Fat: 6g | Protein: 7g | Sodium: 159mg | Fiber: 0g | Carbohydrates: 2g | Sugar: 1g

You Can Eat the Green!

Whole onions, shallots, or the white part of spring onions or scallions are high in FODMAPs because they contain the "O" in FODMAPs, oligosaccharides (fructans). Fructans are made of fructose molecule chains that are completely malabsorbed because the small intestine lacks hydrolases (an enzyme) to break their fructose-fructose bond. The green parts of the scallion, however, are low in FODMAPs and are safe to eat.

Flourless Banana Cinnamon Pancakes

These are the easiest pancakes you will ever make and probably some of the healthiest you'll ever enjoy!

INGREDIENTS | SERVES 1

1 large egg
½ ripe medium banana
1 teaspoon chia seeds
1 teaspoon ground cinnamon
1 tablespoon coconut oil

Looking for Other Fun Combinations for These Pancakes?

Try adding alcohol-free vanilla or almond extract, shredded unsweetened coconut, walnuts, slivered almonds, ground macadamia nuts, pumpkin seeds, pumpkin purée, no-sugar-added dried cranberries.

1. In a glass measuring cup, mix together egg, banana, chia seeds, and cinnamon. Be sure to mash bananas very well or use a blender to mix ingredients until smooth on low speed.

2. Heat oil in a medium skillet over medium heat. Pour a couple of batches of batter onto skillet and cook pancakes until bubbly on top and golden on bottom, about 4 minutes. Flip and cook about 2 more minutes.

Per Serving   Calories: 265 | Fat: 20g | Protein: 8g | Sodium: 72mg | Fiber: 3g | Carbohydrates: 17g | Sugar: 8g

Flourless Vegan Banana Peanut Butter Pancakes

Try these easy and nutritious pancakes, made with healthy fats and yummy banana.

INGREDIENTS | SERVES 1

2 flax eggs (see Chapter 16)
½ ripe medium banana
1 teaspoon chia seeds
1 tablespoon peanut butter
1 tablespoon coconut oil

1. In a glass measuring cup, mix together flax eggs, banana, chia seeds, and peanut butter. Be sure to mash bananas well or use a blender to mix ingredients until smooth on low speed.

2. Heat oil in a medium skillet over medium heat. Pour a couple of batches of batter onto the skillet and cook pancakes until bubbly on top and golden on bottom, about 4 minutes. Flip and cook about 2 more minutes.

Per Serving   Calories: 425 | Fat: 33g | Protein: 18g | Sodium: 215mg | Fiber: 3g | Carbohydrates: 18g | Sugar: 10g

Vegan Buckwheat Crepes

Buckwheat is such a versatile low-FODMAP food! When used as a flour, it tastes delicious in recipes for baked goods as well as breakfast items, like these divine crepes.

INGREDIENTS | SERVES 12

1¼ cups buckwheat flour

3 flax eggs (see Chapter 16)

¼ cup plus 1 tablespoon safflower oil

¾ cup unsweetened almond milk

1¼ cups water

½ teaspoon ground cinnamon

⅛ teaspoon salt

Not a Vegan?

If you're not vegan, you can easily enjoy this recipe by using regular eggs and lactose-free milk.

1. Place flour in a medium bowl. Add flax eggs, ¼ cup oil, milk, water, cinnamon, and salt. Mix to combine.

2. Spread remaining oil in a thin layer in a 9" round non-stick skillet over medium-high heat. Using a ladle or glass measuring cup, slowly pour ¼ cup batter into skillet; swirl around pan.

3. Cook crepe until golden on bottom, 30–45 seconds. Using a wide spatula, turn crepe over; cook 30 more seconds. Keep in mind that crepes can be finicky, so it may take some practice! Transfer to plate. Make more with remaining batter.

4. Crepes may be covered and chilled to use later or for other recipes such as Ham and Cheese Crepes (see recipe in this chapter).

Per Serving Calories: 116 | Fat: 8g | Protein: 4g | Sodium: 50mg | Fiber: 1g | Carbohydrates: 10g | Sugar: 1g

Ham and Cheese Crepes

These crepes are so delicious; they may just take the place of your everyday eggs! For best results make batter ahead of time and refrigerate overnight.

INGREDIENTS | SERVES 5

¾ cup gluten-free all-purpose flour

1½ tablespoons turbinado sugar

¼ teaspoon gluten-free baking powder

6 large eggs, divided

½ cup plus 1 tablespoon lactose-free milk

1 tablespoon butter, melted

¼ teaspoon alcohol-free vanilla extract

¼ teaspoon salt, divided

1 tablespoon safflower oil

10 slices deli ham

½ cup shredded Cheddar cheese

⅛ teaspoon freshly ground black pepper

1 scallion, chopped, green part only

1. Add flour and sugar to a medium bowl or a blender, then add baking powder, 1 egg, milk, butter, vanilla, and ⅛ teaspoon salt; mix until smooth. For the best result, cover batter in an airtight container and refrigerate overnight or up to 1 day. Before using batter, be sure to whisk until smooth and allow it to come to room temperature.

2. Heat a 9" round nonstick skillet over medium-high heat 1 minute then spread oil in a thin layer over surface. Using a ladle or glass measuring cup, slowly pour ¼ cup batter into skillet; swirl around pan.

3. Cook crepe until golden on bottom, 30–45 seconds. Using a wide spatula, turn crepe over; cook 30 more seconds. Keep in mind that crepes can be finicky, so it may take some practice! Transfer to plate and make more with remaining batter.

4. Preheat oven to 350°F.

5. Place 5 crepes on a rimmed baking sheet and fold edges toward center to make a semi-enclosed pocket. Place 2 slices ham on each crepe and add cheese. Crack 1 egg into center of each; sprinkle on ⅛ teaspoon salt and pepper. Bake about 12 minutes. Egg white should be set and yolk should be slightly runny (or cook more according to preference). Top with scallions.

6. Remaining crepes may be covered and chilled to use later or for other recipes.

Per Serving Calories: 339 | Fat: 17g | Protein: 24g | Sodium: 967mg | Fiber: 1g | Carbohydrates: 22g | Sugar: 6g

Pumpkin Spice Crepes

Pumpkin spice makes these crepes deliciously divine! Add some dark chocolate for a delicious treat or fill crepes with turkey and cheese, or lactose-free cream cheese, pumpkin purée, and maple syrup.

INGREDIENTS | SERVES 8

1 cup gluten-free all-purpose flour

2 large eggs

½ cup water

½ cup lactose-free milk

2 tablespoons butter, melted

1 teaspoon molasses

½ teaspoon alcohol-free vanilla extract

1¼ teaspoons pumpkin pie spice

¼ teaspoon salt

1 tablespoon safflower oil

What Substitutions Can I Use to Make This Recipe Vegan?

Instead of using lactose-free milk, use nut milks such as almond or coconut. Instead of regular butter use a vegan buttery spread, and replace eggs with an egg replacement such as flaxseeds (see Chapter 16).

1. Make batter by whisking flour and eggs in a large bowl. Whisk in water and milk and then whisk in remaining ingredients except oil.

2. Spread oil in a thin layer in a 9" round nonstick skillet over medium-high heat. Using a ladle or glass measuring cup, slowly pour ¼ cup batter into skillet; swirl around pan.

3. Cook crepe until golden on bottom, 30–45 seconds. Using a wide spatula, turn crepe and cook 30 more seconds. Keep in mind that crepes can be finicky, so it may take some practice! Transfer to a plate and make more with remaining batter.

4. Crepes may be covered and chilled to use later.

Per Serving   Calories: 110 | Fat: 4g | Protein: 4g | Sodium: 99mg | Fiber: 0g | Carbohydrates: 13g | Sugar: 1g

Coconut Cacao Hazelnut Smoothie Bowl

This nutty and chocolaty bowl will hold you over and keep you smiling for the rest of the day!

INGREDIENTS | SERVES 1

1 tablespoon shredded unsweetened coconut

1 cup unsweetened almond milk

1 frozen medium banana

2 teaspoons raw unsweetened cacao powder

½ tablespoon maple syrup

⅛ teaspoon sea salt

½ cup ice

5 hazelnuts, chopped

1 tablespoon pumpkin seeds

1. Toast coconut in a small skillet over medium heat, stirring frequently until flakes are golden brown. Set aside.

2. Add milk, banana, cacao, maple syrup, and salt to blender with ice and blend until smooth. Add more ice if necessary to make mixture thick and icy.

3. Pour mixture into a serving bowl and top with hazelnuts, pumpkin seeds, and toasted coconut.

Per Serving Calories: 380 | Fat: 15g | Protein: 13g | Sodium: 423mg | Fiber: 7g | Carbohydrates: 54g | Sugar: 31g

Raspberry Banana Mint Chia Pudding

Raspberry and mint go so well together, and make this pudding great for breakfast or the afternoon.

INGREDIENTS | SERVES 2

½ cup canned coconut milk

½ cup unsweetened almond milk

¼ cup chia seeds

1 teaspoon alcohol-free mint extract

1 tablespoon maple syrup

½ medium banana

10 raspberries

2 tablespoons shredded unsweetened coconut

2 whole mint leaves

1. Place milks, chia seeds, mint extract, and maple syrup in a jar and mix well. Cover and refrigerate, mixing every 2 hours until refrigerating overnight.

2. The next day, chop banana into rounds. Place bananas in jar, followed by raspberries, coconut, and mint leaves. Enjoy immediately or refrigerate up to 2 days.

Per Serving Calories: 119 | Fat: 8g | Protein: 3g | Sodium: 31mg | Fiber: 3g | Carbohydrates: 11g | Sugar: 5g

Passionfruit Smoothie Bowl

Passionfruit is native to southern Brazil through Paraguay and northern Argentina. It's a bitter fruit that does well when paired with other sweet ingredients. It is used in drinks, sorbet, tartlets, cakes, bread, and more.

INGREDIENTS | SERVES 1

½ frozen medium banana

1 tablespoon chia seeds

½ cup lactose-free vanilla yogurt

½ teaspoon alcohol-free vanilla extract

1 cup unsweetened almond milk

½ cup ice

Pulp of ½ passionfruit

1 tablespoon almond butter

1 tablespoon shredded unsweetened coconut, toasted

1. Add banana, chia seeds, yogurt, vanilla extract, and milk to a blender with ice and blend until smooth.

2. Pour into a serving bowl and top with passionfruit pulp, almond butter, and toasted coconut.

Per Serving   Calories: 452 | Fat: 19g | Protein: 20g | Sodium: 283mg | Fiber: 6g | Carbohydrates: 52g | Sugar: 36g

Toasting Coconut

To toast coconut, place shredded coconut in a small skillet and heat over medium-high heat. Stir frequently until flakes become golden brown. Remove from heat and set aside. You may also toast coconut in an oven. Heat oven to 350°F. Spread coconut evenly on a rimmed baking sheet, and bake 8 minutes or until light golden brown, stirring occasionally.

Jubilant Muesli Mix

This muesli is packed with healthy fruit, nuts, and seeds to help you start your day right. You can also make this muesli dry without the yogurt and use as a topping for a smoothie bowl, as a snack, or with Banana Coconut Nice Cream (see recipe in Chapter 12).

INGREDIENTS | SERVES 1

2 teaspoons shredded unsweetened coconut

½ medium orange, peeled and chopped

½ tablespoon no-sugar-added dried cranberries

⅓ cup lactose-free vanilla yogurt

⅓ cup quinoa flakes

¼ cup chia seeds

⅛ teaspoon ground nutmeg

¼ teaspoon ground cinnamon

1 teaspoon alcohol-free vanilla extract

⅛ teaspoon sea salt

¼ cup pumpkin seeds

1 tablespoon chopped walnuts

1 teaspoon cacao nibs

1. Place coconut in a small skillet over medium-high heat. Stir frequently until flakes become golden brown. Remove from heat and set aside. You may also toast coconut in oven: Preheat oven to 350°F. Using a rimmed baking sheet, spread out coconut and toast, tossing occasionally until golden, about 5 minutes. Set aside.

2. In a medium bowl, stir together chopped orange, cranberries, yogurt, quinoa, chia seeds, nutmeg, cinnamon, vanilla extract, and salt. Cover and chill overnight. Just before serving, top with pumpkin seeds, walnuts, cacao, and coconut.

Per Serving   Calories: 748 | Fat: 42g | Protein: 30g | Sodium: 364mg | Fiber: 15g | Carbohydrates: 69g | Sugar: 18g

Soaking Nuts

Soaking nuts can be beneficial to those who suffer from IBS or other digestive-related issues. Read more about how to soak nuts in Chapter 16.

Cream of Muesli

Once you have made the basic recipe, you have options for making your muesli even more nutritious and delicious. Enjoy some healthy decadence with a swirl of natural peanut butter topped with sliced banana and a sprinkle of cacao powder.

**INGREDIENTS | MAKES 6½ CUPS
(½ CUP PER SERVING)**

½ cup hulled pumpkin seeds
½ cup hulled sunflower seeds
½ cup shelled walnuts
3 cups gluten-free rolled oats
1 cup gluten-free oat bran
¼ cup buckwheat flour
½ cup finely ground flaxseeds
½ cup finely ground chia seeds
1 tablespoon ground cinnamon
6½ cups lactose-free milk

1. Add all ingredients except milk to a food processor.

2. Pulse 20–30 times. Scrape sides of the work bowl. Pulse 20–30 times more until all seeds and nuts appear chopped to a coarse consistency.

3. For each serving, scoop ½ cup muesli into a small saucepan and add ½ cup milk. Bring to a simmer over medium heat and stir 2–3 minutes.

4. Transfer to a breakfast bowl and serve.

Per Serving Calories: 595 | Fat: 32g | Protein: 24g | Sodium: 124mg | Fiber: 12g | Carbohydrates: 59g | Sugar: 11g

Grinding Seeds

As you follow the low-FODMAP diet, you may find yourself experimenting with some new seeds. Both flaxseeds and chia seeds are good sources of dietary fiber and anti-inflammatory omega-3 fatty acids. Flaxseeds need to be ground before eating. Invest in a little coffee grinder and dedicate it to the easy task of seed grinding.

Eggs Baked in Heirloom Tomatoes

As you cut into these juicy tomatoes, savor the aroma of herbs and the warm baked egg and cheese. If you don't have heirloom tomatoes, choose other large and fresh tomatoes that have nice, thick skins.

INGREDIENTS | SERVES 4

4 large round heirloom tomatoes
3 tablespoons olive oil
1 teaspoon herbes de Provence
¼ teaspoon salt
1 teaspoon freshly ground black pepper
4 large eggs
¼ cup grated Parmesan cheese
¼ cup crumbled feta cheese
2 teaspoons lactose-free milk

1. Preheat oven to 375°F.

2. Slice top off tomatoes and use a paring knife or small spoon to gently remove core and seeds, making sure not to pierce bottoms of tomatoes but cutting enough flesh to leave ample space to drop in egg.

3. Arrange tomatoes so they are snug in an 8" × 8" or larger baking dish lightly greased with cooking spray. Drizzle with olive oil, and add a pinch of herbes de Provence (roughly ⅛ teaspoon each), salt, and pepper.

4. Crack an egg into each tomato. Add in 1 tablespoon each of Parmesan cheese, feta cheese, and ½ teaspoon each of milk.

5. Bake 20 minutes for runny eggs and 30 minutes or more for harder yolks.

Per Serving   Calories: 167 | Fat: 9g | Protein: 13g | Sodium: 575mg | Fiber: 2g | Carbohydrates: 8g | Sugar: 5g

Shakshuka for Two

Shakshuka is believed to have a Tunisian origin and in Israel it is often eaten for breakfast. This version is free of FOMDAPs and is great for breakfast or even dinner with a low-FODMAP serving of Pinot Noir or Pinot Grigio.

INGREDIENTS | SERVES 2

1 tablespoon garlic-infused olive oil
½ cup canned chickpeas, drained and rinsed
½ small chili pepper, seeded and diced
½ large chopped green bell pepper
½ teaspoon smoked paprika
½ teaspoon ground cumin
¼ teaspoon ground turmeric
1/16 teaspoon wheat-free asafetida powder
⅛ teaspoon salt
½ teaspoon freshly ground black pepper
1 (14-ounce) can crushed tomatoes
1 tablespoon tomato paste
1 teaspoon light brown sugar
½ teaspoon rice wine vinegar
½ cup coarsely chopped Swiss chard
½ cup coarsely chopped spinach
½ cup cubed feta cheese
¼ cup crumbled goat cheese
3 large eggs
2 tablespoons chopped fresh cilantro

1. Using a large, wide skillet, heat oil over medium-high heat. Add chickpeas, chili pepper, green bell pepper, paprika, cumin, turmeric, asafetida, salt, and pepper. Cook 5 minutes, stirring occasionally.

2. Add crushed tomatoes, tomato paste, sugar, and vinegar; reduce heat to medium and cook 12–15 minutes or until sauce is slightly thickened. Add chopped greens and cheese and stir.

3. Turn off heat and move skillet to another burner. Make 3 wells in sauce and crack an egg into each indentation. Use a spatula to pull some of egg whites slightly out of wells, being careful not to touch yolks.

4. Place skillet back on hot burner and turn heat to medium-low so sauce is gently simmering. Cook about 10–12 minutes. Cover and cook 3–5 more minutes until eggs are cooked to desired doneness. Top with cilantro.

Per Serving   Calories: 616 | Fat: 35g | Protein: 37g | Sodium: 648mg | Fiber: 13g | Carbohydrates: 40g | Sugar: 19g

Bake Your Shakshuka

After you've made wells for the eggs, you may also heat your oven to 375°F and bake eggs in an ovenproof skillet 8–12 minutes, depending on desired doneness for eggs.

Pesto Eggs Rice Bowl

Make the low-FODMAP Pesto Sauce ahead of time for this recipe.

INGREDIENTS | SERVES 1

½ cup cooked brown rice

⅛ cup Pesto Sauce (see recipe in Chapter 13)

1 hardboiled large egg

⅛ medium avocado

1 tablespoon grated Parmesan cheese

1. Place cooked rice in a soup bowl. Pour pesto over rice and stir until rice is evenly covered.

2. Cut hardboiled egg in half. Place on top of rice and pesto. Place avocado on top. Sprinkle with Parmesan cheese. Enjoy!

Per Serving   Calories: 275 | Fat: 13g | Protein: 14g | Sodium: 297mg | Fiber: 3g | Carbohydrates: 26g | Sugar: 1g

Raspberry Lemon Oatmeal Bars

These are great to make ahead and have for breakfast on the go!

INGREDIENTS | SERVES 12

½ teaspoon turbinado sugar

1¼ cups unsweetened almond milk

½ teaspoon alcohol-free vanilla extract

1 large egg or egg replacer

¼ cup maple syrup

3½ cups gluten-free quick-cooking oats

2 tablespoons lemon juice

2 cups raspberries

1. Preheat oven to 350°F.

2. In a large bowl, whisk together sugar, milk, vanilla, egg, and maple syrup.

3. Add oats, lemon juice, and raspberries. Stir well to combine.

4. Pour into an 9" × 13" baking dish and bake 25 minutes.

Per Serving   Calories: 139 | Fat: 3g | Protein: 5g | Sodium: 21mg | Fiber: 4g | Carbohydrates: 25g | Sugar: 7g

Quinoa, Egg, Ham, and Cheese Breakfast Muffins

This is a super-fun and easy way to make eggs in the morning. Alternatively you can get creative and use different low-FODMAP ingredients to suit different tastes.

INGREDIENTS | SERVES 12

7 large eggs
¼ teaspoon sea salt
¼ teaspoon freshly ground black pepper
1½ cups cooked quinoa
⅓ cup shredded Parmesan cheese
⅓ cup shredded Cheddar cheese
½ cup chopped scallions (green part only)
½ cup chopped parsley
10 black olives, sliced
½ pound breakfast ham, cooked and chopped into small cubes

1. Position a rack in center of oven. Preheat to 400°F.

2. Using cooking spray, coat cups of a 12-cup muffin pan.

3. Add eggs to a large bowl with salt and pepper. Whisk until fluffy.

4. In a medium bowl, combine quinoa, half of the Parmesan and Cheddar cheese, scallions, parsley, olives, and ham.

5. Fill muffin cups about ⅓ full with quinoa mixture. Pour in about ¼ cup eggs into each muffin cup. Sprinkle each with remaining cheese.

6. Bake 20–25 minutes or until golden on top and around edges.

7. Remove cups from pan by carefully sliding a rubber spatula along the sides.

Per Serving   Calories: 161 | Fat: 9g | Protein: 13g | Sodium: 593mg | Fiber: 1g | Carbohydrates: 7g | Sugar: 1g

Mexican Egg Brunch

Expecting company? This low-FODMAP brunch is another easy recipe and only requires 1 bowl and 1 casserole dish.

INGREDIENTS | SERVES 4

2 cups whole corn tortilla chips
1 cup shredded Cheddar cheese
4 whole large eggs
4 egg whites
½ cup salsa
½ cup sliced black olives
2 scallions, chopped, green part only
½ medium avocado, sliced into eighths
½ cup lactose-free sour cream

Not All Casserole Dishes Are Alike

For this recipe choose a clear glass casserole dish, as the glass makes it easier to see when the eggs are cooked through.

1. Preheat oven to 400°F. Grease a 9" × 13" glass casserole dish.

2. Spread tortilla chips in casserole dish. Add half of cheese.

3. In a medium bowl whisk eggs and egg whites until fluffy. Pour eggs into casserole dish.

4. Pour salsa evenly over eggs. Sprinkle on remaining cheese. Sprinkle on black olives and scallions.

5. Bake 15–20 minutes or until eggs look cooked around edges of casserole dish.

6. Top with avocado and sour cream.

Per Serving   Calories: 458 | Fat: 23g | Protein: 20g | Sodium: 564mg | Fiber: 8g | Carbohydrates: 46g | Sugar: 3g

Eggs with Spinach and Chickpeas

Dress up your morning and try something different with eggs. You'll love the flavors of this dish!

INGREDIENTS | SERVES 2

4 tablespoons olive oil, divided

4 cups coarsely chopped baby spinach

⅛ teaspoon asafetida powder

½ teaspoon salt

½ teaspoon freshly ground black pepper

¼ teaspoon smoked paprika

½ cup canned chickpeas, rinsed and drained

2½ cups canned whole San Marzano tomatoes, crushed

3½ cups Vegetable Stock (see recipe in Chapter 4)

2 large eggs

¼ cup crumbled goat cheese

Why Are Canned Chickpeas Allowed on the Low-FODMAP Diet?

Canning allows the oligos–GOS in the chickpeas to leach out into the water of the can, making them lower in FODMAPs. You must rinse and drain them and stick with a ¼-cup serving.

1. Heat 1 tablespoon oil in a large, heavy pan or cast-iron skillet over medium heat. Add spinach, asafetida, salt, and pepper. Cook until spinach is slightly wilted, about 2–3 minutes. Transfer to a medium bowl; set aside.

2. Using the same pan, heat 2 tablespoons oil over medium heat. Add paprika, chickpeas, and tomatoes; stir. Cook 10 minutes.

3. Add 3 cups stock; bring to a simmer. Reduce heat to medium and simmer until sauce is thickened, 15–20 minutes. Add spinach and remaining stock; simmer 8–10 minutes.

4. Heat remaining 1 tablespoon oil in an 8" nonstick skillet over medium-high heat. Crack both eggs into skillet and fry sunny-side up until edges are crispy, about 2–3 minutes. Season eggs with salt and pepper if desired.

5. Place chickpea mixture in serving bowls and top each with a fried egg and goat cheese.

Per Serving Calories: 462 | Fat: 43g | Protein: 22g | Sodium: 2,088mg | Fiber: 7g | Carbohydrates: 26g | Sugar: 9g

Delicioso Breakfast Tacos

Head south of the border for your next breakfast and whip up this satisfying meal in no time.

INGREDIENTS | SERVES 4

4 large eggs
½ cup egg whites
¼ cup lactose-free milk
1 tablespoon chopped fresh cilantro
¼ teaspoon salt
½ teaspoon freshly ground black pepper
4 strips bacon
¼ cup diced green bell pepper
¼ teaspoon ground cumin
4 (8") soft corn tortillas
½ cup shredded light Cheddar cheese
¼ cup lactose-free sour cream
¼ cup salsa

1. In a medium bowl combine eggs, egg whites, milk, cilantro, salt, and pepper. Beat eggs until fluffy.

2. In a 9" skillet over medium-low heat, add bacon strips and once sizzling, turn heat to low. Flip bacon often or until browned. Remove and place between paper towels to soak up excess oil.

3. Turn heat up to medium and add peppers and cumin. Cook until tender, about 3–4 minutes. Pour in egg mixture and gently push, lift, and fold eggs with spatula until set and cooked to desired doneness. Remove from heat and use the edge of your spatula to cut egg mixture into chunks.

4. Warm tortillas in a small skillet or in the microwave 30 seconds. Divide egg mixture among tortillas, then add cheese, bacon, sour cream, and salsa.

Per Serving   Calories: 374 | Fat: 24g | Protein: 20g | Sodium: 846mg | Fiber: 1g | Carbohydrates: 19g | Sugar: 3g

Tomato and Leek Frittata

Onions aren't allowed on the low-FODMAP diet but you can use leek leaves, and they are delicious with eggs. Serve this frittata garnished with some extra goat cheese, tomato slices, and sliced green onions.

INGREDIENTS | SERVES 2

3 teaspoons olive oil, divided

½ cup chopped leek leaves

½ teaspoon sea salt, divided

½ teaspoon freshly ground black pepper, divided

½ cup grape tomatoes

¼ cup capers, rinsed and drained

3 egg whites

1 teaspoon dried herbes de Provence

1 teaspoon dried thyme

2 egg yolks

2 ounces goat cheese, crumbled

1. Preheat oven to 350°F.

2. Heat 2 teaspoons oil in a 10" ovenproof nonstick skillet over medium heat. Add leeks, ¼ teaspoon salt, and ¼ teaspoon pepper. Cook 5 minutes. Stir in grape tomatoes and capers. Cover and cook 3 minutes. Transfer to a small bowl.

3. In a medium bowl, quickly beat egg whites with herbes de Provence, thyme, and remaining salt and pepper. Whisk in egg yolks. Whisk until mixture is fluffy.

4. Brush skillet with remaining olive oil. Add eggs, cooked tomato mixture, and goat cheese. Cook over medium heat 4 minutes. Transfer to oven; bake 15–20 minutes or until eggs are set. To check, cut a small slit in center of frittata.

Per Serving   Calories: 292 | Fat: 22g | Protein: 18g | Sodium: 1,293mg | Fiber: 2g | Carbohydrates: 8g | Sugar: 3g

Cranberry Almond Granola

Throw this delicious, good-for-you granola on top of lactose-free yogurt, rice cereal, or quinoa flakes.

INGREDIENTS | MAKES 2½ CUPS

1 tablespoon whole walnuts

1 tablespoon flaxseeds

3 tablespoons canola oil

3 tablespoons maple syrup

¼ teaspoon alcohol-free vanilla extract

¼ teaspoon alcohol-free almond extract

1 cup gluten-free rolled oats

1 tablespoon slivered almonds

½ teaspoon ground cinnamon

2 tablespoons no-sugar-added dried cranberries

Cranberry Tip

For softer cranberries, place in a small bowl with hot water and let stand 20 minutes. One tablespoon of dried cranberries is low in FODMAPs.

1. Preheat oven to 350°F.

2. Using a food processor or blender, add in walnuts and pulse until ground. Add to a large bowl. Next add flaxseed and pulse until finely ground. Add to same large bowl.

3. In a medium bowl, stir together oil, maple syrup, and vanilla and almond extract.

4. In large bowl, combine walnuts, flaxseed, oats, almonds, and cinnamon. Pour oil mixture over oats and stir well to combine.

5. Spread granola on a rimmed baking sheet and bake 15 minutes. Stir occasionally to ensure granola turns a light brown color.

6. After removing from oven, add cranberries and stir to combine. Store in an airtight container up to 3 weeks.

Per Serving   Calories: 499 | Fat: 28g | Protein: 7g | Sodium: 6mg | Fiber: 7g | Carbohydrates: 57g | Sugar: 23g

Overnight Peanut Butter Pumpkin Spice Oats

You will love digging into these hearty and delicious oats! Perfect before a big day.

INGREDIENTS | SERVES 2

½ cup gluten-free rolled oats

¼ cup unsweetened almond milk

¼ cup pumpkin purée

½ teaspoon pumpkin pie spice

½ teaspoon alcohol-free vanilla extract

½ teaspoon ground cinnamon

1 tablespoon maple syrup

2 tablespoons peanut butter

2 tablespoons chopped walnuts

Overnight Oats Have So Many Possibilities!

Overnight oats are so easy to make and there are several different variations you can try with foods low in FODMAPs. Just always be sure to use a 1:1 ratio for oats and almond milk unless you like your oats runny. Be mindful of the appropriate recommended servings for the low-FODMAP diet to keep your overnight oats low in overall FODMAPs. One ¼-cup serving of oats is low-FODMAP.

1. In a medium bowl, combine oats and almond milk and stir. Add pumpkin purée, pumpkin pie spice, vanilla, cinnamon, and maple syrup. Stir.

2. Spoon half the mixture into 2 small canning jars. Add 1 tablespoon peanut butter on top of oats in each jar. Divide remaining oats on top of peanut butter. Cover with lids. Refrigerate overnight.

3. In the morning, top with walnuts and enjoy! Can be stored in refrigerator up to 3 days.

Per Serving Calories: 270 | Fat: 15g | Protein: 9g | Sodium: 92mg | Fiber: 4g | Carbohydrates: 28g | Sugar: 9g

Overnight Banana Chocolate Oats

For the banana and chocolate lovers out there, these overnight oats can be eaten cold or warmed in the microwave for 30 seconds.

INGREDIENTS | SERVES 1

¼ cup gluten-free rolled oats

2 tablespoons unsweetened almond milk

1 teaspoon unsweetened cocoa powder

½ ripe medium banana, mashed

2 tablespoons lactose-free vanilla yogurt

⅛ teaspoon alcohol-free vanilla extract

2 teaspoons maple syrup

½ teaspoon ground cinnamon

1 ounce dark chocolate, smashed into chunks

1–2 banana slices, for garnish

1. In a medium bowl, combine oats and almond milk and stir. Add cocoa powder, banana, yogurt, vanilla, maple syrup, and cinnamon; stir to combine. Place in a canning jar and cover with lid. Refrigerate overnight.

2. The next day, top with chocolate chunks and banana slices and enjoy! Can be stored in refrigerator up to 3 days.

Per Serving   Calories: 342 | Fat: 11g | Protein: 7g | Sodium: 44mg | Fiber: 7g | Carbohydrates: 60g | Sugar: 34g

Overnight Carrot Cake Oats and Walnuts

Who said you couldn't have cake in the morning?

INGREDIENTS | SERVES 2

3 ounces lactose-free plain yogurt

¼ cup unsweetened almond milk

½ cup gluten-free rolled oats

1 tablespoon chia seeds

¼ cup peeled and shredded carrots

2 tablespoons crushed pineapple

¼ teaspoon alcohol-free vanilla extract

½ tablespoon maple syrup

½ teaspoon ground cinnamon

1 tablespoon walnut halves

1. In a medium bowl, combine yogurt, almond milk, and oats; stir. Add chia seeds, carrots, pineapple, vanilla, maple syrup, and cinnamon and stir to combine. Place in 2 small canning jars and cover with lids. Refrigerate overnight.

2. In the morning top with walnuts and enjoy! Can be stored in refrigerator up to 3 days.

Per Serving   Calories: 342 | Fat: 11g | Protein: 7g | Sodium: 44mg | Fiber: 7g | Carbohydrates: 60g | Sugar: 34g

Amaranth Breakfast

This recipe will make your home smell wonderful! It can be made in a rice cooker if you happen to have one. When serving, feel free to add a few drops of maple syrup and whatever berries you have on hand.

INGREDIENTS | SERVES 4

1 cup amaranth seeds
3 cups water
2 teaspoons ground cinnamon
1 teaspoon alcohol-free vanilla extract
¼ cup lightly chopped pecans

1. Heat a heavy-bottomed saucepan over medium heat and add amaranth. Toast amaranth, stirring occasionally until fragrant, about 5 minutes.

2. Pour in water and bring to a boil. Lower heat and add cinnamon and vanilla. Cover and simmer 20 minutes, stirring occasionally.

3. While amaranth is simmering, place pecans under broiler for 4 minutes to toast.

4. When amaranth has finished cooking, give it a good stir and remove from heat. Serve in bowls topped with pecans.

Per Serving   Calories: 244 | Fat: 20g | Protein: 7g | Sodium: 15mg | Fiber: 8g | Carbohydrates: 12g | Sugar: 2g

Savory Sourdough Strata

Prepared the night before, a strata is an easy weekend brunch main dish.

INGREDIENTS | SERVES 8

1 tablespoon extra-virgin olive oil

10 ounces baby spinach leaves

1 teaspoon sea salt, divided

2 cups Roasted Tomato Sauce (see recipe in Chapter 13)

5 cups cubed (1") gluten-free sourdough bread (crusts removed)

6 large eggs

1½ cups lactose-free milk

1 cup shredded sharp Cheddar cheese, divided

¼ teaspoon freshly ground black pepper

4 slices bacon, cooked, cooled, and chopped

What about Sourdough?

Traditional sourdough is produced through a process of fermentation, which reduces its FODMAP fructan level. However, many commercial sourdough products use baker's yeast to get a rise to save the time needed for the fermentation process. To ensure that the sourdough bread you are eating is low in FODMAP, choose either a gluten-free option or a traditionally prepared artisanal sourdough.

1. Heat oil in a medium skillet over medium heat.

2. Add spinach and pinch of salt, and sauté until wilted. Set aside to cool.

3. Mix cooled spinach with roasted tomato sauce and spread in a thin layer on the bottom of a 9" × 13" baking dish. Top with bread cubes.

4. In a medium bowl, whisk eggs, milk, ½ cup cheese, remaining salt, and pepper. Pour evenly over bread cubes. Hand-turn to coat any dry cubes—ensuring they are all wet. Sprinkle evenly with remaining cheese and bacon. Cover and refrigerate overnight.

5. In the morning, heat oven to 375°F. Bake uncovered 30–40 minutes, or until cheese melts and egg mixture is fully set.

Per Serving   Calories: 265 | Fat: 16g | Protein: 15g | Sodium: 1,002mg | Fiber: 2g | Carbohydrates: 16g | Sugar: 5g

CHAPTER 3

Appetizers

Baba Ghanoush
64

Mini Polenta Pizzas
65

Mini Baked Eggplant Pizza Bites
66

Chicken Lettuce Cups
67

Smoked Salmon Hand Rolls
68

Coconut Shrimp with
Pineapple Sauce
69

Quinoa, Corn, and Zucchini
Fritters
70

Indian-Spiced Mixed Nuts
71

Pão de Queijo (Cheese Bread)
72

Feta Cheese Dip
73

Herbes de Provence Almonds
73

Baked Camembert and
Rosemary
74

Vietnamese Summer Rolls
75

Baba Ghanoush

This low-FODMAP version of Baba Ghanoush is delicious with gluten-free pita bread, gluten-free crackers, or as a spread on a sandwich (see Chapter 6 for recipe).

INGREDIENTS | SERVES 12

2 medium eggplants (about 2 pounds)
1 teaspoon salt
⅓ cup tahini (without added FODMAPs)
⅛ teaspoon wheat-free asafetida powder
2 medium lemons, juiced
½ teaspoon ground cumin
½ teaspoon cayenne pepper
1 tablespoon extra-virgin olive oil
½ teaspoon paprika (for garnish)
2 tablespoons minced fresh flat-leaf parsley (for garnish)

1. Preheat oven to 400°F. Lightly grease a baking sheet with cooking spray.

2. Slice off stem and blossom ends of eggplants. Cut eggplants lengthwise into thin strips, and then cut into cubes. Place cubes in a colander and sprinkle with salt to remove any bitterness. Let stand for 1 hour. Place between paper towels to pat dry.

3. Place eggplant on baking sheet and roast until softened and golden brown, 25–30 minutes.

4. Add tahini, asafetida powder, lemon juice, cumin, cayenne, and olive oil to bowl.

5. Use a fork to mash together mixture until well combined. Sprinkle with paprika and parsley to garnish.

Per Serving Calories: 71 | Fat: 5g | Protein: 2g | Sodium: 206mg | Fiber: 4g | Carbohydrates: 7g | Sugar: 2g

Mini Polenta Pizzas

These mini pizzas are great as appetizers or to serve kids at a birthday party.

INGREDIENTS | SERVES 6

2¼ cups water

1 cup polenta (ground cornmeal)

½ cup freshly grated Parmesan cheese

1/16 teaspoon wheat-free asafetida powder

¼ teaspoon salt

½ teaspoon freshly ground pepper

1 cup shredded mozzarella cheese

6 sun-dried tomatoes, chopped

6 basil leaves, finely chopped

Love Onions and Garlic? Here's Your Substitute

Asafetida powder (also known as asafoetida powder or hing) is used often in Indian vegetarian cooking. It is derived from a species of giant fennel, and has a very unique smell and powerful flavor. It is suitable for the low-FODMAP diet as an onion and garlic replacement. Two tips—make sure you buy a wheat-free version like *Uncle Harry's*. Try just a little bit at a time and adjust the amount accordingly. Using too much can ruin your dish.

1. Preheat oven to 400°F.

2. In a medium saucepan, bring water to a boil. Slowly add polenta, reduce heat to low, and whisk until polenta has thickened, about 5 minutes. Remove from heat, add Parmesan, asafetida, salt, and pepper. Stir to combine.

3. Lightly spray 6 (3½-ounce) ramekins with cooking spray. Add polenta to each cup, filling about ¾ of the way. Create a small well in the center of each cup using your hands or a spoon. Add even amounts of mozzarella, sun-dried tomatoes, and basil to each cup.

4. Place ramekins on a rimmed baking sheet and bake 30 minutes or until cheese becomes slightly browned and bubbly.

Per Serving   Calories: 333 | Fat: 15g | Protein: 18g | Sodium: 610mg | Fiber: 3g | Carbohydrates: 32g | Sugar: 2g

Mini Baked Eggplant Pizza Bites

These baked pizza bites can be very addicting! And because they are baked, not fried, less oil is required, which cuts down on fat, making them a healthier appetizer option.

INGREDIENTS | SERVES 4

2 medium eggplants

½ teaspoon salt

1 large egg

¾ cup gluten-free panko bread crumbs

2 tablespoons dried oregano

2 teaspoons olive oil

½ cup Basic Marinara Sauce (see recipe in Chapter 13)

¼ cup shredded mozzarella cheese

Where to Buy Gluten-Free Panko Bread Crumbs

There are a few brands that carry gluten-free low-FODMAP panko bread crumbs such as Ian's Original. You can buy them from online retailers such as Amazon.

1. Preheat oven to 400°F.

2. Cut top and bottom ends off eggplants, then cut into circle slices. Cut off sides of the circles, leaving square shapes. Place in a colander and toss with ½ teaspoon salt. Let sit for about 10 minutes. Rinse with water.

3. In a small bowl, whisk egg. Place bread crumbs in a shallow bowl and add oregano, stirring well to combine. Dredge eggplant squares in egg, tap off any excess, and then dredge in bread crumbs. Place on a nonstick baking sheet (use nonstick cookware that does not contain toxic or hazardous materials PTFE and PFOA).

4. Slowly drizzle olive oil to cover the tops of each square. Bake 12 minutes.

5. Remove eggplant from oven and spoon marinara sauce onto the center of each square, leaving edges of eggplant uncovered. Sprinkle mozzarella on top of squares. Bake 2–3 minutes or until cheese has melted.

Per Serving Calories: 259 | Fat: 9g | Protein: 11g | Sodium: 653mg | Fiber: 12g | Carbohydrates: 36g | Sugar: 11g

Chicken Lettuce Cups

Be warned—these will go quickly! These cups pair well with fried rice, rice noodles, or most Asian dishes.

INGREDIENTS | SERVES 8

4 pounds ground chicken

⅛ teaspoon finely chopped fresh gingerroot

⅛ teaspoon wheat-free asafetida powder

2 (8-ounce) cans water chestnuts, chopped

¼ cup ground chili powder

2 tablespoons coconut oil

½ cup gluten-free soy sauce (tamari)

2 tablespoons rice wine vinegar

½ cup chopped scallions, green part only

1 tablespoon fresh lime juice

8 inner leaves of iceberg lettuce, chilled and trimmed

1. In a large bowl, add chicken, ginger, asafetida, water chestnuts, and chili powder. Combine well with hands.

2. In a large skillet, heat oil on medium. Add chicken mixture. Move around the pan and use a spatula to cut up into small chunks. Add soy sauce, vinegar, scallions, and lime juice; cook 5–8 minutes or until chicken is cooked through.

3. Stack lettuce leaves on top of one another on a platter. Place chicken mixture in a bowl on the platter with a spoon for serving.

Per Serving Calories: 538 | Fat: 37g | Protein: 40g | Sodium: 1,074mg | Fiber: 1g | Carbohydrates: 8g | Sugar: 2g

Smoked Salmon Hand Rolls

With a little practice, hand rolls can be a great, healthy addition to your diet. Once you master this recipe, try other combinations using different fish and low-FODMAP vegetables.

INGREDIENTS | SERVES 6

6 nori sheets, perforated

1½ cups cooked brown rice, cooled

6 ounces smoked salmon slices

6 tablespoons lactose-free cream cheese

1 medium avocado, cut into eighths

For Beginners

For your first "go" at making hand rolls, consider trying smoked salmon. It is relatively easy to buy, as many larger supermarkets carry it, and if you don't have a fishmonger you trust, it might be harder to find true sushi-grade fish.

1. Tear each nori sheet in half.

2. Moisten your hands and divide rice into 6 portions, forming into balls.

3. Pick up nori sheet and hold shiny side down in the palm of your hand (if you're right-handed, hold nori sheet in left hand and vice versa). Moisten your hand again and place 1 rice ball at a slight angle to far left of sheet; press to a ¼" thickness leaving space between rice and edges of nori sheet; press your index finger into middle to make an indentation the size of your finger.

4. Keep the nori in your hand and add salmon, cream cheese, and avocado. Still holding nori in one hand, use your other hand and tightly roll up bottom left-hand corner on a diagonal, over rice and filling. Create a cone by tightly wrapping opposite right-hand edge around. Fold and tuck to create a cone shape. With a moist finger, place a piece or two of rice on the corner to secure inside edge of nori to outside.

Per Serving Calories: 190 | Fat: 11g | Protein: 8g | Sodium: 269mg | Fiber: 3g | Carbohydrates: 15g | Sugar: 1g

Coconut Shrimp with Pineapple Sauce

Make your own delicious Coconut Shrimp at home!
Great for parties, holidays, or topped on a green salad.

INGREDIENTS | SERVES 8

40 large shrimp (about 2½ pounds)

2½ cups chopped pineapple

2 tablespoons gluten-free fish sauce

1 tablespoon turbinado sugar

⅛ teaspoon wheat-free asafetida powder

1½ teaspoons Sweet Chili Garlic Sauce (see recipe in Chapter 13)

1 tablespoon fresh lime juice

1 cup gluten-free panko bread crumbs

1½ cups shredded unsweetened coconut

½ teaspoon sea salt

2 large eggs

2 egg whites

1. Preheat oven to 425°F.

2. Peel and wash shrimp, leaving tails intact.

3. In a blender or food processor, add pineapple, fish sauce, sugar, asafetida, sweet chili garlic sauce, and lime juice; process 45 seconds or until smooth. Place in a small serving bowl.

4. Combine bread crumbs, coconut, and sea salt in a shallow bowl. In a separate bowl, beat eggs and egg whites until light and airy.

5. Add ¼ batch of shrimp at a time to eggs, tossing to coat. Next, dredge shrimp in bread crumb mixture; place on a baking sheet lined with parchment paper.

6. Bake 12 minutes. Halfway through baking, use tongs to lightly grab shrimp by tails to turn over. Serve shrimp with prepared pineapple sauce.

Per Serving Calories: 202 | Fat: 8g | Protein: 12g | Sodium: 337mg | Fiber: 3g | Carbohydrates: 22g | Sugar: 9g

Quinoa, Corn, and Zucchini Fritters

These fritters are a healthier alternative to deep-fried versions, and they're made with more vegetables!

INGREDIENTS | SERVES 10

1 cup water

½ cup quinoa

3 cups grated zucchini, as much water squeezed out as possible

1 cup frozen corn, thawed and drained

2 teaspoons dried oregano

1/16 teaspoon wheat-free asafetida powder

½ cup gluten-free all-purpose flour

½ teaspoon gluten-free baking powder

2 tablespoons lemon juice

½ teaspoon salt

½ teaspoon freshly ground black pepper

1 tablespoon safflower oil

½ cup freshly grated Parmesan cheese

5 tablespoons lactose-free sour cream

2 tablespoons finely chopped fresh flat-leaf parsley

1. Add water to a small saucepan with quinoa and bring to a boil. Reduce heat to low, cover, and simmer until cooked, about 10–12 minutes. Set aside to cool.

2. Place grated zucchini in a medium bowl and add quinoa, corn, oregano, asafetida, flour, baking powder, lemon juice, salt, and pepper. Mix to combine.

3. Heat oil in a 12" skillet over medium-high heat. Form about ⅓ cup zucchini mixture into a patty. Repeat until all patties are made. Place patties in skillet and cook 5–7 minutes on each side or until golden brown. Work in batches if necessary so edges do not overlap.

4. Garnish each with even amounts of Parmesan cheese, sour cream, and parsley.

Per Serving   Calories: 130 | Fat: 5g | Protein: 7g | Sodium: 330mg | Fiber: 2g | Carbohydrates: 16g | Sugar: 1g

Indian-Spiced Mixed Nuts

These are great to hold over a hungry crowd or to take along as a snack.

INGREDIENTS | MAKES 3¾ CUPS

½ cup almonds

1 cup macadamia nuts

1 cup halved walnuts

1 cup halved pecans

1 teaspoon Himalayan sea salt

¼ teaspoon ground cumin

¾ teaspoon ground cinnamon

¼ teaspoon chili powder

¼ teaspoon ground turmeric

¼ teaspoon ground cardamom

½ teaspoon freshly ground black pepper

½ cup light brown sugar

¼ cup water

1½ tablespoons butter

How Many Nuts in a Low-FODMAP Serving?

On the low-FODMAP diet you can enjoy up to 18 assorted nuts, about 36 grams. Cashews and pistachios are high in FODMAPs and should be avoided. One low-FODMAP serving for almonds, hazelnuts, or Brazil nuts equals 10 nuts; pecans are 10 halves. A low-FODMAP serving for chestnuts or macadamia nuts is 20 nuts and for peanuts it is 32 nuts.

1. Preheat oven to 350°F. Line a baking sheet with aluminum foil and coat with cooking spray.

2. Combine almonds, macadamia nuts, walnuts, and pecans in a large bowl. Add salt, cumin, cinnamon, chili powder, turmeric, cardamom, and black pepper; toss to coat.

3. In a small saucepan over medium heat, heat sugar, water, and butter until butter is melted. Remove from heat. Carefully and slowly pour butter mixture over bowl of nuts; stir to coat.

4. Transfer nuts to prepared baking sheet, spreading nuts evenly into a single layer. Bake 10 minutes.

5. Remove and stir nuts, ensuring every nut gets coated and keeping all nuts in a single layer. Return to oven and bake 7 minutes. Allow nuts to cool before serving in a bowl.

Per Serving Calories: 225 | Fat: 20g | Protein: 4g | Sodium: 150mg | Fiber: 3g | Carbohydrates: 11g | Sugar: 8g

Pão de Queijo (Cheese Bread)

Pão de Queijo is a small cheesy roll, and is a popular snack and breakfast food in Brazil. They're also great served alongside your favorite stew or roast.

INGREDIENTS | MAKES 2 DOZEN

1 cup lactose-free milk
½ cup coconut oil
1 teaspoon sea salt
2 cups tapioca starch
2 large eggs
1½ cups grated Parmesan cheese

1. Preheat oven to 450°F.

2. Combine milk, oil, and salt in a medium saucepan. Whisk occasionally, and bring to a slow boil over medium heat. Once you see large bubbles, remove pan from heat.

3. Add flour to saucepan; stir until well combined. Dough should have a gelatinous texture.

4. Transfer dough to bowl of stand mixer with a paddle attachment. At medium speed, beat dough for 5–7 minutes or until smooth.

5. Whisk eggs together in a small bowl. On medium speed, add eggs slowly to dough. Use a spatula to scrape down any dough stuck to sides of bowl.

6. Add cheese and beat on medium speed until fully incorporated. Dough should be very sticky, stretchy, and soft.

7. Use a tablespoon measure or ice cream scoop to make rounded balls and place on a parchment-lined baking sheet. Space balls of dough 1–2" apart. Dip your fingers in a bowl of olive oil to keep dough from sticking to your hands.

8. Place in oven. Turn down heat to 350°F. Bake 25–30 minutes. Remove once outsides are dry and are just starting to color. You'll see orange flecks of color.

Per Serving   Calories: 225 | Fat: 20g | Protein: 4g | Sodium: 150mg | Fiber: 3g | Carbohydrates: 11g | Sugar: 8g

Feta Cheese Dip

This creamy and sultry dip tastes so good with gluten-free pita bread, crackers, or crunchy vegetables.

INGREDIENTS | MAKES 1 CUP

⅓ cup crumbled feta cheese

¼ cup lactose-free cream cheese

3 tablespoons Basic Mayonnaise (see recipe in Chapter 13)

¼ cup chopped black olives

1 tablespoon lemon juice

1/16 teaspoon wheat-free asafetida powder

¼ teaspoon dried oregano

¼ teaspoon dried dill

¼ teaspoon dried thyme

1 teaspoon freshly ground black pepper

Combine all ingredients in a large bowl. Mix well with to combine or use a stand mixer.

Per Serving (¼ cup)   Calories: 132 | Fat: 12g | Protein: 4g | Sodium: 327mg | Fiber: 1g | Carbohydrates: 3g | Sugar: 1g

Herbes de Provence Almonds

These savory roasted almonds are too good to be true and very easy to make.

INGREDIENTS | MAKES 1 CUP

1½ tablespoons butter

1½ teaspoons herbes de Provence, crushed

½ teaspoon sea salt

⅛ teaspoon paprika

1 cup raw almonds

1. Preheat oven to 350°F.

2. Melt butter in microwave 20–45 seconds (microwave ovens vary) or melt in a small saucepan. Mix herbes de Provence, salt, and paprika into butter and stir to combine. Add almonds and toss to coat.

3. Scatter almonds evenly on a rimmed baking sheet.

4. Bake 10–12 minutes, stirring halfway through baking. Nuts are done when toasted and fragrant.

5. Remove from oven and serve warm.

Per Recipe   Calories: 699 | Fat: 64g | Protein: 20g | Sodium: 1,182mg | Fiber: 12g | Carbohydrates: 21g | Sugar: 4g

Baked Camembert and Rosemary

Thankfully on the low-FODMAP diet you can enjoy such heavenly things as Camembert cheese! Stick to 2 wedges (about 1.41 ounces) for a low-FODMAP serving.

INGREDIENTS | SERVES 7

8 ounces Camembert, in box

5 sprigs rosemary

2 tablespoons dry white wine

1 tablespoon maple syrup

½ teaspoon freshly ground black pepper

12–18 thin slices gluten-free baguette

2 tablespoons garlic-infused extra-virgin olive oil, divided

1 teaspoon coarse sea salt

1. Remove cheese from refrigerator 1 hour before cooking and bring to room temperature.

2. Preheat oven to 315°F. Take cheese out of box and unwrap.

3. Pull base up out of box and remove any wax paper from box. Push base into box and rest cheese on top. Lay on a rimmed baking sheet. Make a few slits on top of cheese. Place rosemary inside slits; pour wine and maple syrup into slits and on top of cheese. Sprinkle on black pepper.

4. Bake 20 minutes; after 12 minutes, add sliced baguette to baking sheet and drizzle bread with 1 tablespoon oil and sprinkle with salt.

5. Remove cheese from oven and allow to cool. Drizzle cheese with remaining oil. Serve with baguettes.

Per Serving   Calories: 383 | Fat: 13g | Protein: 16g | Sodium: 1,142mg | Fiber: 3g | Carbohydrates: 49g | Sugar: 4g

Vietnamese Summer Rolls

Rolling up summer rolls may take a little practice, but once you've got it down, you'll love making these rolls as appetizers, snacks, or lunch.

INGREDIENTS | MAKES 16

½ cup water

3 tablespoons lime juice

2 tablespoons light brown sugar

2½ tablespoons gluten-free fish sauce

⅛ teaspoon wheat-free asafetida powder

¼ teaspoon red pepper flakes (optional)

4 ounces rice vermicelli noodles

¾ pound boneless pork loin or shoulder

24 medium shrimp

14 ounces firm tofu

16 rice paper sheets

8 large leaves Bibb lettuce, halved

16 small sprigs cilantro

32 fresh mint leaves

32 Thai basil or regular basil leaves

3 medium scallions, chopped, green part only

1 cup bean sprouts

1. In a small serving bowl, whisk together water with lime juice, sugar, fish sauce, and asafetida. Whisk in red pepper flakes if they do not bother your gut. Set sauce aside to dip rolls.

2. Soak rice noodles in room temperature water at least 1 hour or bring about 5 cups water to a boil in a medium pot and add noodles; remove from heat, cover, and soak 15 minutes. Since noodles are very fine, use a sieve instead of a colander to drain. Gently press paper towels into sieve to soak up any excess water.

3. Bring a medium pot of water to boil and add pork. Reduce heat to medium and cook about 15–25 minutes or until pork is cooked through. Remove from water and allow to cool. Slice into thin strips. Set aside.

4. Boil shrimp for 2–3 minutes or until opaque. Keep shell on shrimp and use a sharp knife to split shrimp in half along the back. Once cut in half, remove shell and tail and devein.

5. Drain and pat tofu dry. Cut block in half, then slice into thirds.

6. Fill a large pot with water and heat until hot but not boiling. Press 1 rice paper sheet into warm water with your hand and then remove as soon as it has been completely submerged. Tap off any excess water, then transfer to clean work surface. Smooth out with hand.

7. In middle of rice paper sheet, arrange half lettuce leaf, 1 sprig cilantro, 2 mint leaves, 2 basil leaves, a few scallion tips, a few sprouts, and some rice noodles.

8. Fold up bottom third of rice paper sheet over contents of roll, tuck in tightly, and then tuck in sides. Lay down a couple pieces of pork and top with a couple pieces of tofu. On upper-most third of rice paper sheet, layer 3 pieces of shrimp. Continue rolling up tightly, enclosing shrimp.

9. Serve with dipping sauce and enjoy!

Per Serving Calories: 92 | Fat: 2g | Protein: 8g | Sodium: 255mg | Fiber: 1g | Carbohydrates: 11g | Sugar: 2g

CHAPTER 4

Soups and Salads

Easy Onion- and Garlic-Free Chicken Stock
78

Seafood Stock
79

Roman Egg Drop Soup
80

Chicken and Dumplings Soup
81

Vegetable Stock
82

Potato Soup
82

Red Pepper Soup
83

Carrot and Ginger Soup
84

Lentil Chili
85

Coconut Curry Lemongrass Soup
86

Greek Pasta Salad
87

Fennel Pomegranate Salad
88

Glorious Strawberry Salad
88

Orange, Red, and Green Buckwheat Salad
89

Citrus Fennel and Mint Salad
89

Abundantly Happy Kale Salad
90

Moroccan-Inspired Carrot Ginger Soup
91

Beef with Buckwheat Soup
92

Slow Cooker Chicken Tagine
93

Vegan Carrot, Leek, and Saffron Soup
94

Fish Curry
95

Chicken Tortilla Soup
96

Kale Sesame Salad with Tamari-Ginger Dressing
97

Warm Basil and Walnut Potato Salad
98

Lemon Kale Salad
99

Zucchini Ribbon Salad with Goat Cheese, Pine Nuts, and Pomegranate
99

Prosciutto di Parma Salad
100

Baked Papaya and Chicken Salad with Cilantro-Lime Dressing
101

Mom's Chicken Salad
102

Butter Lettuce Salad with Poached Egg and Bacon
103

Filet Mignon Salad
104

Easy Onion- and Garlic-Free Chicken Stock

This is a great low-FODMAP staple to have ready-made for soups, sauces, rice and other low-FODMAP dishes included in this book.

INGREDIENTS | MAKES 2 QUARTS

1 (2-pound) ready-made rotisserie chicken

2 quarts cold water

2 medium carrots, peeled and cut into chunks

1 medium stalk celery with leaves, cut into chunks

1 large bok choy stalk with leaves, cut into chunks

½ teaspoon dried or fresh rosemary

½ teaspoon dried or fresh thyme

4–5 sprigs fresh parsley

2 dried bay leaves

8 whole peppercorns

1. Remove meat from rotisserie chicken and set aside to use for sandwiches, stir-fry, chicken salad, or other recipes.

2. Place chicken carcass in a 4- to 6-quart slow cooker and make sure it is fully covered with water.

3. Place vegetables and spices in slow cooker.

4. Set slow cooker to low and cook 6–8 hours.

5. Use tongs to transfer and discard chicken bones from slow cooker. Place a large sieve over a large bowl. Drain contents from slow cooker through sieve. Discard large vegetable pieces. Skim fat from surface of stock using a large spoon.

6. Cool completely, divide into a few small glass jars or plastic containers, and refrigerate up to 1 week or freeze up to 3 months.

Per Serving (1 quart)   Calories: 566 | Fat: 14g | Protein: 96g | Sodium: 437mg | Fiber: 2g | Carbohydrates: 7g | Sugar: 3g

Seafood Stock

When making Vietnamese Summer Rolls (see recipe in Chapter 3), save the shrimp shells to make this stock. It freezes well, so you'll always have this low-FODMAP pantry essential on hand.

INGREDIENTS | MAKES 6 CUPS

2 tablespoons extra-virgin olive oil

2 cloves garlic, peeled and slightly crushed

1 medium yellow onion, peeled and quartered

2 large carrots, peeled and diced

1 medium zucchini, trimmed and diced

12 large raw shrimp shells

6 cups water

½ cup Tomato Paste (see recipe in Chapter 13)

½ cup dry white wine

1 tablespoon sea salt

1 teaspoon freshly ground black pepper

Cooking with Wine

Although both drinking wine and cooking wines are permitted on the low-FODMAP diet, keep in mind that cooking wines typically have high sodium levels that may affect the flavor of the dish.

1. Heat oil over medium-low heat in a large skillet. Add garlic and onion and sauté, stirring constantly until garlic is softened and brown at edges, about 5 minutes. Remove and discard garlic and onion, leaving oil.

2. Increase heat to medium-high, add carrots and zucchini, and sauté 5 minutes.

3. Add shrimp shells, water, tomato paste, wine, salt, and pepper and stir until paste is completely dissolved.

4. Bring just to a boil, then reduce heat to low and simmer 45 minutes, uncovered.

5. Remove from heat and allow stock to cool. Using a slotted spoon, remove and discard shells and large solids. Using a mesh sieve over a large bowl, strain remaining solids and reserve stock.

6. Transfer stock to a container for refrigerator storage for 3–4 days.

Per Serving (1 cup)   Calories: 113 | Fat: 5g | Protein: 5g | Sodium: 1,400mg | Fiber: 2g | Carbohydrates: 10g | Sugar: 6g

Roman Egg Drop Soup

A popular soup in Rome, Roman Egg Drop Soup, or Stracciatella alla Romana, is a delicious soup for the cold winter months, or traditionally, a soup to have with family during Easter.

INGREDIENTS | SERVES 8

8 cups Easy Onion- and Garlic-Free Chicken Stock (see recipe in this chapter)

½ teaspoon kosher salt, divided

4 cups packed spinach leaves, shredded

4 large eggs

½ cup grated Parmigiano-Reggiano, divided

½ teaspoon freshly ground black pepper

¼ teaspoon ground nutmeg

3 tablespoons chopped fresh Italian parsley

1. In a medium pot, bring stock to a simmer with ¼ teaspoon salt. After 3–4 minutes, add spinach and cook until tender, about 3 minutes.

2. Meanwhile, in a medium bowl, whisk together eggs, ¼ cup cheese, remaining ¼ teaspoon salt, and pepper.

3. Add a ⅓ of egg mixture to stock and spinach, and continuously whisk. Add nutmeg, remaining eggs in 2 more batches, and allow soup to return to a boil. If any large clusters of eggs form, whisk until you see more shreds of eggs. Serve soup with remaining cheese and garnish with parsley.

Per Serving   Calories: 154 | Fat: 7g | Protein: 12g | Sodium: 710mg | Fiber: 1g | Carbohydrates: 10g | Sugar: 4g

Chicken and Dumplings Soup

A take on the traditional recipe, this gluten-free version will leave you just as satisfied.

INGREDIENTS | SERVES 6

1 whole (3-pound) chicken
2 bay leaves
6–8 cups water
2 tablespoons garlic-infused olive oil
5 large carrots, peeled and sliced
2 medium stalks celery, sliced
1 teaspoon dried thyme
¼ teaspoon salt
3 whole peppercorns
2 cups gluten-free all-purpose flour
¼ teaspoon xanthan gum
2 teaspoons gluten-free baking powder
1 teaspoon plus 1 tablespoon finely chopped fresh flat-leaf parsley, divided
¾ teaspoon salt
2 large eggs, beaten
2 tablespoons butter, melted
¾ cup plus 2 tablespoons lactose-free milk

1. Put whole chicken in a large pot and add bay leaves and 6–8 cups water, or enough to cover chicken. Bring to a boil and then simmer with lid on about 1 hour, skimming off any foam. After 1 hour, remove chicken and allow to cool. Keep remaining broth in pot. Once chicken is cool, peel off skin and tear meat off bones. Set meat aside.

2. Heat oil in a large saucepan and sauté carrots and celery 5 minutes.

3. Drain broth from chicken pot through a colander into another large pot or a bowl. Discard any remaining bones and bay leaves and add drained broth to pan with vegetables and add in thyme, salt, and peppercorns. Bring to a simmer.

4. To make dumplings: combine flour, xanthan gum, baking powder, 1 teaspoon parsley, and salt in a medium bowl. Add beaten eggs, butter, and milk; gently mix to combine with a spoon. Mix just until mixture comes together nicely and stays moist. (Overmixing may make dumplings too dense.)

5. Using a soupspoon, spoon out even-sized portions of dough and drop into soup. Cover soup and simmer 20 minutes.

6. Garnish with 1 tablespoon parsley and serve.

Per Serving   Calories: 530 | Fat: 14g | Protein: 56g | Sodium: 856mg | Fiber: 3g | Carbohydrates: 41g | Sugar: 5g

Vegetable Stock

*Use this as a base for other low-FODMAP soups and recipes,
and especially for vegetarian and vegan dishes.*

INGREDIENTS | MAKES 2 QUARTS

1 tablespoon garlic-infused olive oil

½ medium stalk celery, cut into chunks

2 medium stalks bok choy stalks, cut into chunks

2 large carrots, peeled and cut into chunks

1 small fennel bulb, cut into chunks

4 quarts cold water

6 sprigs flat-leaf parsley

1 bay leaf

1 teaspoon whole black peppercorns

1. Heat oil in a large stockpot over medium-high heat. Add celery, bok choy, carrots, and fennel and cook, stirring occasionally until vegetables begin to soften, 5–7 minutes.

2. Add water, parsley, bay leaf, and peppercorns. Bring to a boil; reduce heat and simmer until stock is reduced by half, 1–1½ hours.

3. Strain stock through a fine-mesh sieve into a large bowl; discard solid vegetables and peppercorns. Store in an airtight container in refrigerator for 4–5 days or in freezer for 4–6 months.

Per Serving (1 quart) Calories: 133 | Fat: 7g | Protein: 3g | Sodium: 187mg | Fiber: 6g | Carbohydrates: 17g | Sugar: 4g

Potato Soup

Top this soup with some additional Cheddar cheese and sliced green onions for an attractive presentation.

INGREDIENTS | SERVES 4

6 medium russet potatoes, peeled and cut into cubes

¼ cup butter

½ cup gluten-free all-purpose flour

6 cups lactose-free milk

⅛ teaspoon salt

¼ teaspoon cracked black pepper

¼ pound grated Cheddar cheese

¼ pound grated Parmesan cheese

1 green onion, green part only, diced

1. Boil potatoes in a large pot until tender, about 15 minutes. Drain and add potatoes to a food processor; blend until smooth.

2. In a large saucepan, melt butter over medium heat. Add flour and cook about 1 minute, stirring continuously.

3. Add 3 cups milk to pan with salt and pepper; stir until there are no lumps. Add potatoes and remaining milk and increase heat to medium-high; bring to a rolling boil, stirring constantly.

4. After boiling, turn heat off and add cheese and green onion. Stir until cheese is melted. Serve immediately.

Per Serving Calories: 504 | Fat: 21g | Protein: 24g | Sodium: 733mg | Fiber: 5g | Carbohydrates: 54g | Sugar: 16g

Red Pepper Soup

Surprisingly, a few drops of vanilla enhances the savory flavors of this delightful soup. Serve it warm in winter—sans the toppings—or cool, as described, in the summer months.

INGREDIENTS | SERVES 6

1 tablespoon extra-virgin olive oil

3 medium red bell peppers, seeded and diced

1 large red potato, peeled and diced

1 cup peeled and diced carrot

1 large parsnip, peeled and diced

6 cups water

¼ teaspoon sea salt

⅛ teaspoon freshly ground black pepper

⅛ teaspoon alcohol-free vanilla extract

¾ cup canned coconut milk, refrigerated

¼ cup chopped fresh chives, divided

1. Heat oil over medium-low heat in a large stockpot.

2. Add vegetables and sauté 10 minutes. Add water. Bring to a boil, lower heat, and simmer uncovered 2–3 hours until vegetables are very tender. Season with salt and pepper. Stir in vanilla. Remove from heat and let cool completely.

3. Once cool, purée soup in batches in a food processor or blender.

4. Fill 6 individual serving bowls with 1 cup soup each. Swirl in 2 tablespoons coconut milk and sprinkle each with a heaping ½ tablespoon chives.

Per Serving Calories: 161 | Fat: 9g | Protein: 3g | Sodium: 130mg | Fiber: 4g | Carbohydrates: 20g | Sugar: 5g

Carrot and Ginger Soup

This elegant soup is sure to be soothing to your whole system. Feel free to substitute Vegetable Stock (see recipe in this chapter) for a vegetarian version.

INGREDIENTS | SERVES 6

2 tablespoons pumpkin seeds

2 tablespoons extra-virgin olive oil

1 pound carrots, peeled and thinly sliced

1 (2") piece gingerroot, peeled and grated

4 cups Easy Onion- and Garlic-Free Chicken Stock (see recipe in this chapter)

¼ cup freshly squeezed orange juice

2 teaspoons grated orange zest

⅛ teaspoon sea salt

⅛ teaspoon freshly ground black pepper

1. Toast pumpkin seeds on a rimmed baking sheet under broiler 3 minutes. Set aside.

2. Heat oil in a large stockpot over medium-low heat. Add carrots and ginger and sauté 5 minutes, stirring frequently.

3. Add stock. Turn heat to high and bring just to a boil, then lower heat and simmer, uncovered, 20 minutes or until carrots are soft.

4. Purée the soup in a blender or food processor. Return to pot.

5. Stir in orange juice, zest, salt, and pepper.

6. Serve soup in bowls garnished with pumpkin seeds.

Per Serving   Calories: 150 | Fat: 8g | Protein: 6g | Sodium: 330mg | Fiber: 2g | Carbohydrates: 14g | Sugar: 7g

Lentil Chili

Who says you can't enjoy a little chili? This chili replaces high-FODMAP beans with canned lentils. Yum!

INGREDIENTS | SERVES 4

1 tablespoon olive oil

1 medium stalk celery, diced

1 large carrot, peeled and diced, or 1 cup store-bought shredded carrots

1 large red bell pepper, seeded and chopped

4 cups Vegetable Stock (see recipe in this chapter)

2 teaspoons chili powder

1 teaspoon ground cumin

2 cups canned lentils, drained and thoroughly rinsed

3 Roma tomatoes, diced

¼ cup chopped fresh cilantro

2 cups baby spinach

½ cup lactose-free sour cream (optional)

1. Heat a large pot over medium-high heat and add olive oil.

2. Once hot, add celery, carrot, and bell pepper; sauté about 5 minutes, stirring frequently.

3. Stir in ¼ cup stock.

4. Add chili powder and cumin and stir; cook 1 minute.

5. Add lentils, tomatoes, cilantro, and remaining stock. Once boiling, reduce heat to medium-low and simmer 25 minutes partially covered.

6. Uncover and cook 8 minutes longer. Add spinach and stir, cooking another 2 minutes.

7. Top with sour cream if using and serve.

Per Serving   Calories: 236 | Fat: 8g | Protein: 12g | Sodium: 614mg | Fiber: 11g | Carbohydrates: 32g | Sugar: 8g

Coconut Curry Lemongrass Soup

Coconut and lemongrass make this soup both mild and refreshing.

INGREDIENTS | SERVES 4

1 tablespoon coconut oil

2 green onions, chopped, green part only

1 cup thinly sliced bok choy

2 medium red bell peppers, seeded and thinly sliced

1/16 teaspoon wheat-free asafetida powder

1 (1") piece gingerroot, peeled and thinly sliced

4 cups Easy Onion- and Garlic-Free Chicken Stock (see recipe in this chapter)

1 cup canned coconut milk

2 teaspoons curry powder

1 tablespoon gluten-free fish sauce

4 medium stalks lemongrass

9 ounces thin rice noodles

3 small skinless, boneless chicken breasts (about 1½ pounds), sliced thin

1 tablespoon fresh lime juice

1. Heat coconut oil in a large pot over medium-high heat. Add green onions, bok choy, bell peppers, asafetida, and ginger; stirring occasionally, cook until red peppers are softened, about 8 minutes.

2. Add chicken stock, coconut milk, curry powder, and fish sauce; cover and bring to a boil.

3. Meanwhile, trim top and base of lemongrass stalks; use only bottom 4". Peel off any dry or tough outer layers before finely chopping or mincing. Add lemongrass and noodles to pot; simmer uncovered until noodles are al dente, about 3 minutes.

4. Add chicken and simmer until just cooked through, about 3 more minutes. Stir in lime juice.

Per Serving   Calories: 525 | Fat: 23g | Protein: 48g | Sodium: 716mg | Fiber: 3g | Carbohydrates: 68g | Sugar: 7g

Greek Pasta Salad

When you need a little Greek fix, this pasta salad will do the trick!
This recipe is great for barbecues or a make-ahead lunch.

INGREDIENTS | SERVES 6

1 (12-ounce) package gluten-free rice spiral pasta
¼ cup garlic-infused olive oil
¼ cup extra-virgin olive oil
1 large lemon, juiced
⅓ cup rice wine vinegar
2 teaspoons dried oregano
⅛ teaspoon sea salt
¼ teaspoon freshly ground black pepper
1 (10-ounce) bag fresh spinach, rinsed, drained, and coarsely chopped
8 ounces feta cheese, crumbled
1 pint grape tomatoes, halved
½ cup pitted Kalamata olives

1. Cook pasta according to package directions; drain and rinse.

2. Make dressing: In a large bowl, whisk together oils, lemon juice, vinegar, oregano, salt, and pepper.

3. Add spinach, feta, tomatoes, and olives to the bowl.

4. Add pasta and toss gently until evenly coated. Can be made ahead and covered in refrigerator up to 1 day.

Per Serving   Calories: 495 | Fat: 26g | Protein: 9g | Sodium: 610mg | Fiber: 3g | Carbohydrates: 55g | Sugar: 3g

Fennel Pomegranate Salad

You will love all the flavors in this salad, from the burst of flavor from the pomegranate seeds, to the mellow fennel and goat cheese, to the tangy lemon juice and earthy olive oil!

INGREDIENTS | SERVES 2

3 small fennel bulbs, thinly sliced

¼ medium stalk celery, sliced into thin slivers

½ cup coarsely chopped fresh parsley

½ cup pomegranate seeds, divided

¼ cup fresh lemon juice

¼ cup extra-virgin olive oil

¼ teaspoon salt

½ teaspoon freshly ground black pepper

½ cup crumbled goat cheese

1. Toss fennel, celery, parsley, and ¼ cup pomegranate seeds in a large bowl.

2. Add lemon juice and oil and toss to coat. Add salt and pepper.

3. Serve topped with goat cheese and remaining pomegranate seeds.

Per Serving   Calories: 394 | Fat: 30g | Protein: 12g | Sodium: 400mg | Fiber: 14g | Carbohydrates: 23g | Sugar: 1g

Glorious Strawberry Salad

This salad can be made into an entrée salad by adding grilled chicken to serve two or it can make an excellent addition to a chicken, beef, or fish entrée. Pair this salad with a glass of Beaujolais Nouveau (please see note on alcohol in Appendix B)!

INGREDIENTS | SERVES 4

6 cups fresh baby spinach

½ cup sliced strawberries

¼ cup whole walnuts

¼ cup chopped fresh basil

½ cup crumbled goat cheese

¼ teaspoon sea salt

1 tablespoon freshly ground black pepper

3 tablespoons rice wine vinegar

⅔ cup extra-virgin olive oil

½ medium avocado, cut into eighths

1. In a large salad bowl toss together spinach, strawberries, walnuts, basil, goat cheese, salt, and pepper.

2. In a small bowl whisk together vinegar and oil. Drizzle over salad and toss salad again.

3. Serve on individual salad plates and top each with avocado.

Per Serving   Calories: 478 | Fat: 48g | Protein: 6g | Sodium: 396mg | Fiber: 4g | Carbohydrates: 8g | Sugar: 2g

Orange, Red, and Green Buckwheat Salad

Colorful, flavorful, and healthy, this salad is great for lunch or holiday gatherings.

INGREDIENTS | SERVES 4

2 tablespoons maple syrup

2 tablespoons rice wine vinegar

1 tablespoon balsamic vinegar

¼ cup extra-virgin olive oil

¼ teaspoon sea salt

2 cups buckwheat, cooked and rinsed

½ pound sweet potatoes, peeled, roasted and cubed

2 tablespoons no-sugar-added dried cranberries

2 cups arugula

2 cups mesclun greens

¼ cup slivered almonds

1. In a small bowl, whisk together dressing ingredients: maple syrup, rice wine vinegar, balsamic vinegar, extra-virgin olive oil, and salt. Set aside.

2. In a large bowl, combine buckwheat, sweet potatoes, cranberries, arugula, mesclun greens, and almonds. Drizzle with dressing and toss gently.

Per Serving Calories: 447 | Fat: 18g | Protein: 10g | Sodium: 190mg | Fiber: 9g | Carbohydrates: 66g | Sugar: 13g

Citrus Fennel and Mint Salad

This refreshing salad is perfect for a sunny brunch, a barbecue, or paired with a beef entrée.

INGREDIENTS | SERVES 2

1 large navel orange, peeled and sectioned

1 cup fennel bulb slices

1 medium carrot, peeled and shaved

2 radishes, finely sliced

2 tablespoons coarsely chopped fresh mint leaves

2 tablespoons extra-virgin olive oil

1 tablespoon lime juice

⅛ teaspoon Himalayan salt

¼ teaspoon freshly ground black pepper

1. Add orange to a medium serving bowl.

2. Add fennel, carrot, and radishes to bowl.

3. Add mint to a small bowl with oil, lime juice, salt, and pepper. Whisk well to combine. Pour into serving bowl with rest of ingredients and toss to combine.

Per Serving Calories: 185 | Fat: 14g | Protein: 2g | Sodium: 197mg | Fiber: 4g | Carbohydrates: 16g | Sugar: 8g

Abundantly Happy Kale Salad

This salad is a low-FODMAP phytonutrient and vitamin powerhouse! It's also very easy to make.

INGREDIENTS | SERVES 5

9 large leaves curly kale, thinly shredded (ribs and stems removed)

½ teaspoon sea salt

3 tablespoons extra-virgin olive oil, divided

Juice of 1 large lemon

1 cup shredded butter lettuce

1 medium stalk celery, diced

1 medium yellow bell pepper, seeded and diced

1 medium carrot, peeled and grated

1 tablespoon hemp seeds

1 tablespoon pumpkin seeds

1 tablespoon chopped walnuts

2 cups shredded common (green) cabbage

2 radishes, sliced very thin

1 cup sliced fennel bulb

1 cup fresh blueberries

1. Add kale to a medium bowl and sprinkle salt and 2 tablespoons oil on top. Massage leaves with hands until leaves begin to darken and soften.

2. Add remaining oil and remaining ingredients and toss gently. Keep covered in refrigerator up to 3 days.

Per Serving   Calories: 163 | Fat: 11g | Protein: 4g | Sodium: 289mg | Fiber: 5g | Carbohydrates: 17g | Sugar: 6g

Moroccan-Inspired Carrot Ginger Soup

A soothing, very flavorful, and delicious spiced soup.

INGREDIENTS | SERVES 4

1 tablespoon coconut oil

2 tablespoons peeled and minced fresh gingerroot

8 large carrots, peeled and roughly chopped

2 small zucchini, peeled and roughly chopped

1 teaspoon ground turmeric

1 teaspoon paprika

¼ teaspoon ground cumin

½ teaspoon ground coriander

½ teaspoon ground cinnamon

4 cups Vegetable Stock (see recipe in this chapter)

1 cup canned coconut milk

⅛ teaspoon sea salt

¼ teaspoon freshly ground black pepper

1. Heat oil in a large saucepan over medium-high heat.

2. Add ginger and cook 4 minutes.

3. Add carrots, zucchini, turmeric, paprika, cumin, coriander, and cinnamon, and cook until carrots are tender, about 6–8 minutes.

4. Pour in stock and bring to a boil; lower heat to low and simmer, partially covered, for 25–30 minutes.

5. Place soup in a blender and purée.

6. Return to saucepan and add coconut milk, salt, and pepper. Serve immediately.

Per Serving   Calories: 230 | Fat: 16g | Protein: 3g | Sodium: 736mg | Fiber: 5g | Carbohydrates: 22g | Sugar: 10g

Beef with Buckwheat Soup

This comforting soup takes a little less than an hour to whip up and is very easy to make.

INGREDIENTS | SERVES 4

1¼ pounds stew beef

4 quarts Easy Onion- and Garlic-Free Chicken Stock (see recipe in this chapter)

¾ teaspoon paprika

¾ teaspoon gluten-free Worcestershire sauce

3 bay leaves

⅛ teaspoon salt

½ teaspoon freshly ground black pepper

1 cup buckwheat groats

2 large yellow potatoes, diced

2 large carrots, peeled and diced

½ medium stalk celery, diced

1 tablespoon olive oil

¼ cups fresh dill

1. Place meat in a large pot with chicken stock. Add paprika, Worcestershire, bay leaves, salt, and pepper. Bring to a boil and then turn heat to medium and cook 40 minutes, uncovered.

2. Add buckwheat and potatoes; cook 15 minutes.

3. Sauté carrots and celery in oil in a medium skillet over medium heat until carrots are softened, about 6–8 minutes. Add to soup. Simmer 5 minutes.

4. Add dill to soup and serve.

Per Serving Calories: 450 | Fat: 13g | Protein: 31g | Sodium: 789mg | Fiber: 6g | Carbohydrates: 52g | Sugar: 10g

Slow Cooker Chicken Tagine

Tagine is a stew that originated in Morocco and is also found in other areas of Northern Africa. It's also known as tavas in Cypriot cuisine. Enjoy this easier version of a more traditional tagine recipe.

INGREDIENTS | SERVES 4

1½ tablespoons sweet paprika

1 teaspoon ground cinnamon

1½ tablespoons ground coriander

½ tablespoon ground turmeric

2 teaspoons ground cardamom

1½ teaspoons ground allspice

⅛ teaspoon wheat-free asafetida powder

¼ teaspoon sea salt

¼ teaspoon freshly ground black pepper

1 tablespoon olive oil

4 (5-ounce) skinless, boneless chicken thighs, halved

½ tablespoon ground ginger

½ tablespoon saffron

1 (14-ounce) can whole tomatoes

⅓ cup canned chickpeas, thoroughly drained and rinsed

4 cups Easy Onion- and Garlic-Free Chicken Stock (see recipe in this chapter)

1 preserved lemon, chopped into wedges (optional)

1 tablespoon chopped fresh flat-leaf parsley

1. In a small skillet, toast paprika, cinnamon, coriander, turmeric, cardamom, and allspice until fragrant, about 2 minutes. Set aside and allow to cool.

2. Once cooled, sprinkle spice mixture, along with asafetida, salt, and pepper on both sides of chicken.

3. In a large skillet, heat oil over medium heat. Add chicken thighs and sear until browned. Add chicken to a 4- to 6-quart slow cooker.

4. Add ginger to skillet. Cook and stir 2 minutes. Remove from heat.

5. Add ginger, saffron, tomatoes, chickpeas, and chicken stock to slow cooker. Cook on high 3–4 hours. Garnish with preserved lemon and/or parsley.

Per Serving Calories: 155 | Fat: 7g | Protein: 15g | Sodium: 350mg | Fiber: 4g | Carbohydrates: 9g | Sugar: 3g

Vegan Carrot, Leek, and Saffron Soup

This type of soup would usually call for heavy cream,
but here it is replaced with luscious coconut cream.

INGREDIENTS | SERVES 4

2 tablespoons butter

2 medium leeks, coarsely chopped, leaves only

1 medium red bell pepper, seeded and diced

1 pound carrots, peeled and sliced

1 tablespoon ground coriander

¼ teaspoon cayenne pepper

½ teaspoon ground turmeric

½ teaspoon plus 2 teaspoons saffron

4 cups Vegetable Stock (see recipe in this chapter)

⅛ teaspoon salt

¼ teaspoon white pepper

½ cup canned coconut cream or full-fat coconut milk

1. Melt butter in a medium saucepan over medium heat. Add leeks and cook 7 minutes or until translucent.

2. Add bell pepper and carrots, and cook another 5–7 minutes or until carrots soften just slightly.

3. Add coriander, cayenne, turmeric, and ½ teaspoon saffron and stir. Cook 1 minute. Add stock, salt, and pepper and bring to a boil. Reduce heat to low and cover. Cook 20–35 minutes or until vegetables are very tender.

4. Remove soup from heat and let cool to room temperature. Using a blender or food processor, purée soup in batches.

5. Serve in soup bowls with a swirl of cream in each and garnished with the remaining saffron.

Per Serving   Calories: 257 | Fat: 12g | Protein: 2g | Sodium: 717mg | Fiber: 5g | Carbohydrates: 37g | Sugar: 28g

Ready-Made Coconut Cream

Coconut cream is a delicious and healthy way to substitute heavy cream. If you do not have coconut cream on hand, here is how to make it: Chill a can of coconut milk in the refrigerator for 24 hours or more. Carefully open the can and scoop out the thick cream on top. Do not scoop up liquid at bottom of can. Keep the liquid and use for smoothies. You can also buy it on Amazon.com or in most natural foods stores and some large chain supermarkets. It's great to always have a can of coconut milk in the refrigerator so you can use it for other low-FODMAP recipes such as Coconut Whipped Cream (see recipe in Chapter 12) or Fish Curry (see recipe in this chapter).

Fish Curry

Dinner for one tonight? Make this super-simple and pleasing dish for yourself.
It's so good, you'd never want to share it anyhow!

INGREDIENTS | SERVES 1

1 medium carrot, peeled and chopped into chunks

2 cups chicken broth

¼ teaspoon gluten-free fish sauce

1 (13.5-ounce) can coconut milk, refrigerated overnight

1 Roma tomato or vine-ripe tomato, diced

½ small stalk celery, diced

1 tablespoon curry powder

¼ teaspoon ground cumin

¼ teaspoon ground coriander

½ teaspoon ground turmeric

¼ teaspoon freshly grated gingerroot

2 tablespoons roughly chopped cilantro

¹⁄₁₆ teaspoon wheat-free asafetida powder

½ pound tilapia or other thick fish fillet, cut into large chunks

1. Boil carrot in a small saucepan with water until softened just slightly. Discard water and add chicken broth (you can also use vegetable stock) and fish sauce.

2. Carefully open coconut milk can and scoop out thick cream on top; add to pot with carrots and broth. (Do not scoop up liquid at bottom of can; use cream only.) Add tomato, celery, curry powder, cumin, coriander, and turmeric.

3. Bring to a boil and then cover; simmer 20 minutes stirring every 5–7 minutes.

4. Stir in ginger, cilantro, and asafetida. Add fish and stir to cover every piece with liquid.

5. Cook 5 minutes to achieve nice flaky pieces of fish, and serve.

Per Serving   Calories: 997 | Fat: 36g | Protein: 56g | Sodium: 1,871mg | Fiber: 6g | Carbohydrates: 116g | Sugar: 28g

Chicken Tortilla Soup

This flavorful soup is similar to one you would be served at an authentic Mexican restaurant.

INGREDIENTS | SERVES 2

1/16 teaspoon wheat-free asafetida powder

2½ tablespoons chopped fresh cilantro

½ cup canned tomatoes

¼ cup plus 1 tablespoon safflower oil

¼ teaspoon ground coriander

¼ teaspoon ground cumin

¼ teaspoon dried oregano

2 cups chicken stock

¼ teaspoon chili powder

¼ pound skinless, boneless chicken breast, cut into thin strips

⅛ teaspoon salt

½ teaspoon freshly ground black pepper

2 hard corn tortilla shells

¼ avocado, sliced in half

½ ounce Cheddar cheese, shredded

1 teaspoon fresh lime juice

1. In a blender or food processor, combine asafetida, cilantro, and tomatoes and process until smooth.

2. Heat 1 tablespoon oil in a medium skillet over medium-high heat. Add tomato mixture, coriander, cumin, and oregano. Cook about 6–7 minutes or until mixture becomes thickened; stir often.

3. Set a large saucepan over medium-low heat and add tomato mixture, stock, and chili powder. Partially cover pan and simmer about 20 minutes, stirring occasionally.

4. Add chicken, salt, and pepper and simmer 20–25 minutes longer. Chicken should be slightly opaque.

5. Ladle soup into 2 bowls. Crush 1 tortilla into each bowl with your hands, or crush on a plate using a wooden spoon and then add to soup. Top each serving with half the avocado and cheese, and sprinkle with lime juice. Serve immediately.

Per Serving Calories: 585 | Fat: 45g | Protein: 22g | Sodium: 698mg | Fiber: 4g | Carbohydrates: 26g | Sugar: 6g

Kale Sesame Salad with Tamari-Ginger Dressing

This umami salad is great on its own or when paired with chicken.

INGREDIENTS | SERVES 2

1½ tablespoons sesame seeds

4 cups shredded kale (thick ribs and stems removed)

3 tablespoons extra-virgin olive oil, divided

1 tablespoon chopped scallion, green part only

½ cup peeled and julienned carrots

1 tablespoon rice wine vinegar

½ tablespoon finely grated gingerroot

½ tablespoon gluten-free soy sauce (tamari)

1 teaspoon lime juice

1/16 teaspoon wheat-free asafetida powder

¼ medium avocado, sliced in half

2 tablespoons chopped fresh basil

1. Using a small skillet set over medium-high heat, toast sesame seeds until golden brown, about 1 minute. Stir continuously to keep seeds from burning. Set aside.

2. Place kale in a large salad bowl. Add 1 tablespoon olive oil and massage with hands until kale leaves become soft. Add scallion and carrots and toss to combine.

3. Make dressing in a small bowl by whisking together vinegar, ginger, soy sauce, lime juice, and asafetida.

4. Pour dressing over kale and stir again to combine. Divide into 2 salad bowls and top each with sesame seeds, 1 slice avocado, and 1 tablespoon basil.

Per Serving   Calories: 344 | Fat: 28g | Protein: 7g | Sodium: 306mg | Fiber: 6g | Carbohydrates: 21g | Sugar: 1g

Warm Basil and Walnut Potato Salad

Making steak or chicken? Going to a barbecue? Try this fancier version of potato salad.

INGREDIENTS | SERVES 4

¼ cup packed fresh basil leaves

1 tablespoon small walnut pieces

¼ teaspoon kosher salt, divided

½ teaspoon freshly ground black pepper

1½ tablespoons extra-virgin olive oil

4 medium Yukon Gold or other yellow potatoes, peeled

Zest of 1 medium lemon

1. Using a food processor, combine basil, walnuts, ⅛ teaspoon salt, and pepper. Process until it becomes a paste. With processor running, gradually add olive oil. Set aside.

2. Place potatoes in a medium pot. Stir in ⅛ teaspoon salt and enough water to cover tops of potatoes.

3. Bring water to boil over medium-high heat; cook until potatoes are tender, about 15 minutes. A knife inserted into potato should pierce through easily. Drain potatoes. Transfer to a cutting board and cut into chunks.

4. Place potatoes in a serving bowl and pour on basil-walnut sauce. Toss gently to coat potatoes and add lemon zest. Serve immediately or cover and refrigerate up to 3 days.

Per Serving Calories: 204 | Fat: 6g | Protein: 4g | Sodium: 160mg | Fiber: 5g | Carbohydrates: 34g | Sugar: 3g

Lemon Kale Salad

Light, lemony, and fresh, this salad is great for lunch or served along with an entrée.

INGREDIENTS | SERVES 4

10 ounces kale leaves, coarsely chopped (thick ribs and stems removed)
¼ teaspoon sea salt
½ cup extra-virgin olive oil
½ teaspoon freshly ground black pepper
Juice of 2 medium lemons
¼ cup slivered almonds

1. Place kale in a large salad bowl. Add salt and olive oil and massage with hands until kale leaves become soft.

2. Add pepper, lemon juice, and almonds. Stir well to combine.

Per Serving   Calories: 415 | Fat: 42g | Protein: 5g | Sodium: 72mg | Fiber: 3g | Carbohydrates: 9g | Sugar: 1g

Zucchini Ribbon Salad with Goat Cheese, Pine Nuts, and Pomegranate

A delicate, mild, and slightly sweet salad that is great for lunch or as a side.

INGREDIENTS | SERVES 8

4 large zucchini
¼ teaspoon kosher salt
⅛ teaspoon coarse sea salt
¼ cup extra-virgin olive oil
3 tablespoons rice wine vinegar
Juice of 1 large lemon
2 tablespoons fresh parsley
¼ cup pine nuts
½ cup pomegranate seeds
½ teaspoon freshly ground black pepper
¾ cup crumbled goat cheese

1. Peel zucchini and use a mandoline, a spiralizer with a straight blade, or a vegetable peeler to make thin ribbons. Place zucchini in a colander and sprinkle with kosher salt. Let sit 25–30 minutes, then lay on paper towels.

2. Meanwhile, in a large salad bowl, add oil, vinegar, lemon juice, parsley, pine nuts, pomegranate seeds, sea salt, and pepper. Add zucchini and toss well to combine. Cover with plastic wrap and refrigerate 4–6 hours.

3. Remove salad from refrigerator. Toss again. Top with goat cheese and toss gently. Serve.

Per Serving   Calories: 185 | Fat: 14g | Protein: 2g | Sodium: 197mg | Fiber: 4g | Carbohydrates: 16g | Sugar: 8g

Prosciutto di Parma Salad

You will love this light and easy low-FODMAP lunch or dinner salad!

INGREDIENTS | SERVES 2

For the salad:

2 cups mix of baby spinach and arugula

25 blueberries

15 macadamia nuts, halved

6 slices prosciutto di Parma

⅛ teaspoon sea salt

1 cup crumbled goat cheese

¼ teaspoon freshly ground black pepper

For the dressing:

1 tablespoon rice wine vinegar

1 tablespoon extra-virgin olive oil

1 tablespoon maple syrup

1. Layer baby spinach, arugula, blueberries, nuts, and prosciutto in a medium bowl. Sprinkle with salt.

2. Make dressing by whisking together rice vinegar, oil, and maple syrup in a small bowl.

3. Pour dressing over salad and cover bowl with a lid or plastic wrap. Shake until well-coated.

4. Add crumbled goat cheese and black pepper and serve.

Per Serving (Salad)   Calories: 546 | Fat: 41g | Protein: 33g | Sodium: 1,461mg | Fiber: 4g | Carbohydrates: 11g | Sugar: 4g

Per Serving (Dressing)   Calories: 87 | Fat: 7g | Protein: 0g | Sodium: 1mg | Fiber: 0g | Carbohydrates: 7g | Sugar: 6g

Baked Papaya and Chicken Salad
with Cilantro-Lime Dressing

This is an excellent salad for a barbecue or when you're simply in a tropical mood!

INGREDIENTS | SERVES 2

1 (1-pound) papaya
1 teaspoon ground cinnamon
1 teaspoon dark brown sugar
1 teaspoon turbinado sugar
1 pound boneless, skinless chicken breasts
1/16 teaspoon salt
1/4 teaspoon freshly ground black pepper
1 tablespoon coconut oil
1/4 cup roughly chopped fresh cilantro
1 cup watercress
1 cup arugula
1 cup chopped romaine lettuce
1/2 cup torn mint leaves
1/3 cup torn basil leaves
3 tablespoons sesame oil
1 tablespoons lime juice
1 teaspoon gluten-free soy sauce (tamari)
1/4 teaspoon gluten-free fish sauce
1 handful fresh cilantro, finely chopped
1/2 teaspoon maple syrup

Can't Have Soy?

Coconut aminos are a soy-free and gluten-free alternative to gluten-free soy sauce. As of this publishing, coconut aminos have not been formally analyzed for their FODMAP content but might be tolerable for most. Coconut aminos are salty and slightly sweet in flavor, resembling light soy sauce or tamari.

1. Preheat oven to 350°F.

2. Cut papaya in half and clean out seeds with a spoon. Cut off both ends of papaya. Put papaya on its side and carefully remove skin with a paring knife. Cut both halves into slices of medium thickness. Sprinkle all sides with cinnamon and sugars and place in a 9" × 13" baking dish. Bake 15–20 minutes or until papaya is heated through.

3. Season chicken with salt and pepper. Heat oil in a medium skillet over medium-high heat. Sear chicken on both sides, about 6–7 minutes per side. Cut into thickest part of chicken to ensure it is no longer pink. An instant-read thermometer through the thickest part of the chicken should register 165°F. Set chicken aside on a cutting board.

4. In a large salad bowl mix together roughly chopped cilantro, watercress, arugula, romaine, mint, and basil.

5. Make dressing by whisking together sesame oil, lime juice, soy sauce, fish sauce, finely chopped cilantro, and maple syrup in a small bowl.

6. Cut chicken into thin slices. Add chicken to salad bowl along with papaya and pour on dressing. Toss well to combine. Serve.

Per Serving Calories: 601 | Fat: 33g | Protein: 53g | Sodium: 523mg | Fiber: 5g | Carbohydrates: 22g | Sugar: 13g

Mom's Chicken Salad

Moms seem to make the best sandwiches, and this chicken salad definitely tastes just like home. Serve it on top of a green salad or as a sandwich.

INGREDIENTS | SERVES 4

1½ pounds boneless, skinless chicken breasts

2 cups Easy Onion- and Garlic-Free Chicken Stock (see recipe in this chapter)

⅛ teaspoon salt, divided

½ teaspoon dried thyme

1 cup Basic Mayonnaise (see recipe in Chapter 13)

½ medium stalk celery, diced

1½ teaspoons finely chopped fresh tarragon

¼ teaspoon freshly ground black pepper

1. In a 2–4-quart saucepan with a lid, arrange chicken breasts in a single layer and set to medium-high heat. Pour in chicken stock, ¹⁄₁₆ teaspoon salt, and thyme. If stock is not covering chicken breasts completely, add some water.

2. Bring to a boil, then reduce heat to low and cover pot; poach chicken 8–12 minutes. Check chicken after 8 minutes. If it is opaque throughout, it is ready. An instant-read thermometer placed in thickest part of meat should register 165°F. Transfer chicken with a slotted spoon to a plate and cover with plastic wrap. Chill in refrigerator 20–30 minutes.

3. Remove chicken from plastic wrap and cut into cubes, removing any white film that might still remain.

4. Add chicken, mayonnaise, celery, tarragon, remaining salt, and pepper to a medium serving bowl. Stir well to combine. Chill in the refrigerator until ready to serve.

Per Serving   Calories: 631 | Fat: 50g | Protein: 39g | Sodium: 710mg | Fiber: 1g | Carbohydrates: 6g | Sugar: 2g

Butter Lettuce Salad with Poached Egg and Bacon

You'll love these perfectly poached eggs with delicate butter lettuce and thick bacon.

INGREDIENTS | SERVES 4

4 slices thick-cut bacon
1 tablespoon fresh lemon juice
2 teaspoons Dijon mustard
2 tablespoons extra-virgin olive oil
½ teaspoon freshly ground black pepper
1 tablespoon rice wine vinegar
4 large eggs
4 cups butter lettuce

1. Preheat oven to 400°F.

2. Line a rimmed baking sheet with parchment paper and place bacon on top of paper. Bake 15–18 minutes or until crisp and browned, rotating baking sheet once. Drain bacon strips on a plate with paper towels. Once cool enough to handle, cut bacon into ½" strips.

3. In a small bowl combine lemon juice, mustard, oil, and pepper. Stir well to combine.

4. Pour cold water into a large saucepan until there is at least 4" of water. Add vinegar and bring to a boil over medium heat, then reduce heat to low.

5. Crack 1 egg into a small shallow bowl. Stir water in saucepan continuously to create a whirlpool. Gently pour egg into water. Cook 3–4 minutes until firm. Remove egg from water with a slotted spoon. Skim any remaining foam from water. Repeat with remaining eggs.

6. Place lettuce and bacon in a large salad bowl. Pour in lemon-mustard dressing. Toss well to combine. Divide among 4 plates. Gently add 1 egg to each plate and serve.

Per Serving   Calories: 223 | Fat: 20g | Protein: 9g | Sodium: 324mg | Fiber: 0g | Carbohydrates: 1g | Sugar: 1g

Filet Mignon Salad

*Grilled filet mignon, probably the most tender and popular cut of beef,
is dressed to the nines in greens, tomatoes, and goat cheese in this salad.*

INGREDIENTS | SERVES 2

¼ large head romaine lettuce, chopped (stems removed)

½ large head Belgian endive (about 1½ cups), thinly sliced crosswise

¼ cup chopped fresh basil

1½ cups baby arugula

2 teaspoons maple syrup

½ cup rice wine vinegar

1½ tablespoons lemon juice

½ teaspoon sea salt

½ teaspoon freshly ground black pepper

½ cup plus ½ tablespoon olive oil

1 tablespoon unsalted butter

½ pound filet mignon

2 ounces crumbled goat cheese

8 cherry tomatoes, halved

1. In a large salad bowl combine romaine, endive, basil, and arugula.

2. In a food processor or blender, add maple syrup, vinegar, lemon juice, salt, and pepper. With machine running on low speed, slowly blend in ½ cup oil. Set aside.

3. Melt butter with ½ tablespoon olive oil in a medium cast-iron skillet or stainless steel skillet over medium heat. Add filet mignon and cook 5–7 minutes on each side or longer depending on desired degree of doneness. Allow to stand 5 minutes. Slice into strips of medium thickness.

4. Add filet mignon, goat cheese, and cherry tomatoes to salad bowl. Pour in dressing. Toss well to coat, and serve.

Per Serving   Calories: 449 | Fat: 45g | Protein: 16g | Sodium: 381mg | Fiber: 2g | Carbohydrates: 6g | Sugar: 4g

CHAPTER 5

Vegetables and Sides

Herbed Mashed Potatoes
106

Coconut Rice
106

Swiss Chard with Pine Nuts and
Parmesan
107

Herbed Yellow Squash
108

Mediterranean Buckwheat Salad
109

Roasted Parsnips with Rosemary
109

Garlicky Parsnip and Carrot Fries
110

Swiss Chard with Cranberries
and Pine Nuts
110

Potato and Kale Gratin
111

Toasted Coconut Almond Millet
112

Root-a-Burgers
113

Confetti Corn
114

Zoodles with Pesto
114

Sweet Potato with Maple Yogurt
and Pumpkin Seeds
115

Roasted Maple Dill Carrots
116

Hasselback Potatoes
117

Lemon Pepper Green Beans
118

Sesame and Ginger Bok Choy
118

Spaghetti Squash with Goat
Cheese
119

Quinoa Tabbouleh
119

Herbed Mashed Potatoes

Simply luscious, these potatoes are great on their own or paired with beef or fish. Serve these potatoes with an added pat of butter on top to kick up the creamy, delicious flavor.

INGREDIENTS | SERVES 4

1½ pounds Yukon Gold potatoes, peeled and cut into quarters

½ teaspoon salt

1 tablespoon lactose-free milk

2 tablespoons unsalted butter

1/16 teaspoon wheat-free asafetida powder

½ tablespoon dried oregano

½ tablespoon dried thyme

½ tablespoon dried rosemary

½ tablespoon freshly ground black pepper

1. Heat a large saucepan or pot over high heat.

2. Add potatoes, salt, and enough cold water to cover tops of potatoes. Once boiling, reduce heat to low, cover, and cook potatoes about 15 minutes. When potatoes are done, drain water and place potatoes back in pot.

3. Add milk, butter, and start to mash with potato masher. After about 1 minute of mashing, add asafetida, oregano, thyme, rosemary, and pepper. Continue mashing to desired consistency.

Per Serving Calories: 176 | Fat: 6g | Protein: 3g | Sodium: 308mg | Fiber: 5g | Carbohydrates: 29g | Sugar: 2g

Coconut Rice

This recipe pairs well with Asian dishes such as soups and stir-fries, or you could have it with chicken or fish.

INGREDIENTS | SERVES 2

1 tablespoon coconut oil

½ teaspoon grated fresh gingerroot

2 cups cooked jasmine rice

1 (13.5-ounce) can coconut milk

¼ cup shredded unsweetened coconut

¼ teaspoon Himalayan salt

1 tablespoon lime juice

1. In a 6" skillet, heat oil over medium heat. Once oil is shimmering, add ginger and cook 2–3 minutes.

2. Add cooked rice, coconut milk, shredded coconut, and salt. Cook and stir until rice mixture is heated through, 5–7 minutes.

3. Stir in lime juice and remove from heat.

Per Serving Calories: 523 | Fat: 34g | Protein: 7g | Sodium: 314mg | Fiber: 2g | Carbohydrates: 50g | Sugar: 1g

Swiss Chard with Pine Nuts and Parmesan

Here is a nice leafy and mild side dish that goes very well with fish.

INGREDIENTS | SERVES 4

2 tablespoons unsalted butter

2 tablespoons garlic-infused olive oil

1 bunch Swiss chard, stems and center ribs cut out and chopped together, leaves coarsely chopped separately

½ cup dry white wine

1 tablespoon fresh lemon juice

3 tablespoons pine nuts

Pinch sea salt (optional)

2 tablespoons freshly grated Parmesan cheese

½ teaspoon freshly ground black pepper

1. Melt butter with oil in a large skillet over medium-high heat.

2. Add chard stems and white wine and simmer until stems begin to soften, about 5 minutes.

3. Stir in chard leaves and cook until wilted.

4. Stir in lemon juice and pine nuts and cook about 30 seconds.

5. Add salt if using.

6. Using tongs, immediately transfer half of leaves and stems to a serving plate, add half of Parmesan cheese, then the rest of leaves and stems and Parmesan cheese.

7. Top with freshly ground black pepper.

Per Serving Calories: 232 | Fat: 21g | Protein: 4g | Sodium: 152mg | Fiber: 1g | Carbohydrates: 4g | Sugar: 1g

Herbed Yellow Squash

This dish is best made when squash are in season.
A little butter and some herbs make this squash delicious.

INGREDIENTS | SERVES 2

1½ pounds yellow squash

1 tablespoon butter

½ cup chicken broth

3 sprigs fresh thyme

1 tablespoon chopped fresh rosemary

¼ teaspoon salt

2 tablespoons chopped fresh flat-leaf parsley

½ teaspoon freshly ground black pepper

1. Place squash on a cutting board and cut into ¼" circles.

2. Heat butter in a small skillet over medium-high heat and sauté squash about 1 minute.

3. Add chicken broth, thyme, rosemary, and salt; bring to a simmer.

4. Partially cover and reduce heat to low. Cook until tender, about 6–8 minutes, stirring occasionally.

5. Add parsley and pepper. Serve.

Per Serving Calories: 150 | Fat: 8g | Protein: 5g | Sodium: 567mg | Fiber: 5g | Carbohydrates: 18g | Sugar: 12g

Mediterranean Buckwheat Salad

Earthy and healthy buckwheat gets a taste of the Mediterranean with this super-filling salad!

INGREDIENTS | SERVES 3

1½ cups buckwheat groats

¼ cup canned chickpeas, drained and rinsed

12 black olives, pitted and quartered

1 cup chopped broccoli florets

1 tablespoon chopped fresh dill

6 leaves fresh basil, chopped

Juice of 1 large lemon

½ cup crumbled feta cheese

1 tablespoon extra-virgin olive oil

½ teaspoon salt

½ teaspoon freshly ground black pepper

1. In a large saucepan of boiling salted water, cook buckwheat until tender, 10–15 minutes. Drain and rinse well under cold water, rinsing away any pinkish-red film (or mucilage). Spread out on a baking sheet and allow to dry.

2. Once buckwheat is cooled and dry, add to a large mixing bowl along with remaining ingredients. Mix until well combined.

3. Serve immediately or refrigerate for a few hours (or overnight). Refrigerating allows flavors to soak into buckwheat.

Per Serving   Calories: 439 | Fat: 14g | Protein: 15g | Sodium: 908mg | Fiber: 11g | Carbohydrates: 69g | Sugar: 2g

Roasted Parsnips with Rosemary

Parsnips are another great option to add to your low-FODMAP diet and children like them too, especially when roasted.

INGREDIENTS | SERVES 4

2 tablespoons olive oil

2 teaspoons chopped fresh rosemary

2 teaspoons chopped fresh parsley

2 teaspoons fresh dill

¼ teaspoon sea salt

¼ teaspoon freshly ground black pepper

1½ pounds parsnips, peeled and cut diagonally into 1"-thick slices

1 tablespoon lemon juice

1. Preheat oven to 450°F.

2. In a large bowl add olive oil, rosemary, parsley, dill, salt, and pepper.

3. Add parsnips to bowl and toss to coat with other ingredients.

4. Place on a rimmed baking sheet and roast 20 minutes, flipping parsnips halfway through roasting. When done, sprinkle with lemon juice and serve.

Per Serving   Calories: 187 | Fat: 7g | Protein: 2g | Sodium: 165mg | Fiber: 8g | Carbohydrates: 31g | Sugar: 8g

Garlicky Parsnip and Carrot Fries

A fun and delicious treat for the family or a gathering.

INGREDIENTS | SERVES 6

2 tablespoons garlic-infused olive oil

1/8 teaspoon wheat-free asafetida powder

2 teaspoons chopped fresh flat-leaf parsley

1/2 teaspoon coarse salt

5 medium carrots, peeled and cut diagonally into 1"-thick slices

3 medium parsnips, peeled and cut diagonally into 1"-thick slices

1. Preheat oven to 400°F.

2. In a large bowl combine oil, asafetida, parsley, and salt. Add carrots and parsnips to bowl and toss well to coat.

3. Place on a rimmed baking sheet and roast 20 minutes, flipping pieces halfway through roasting. Parsnips and carrots should be crisp and golden brown.

Per Serving   Calories: 86 | Fat: 5g | Protein: 1g | Sodium: 235mg | Fiber: 3g | Carbohydrates: 11g | Sugar: 4g

Swiss Chard with Cranberries and Pine Nuts

This recipe was inspired by Sicilian-style greens, normally consisting of spinach, currants, and pine nuts. Cranberries are allowed on the low-FODMAP diet; it's best to buy ones without added sugar.

INGREDIENTS | SERVES 4

1/8 teaspoon salt, divided

2½ pounds Swiss chard

1 tablespoon garlic-infused olive oil

3 tablespoons pine nuts

1/8 teaspoon wheat-free asafetida powder

3 tablespoons no-added-sugar cranberries

1/4 teaspoon freshly ground black pepper

1. Fill a medium bowl with ice water. Add 1/16 teaspoon salt to a large pot of water and boil. Add chard. Cook until tender, about 2 minutes. Transfer chard to bowl of ice water and let sit 5 minutes. Drain in a colander and squeeze out as much water as possible. Remove stems and veins and keep leaves. Chop coarsely.

2. Heat garlic-infused olive oil over medium heat in a large, heavy skillet or cast-iron pan.

3. Add pine nuts and asafetida powder and cook 2–3 minutes.

4. Add chard and cranberries and cook until heated through, 2–3 minutes. Season with remaining salt and pepper.

Per Serving   Calories: 181 | Fat: 14g | Protein: 6g | Sodium: 680mg | Fiber: 6g | Carbohydrates: 13g | Sugar: 3g

Potato and Kale Gratin

This makes for a satisfying, comforting weekend dish, or it's also great for the holidays.

INGREDIENTS | SERVES 4

1 large bunch kale (about ½ pound), chopped (thick ribs and stems removed)

½ cup lactose-free milk

1 teaspoon sea salt

½ teaspoon freshly ground black pepper

2 tablespoons butter, cut into pieces, plus more for buttering

1 pound Yukon Gold potatoes, sliced very thin

½ cup grated Parmesan cheese

1 tablespoon fresh thyme leaves

1. Preheat oven to 400°F and place a rack in the middle.

2. Bring a large pot of water to a boil and add kale. Boil 2–3 minutes, or until leaves are wilted. Drain in a colander, squeezing out excess water. Set aside.

3. In a medium bowl whisk together milk, salt, and pepper. Set aside.

4. Grease a 9" × 13" baking dish with butter. Layer about half of potato slices evenly on bottom. Top with kale, then with half of Parmesan. Layer remaining potatoes on top and sprinkle with remaining Parmesan.

5. Pour milk mixture over potatoes. Sprinkle on thyme. Scatter butter pieces on top of potatoes.

6. Bake, covered with aluminum foil, 25 minutes. Remove foil and bake another 25 minutes or until potatoes are tender and cheese is golden brown.

Per Serving Calories: 86 | Fat: 5g | Protein: 1g | Sodium: 235mg | Fiber: 3g | Carbohydrates: 11g | Sugar: 4g

Toasted Coconut Almond Millet

Missing couscous on a low-FODMAP diet?
Give delicious, versatile millet a try. You are sure to love its sweet, nutty flavor.

INGREDIENTS | SERVES 4

1 cup millet
1½ cups water
¼ cup orange juice
⅛ teaspoon alcohol-free vanilla extract
⅛ teaspoon freshly ground black pepper
½ teaspoon sea salt
½ cup sliced almonds
¼ cup shredded unsweetened coconut
Coconut oil spray
1 teaspoon pure maple syrup

Meet Millet

Here is another gluten-free grain that you will want to get to know as you follow the low-FODMAP diet. Millet is packed with fiber. It is also a good source of protein, B vitamins, copper, magnesium, manganese, and phosphorus. Millet can be used for baking or cooked like rice.

1. Heat a medium saucepan over medium heat. Add millet and sauté 2–3 minutes or until fragrant.

2. Add water, orange juice, vanilla, pepper, and salt. Bring just to a boil and then reduce heat to low. Simmer, covered, 25–30 minutes or until all water is absorbed.

3. Meanwhile, preheat broiler. Line a baking sheet with foil. Toss almonds with coconut on the baking sheet. Spray with coconut oil spray and toss to coat. Broil 1–2 minutes or until mixture starts to turn light brown. Remove from broiler, transfer to a bowl, and toss with maple syrup.

4. When millet is cooked, fluff with a fork. Divide evenly among serving plates and sprinkle with toasted coconut mixture.

Per Serving Calories: 287 | Fat: 10g | Protein: 8g | Sodium: 301mg | Fiber: 6g | Carbohydrates: 43g | Sugar: 3g

Root-a-Burgers

You can't put high-FODMAP mushrooms on top of these burgers, but a drizzle of black truffle oil before and after grilling provides a similar—more dramatic—earthy flavor.

INGREDIENTS | SERVES 6

2 medium parsnips, peeled and cut into ½" rounds

2 medium carrots, peeled and cut into ½" rounds

1 teaspoon grapeseed oil

2 teaspoons salt, divided

½ teaspoon freshly ground black pepper, divided

2 slices gluten-free bread, toasted

1 cup canned lentils, drained and rinsed well

1 large egg

1 cup freshly grated Parmesan cheese

1 teaspoon black truffle oil

What Is Truffle Oil?

Truffles are a type of fungi, often found near the roots of trees; not all are edible. Truffle oil adds the taste of truffles to cooking. White truffle oil provides a fairly light, herby taste while black truffle oil has a stronger, earthy taste. Some truffle oils are made from synthetic ingredients; true oil is more expensive. Although neither one has been specifically tested for FODMAP content, typically oils are low in FODMAPs.

1. Preheat oven to 400°F. Line a baking sheet with parchment paper.

2. In a large bowl, toss parsnips and carrots with grapeseed oil, 1 teaspoon salt, and ¼ teaspoon pepper. Spread on baking sheet and bake 30 minutes. Set aside to cool.

3. In a food processor, pulse toast to a crumb consistency. Transfer to a bowl.

4. Add roasted vegetables to food processor and pulse until there are no major lumps. Add remaining salt and pepper, toasted bread crumbs, lentils, egg, and cheese. Pulse to combine.

5. Transfer to a workspace and form 6 equal patty rounds.

6. Refrigerate patties 12–24 hours before grilling or broiling on surface coated with truffle oil. Cook patties 3–4 minutes on each side; drain on paper towels.

Per Serving   Calories: 265 | Fat: 12g | Protein: 19g | Sodium: 1485mg | Fiber: 2g | Carbohydrates: 21g | Sugar: 3g

Confetti Corn

It's easy to eat a rainbow when this dish is part of your menu.
Fresh corn and basil turn this colorful side into a real taste of summer.

INGREDIENTS | SERVES 4

2 medium ears corn, shucked and cooked
1 tablespoon butter
½ cup finely diced red bell pepper
½ cup finely diced yellow bell pepper
½ cup finely diced orange bell pepper
½ cup finely diced green bell pepper
½ teaspoon sea salt
⅛ teaspoon ground red pepper flakes
¼ cup chopped fresh basil leaves

1. Cut kernels off cobs into a medium bowl.

2. Melt butter in a large skillet over medium-low heat.

3. Add bell peppers, salt, and pepper; sauté, stirring occasionally, 8–10 minutes.

4. Add corn kernels to pepper mixture and sauté 3–5 minutes more, stirring occasionally.

5. Transfer to a serving dish and garnish with basil.

Per Serving   Calories: 104 | Fat: 4g | Protein: 3g | Sodium: 301mg | Fiber: 3g | Carbohydrates: 19g | Sugar: 4g

Zoodles with Pesto

Making "zoodles," or zucchini noodles, is not only fun, but a healthy way to enjoy pasta recipes.

INGREDIENTS | SERVES 3

¾ cup fresh basil leaves
2 tablespoons garlic-infused olive oil
¼ cup pine nuts
2 tablespoons extra-virgin olive oil
½ cup freshly grated Parmesan cheese
¼ teaspoon sea salt, divided
¼ teaspoon freshly ground black pepper, divided
1 pound zucchini
1 tablespoon olive oil

1. For pesto sauce: Combine basil, garlic oil, and pine nuts in a food processor and pulse until coarsely chopped. Add extra-virgin olive oil, cheese, 1/16 teaspoon salt, and ⅛ teaspoon pepper and process until fully incorporated and smooth.

2. Use a tool such as the Veggetti Spiral Vegetable Slicer and follow directions or use a vegetable peeler to make long, thin slices of zucchini.

3. Heat olive oil in a medium sauté pan. Add zucchini noodles, 1/16 teaspoon salt, and ⅛ teaspoon pepper to pan and stir 3–5 minutes, or until noodles are just tender. Serve with pesto sauce.

Per Serving   Calories: 491 | Fat: 44g | Protein: 18g | Sodium: 445mg | Fiber: 4g | Carbohydrates: 10g | Sugar: 4g

Sweet Potato with Maple Yogurt and Pumpkin Seeds

This can be a wonderful side dish or even a new morning breakfast item. Enjoy!

INGREDIENTS | SERVES 2

1 medium sweet potato
½ tablespoon butter or vegan substitute
¼ teaspoon ground cinnamon
3 tablespoons lactose-free vanilla yogurt
1 tablespoon maple syrup
⅛ teaspoon salt
1 tablespoon pumpkin seeds

How Much Sweet Potato Is Low-FODMAP?

A ¾-cup serving of sweet potato or more is high in the polyol mannitol and intake should be limited if you have an issue with malabsorption of mannitol. Learn more about hydrogen breath testing in Chapter 1.

1. Bake sweet potato quickly by placing in microwave (cook time varies for different microwaves) or bake in oven. For baking, preheat oven to 350°F. Cut a slit down middle of potato, add butter and cinnamon, and wrap in tinfoil. Place on baking sheet and bake 1–1½ hours or until tender.

2. Remove potato from oven and carefully pull away tinfoil. Split potato in half to make 2 servings.

3. In a small bowl, mix together yogurt, maple syrup, and salt. Place a dollop on top of each potato half. Sprinkle with pumpkin seeds.

Per Serving   Calories: 153 | Fat: 5g | Protein: 4g | Sodium: 201mg | Fiber: 2g | Carbohydrates: 24g | Sugar: 12g

Roasted Maple Dill Carrots

Looking for a side to go with a hearty meal? These carrots are the perfect accompaniment. You can also swap out maple syrup and cinnamon for lemon juice and another herb.

INGREDIENTS | SERVES 6

2 pounds carrots
2 tablespoons extra-virgin olive oil
2 tablespoons pure maple syrup
1½ teaspoons ground cinnamon
1 teaspoon sea salt
1½ tablespoons fresh dill

1. Preheat oven to 450°F. Grease a rimmed baking sheet with cooking spray.

2. Peel carrots and then cut lengthwise down middle. Cut again so each piece is about 3" long.

3. Add carrots to a large bowl and toss with oil, maple syrup, cinnamon, and salt.

4. Place carrots on prepared baking sheet cut side down and spread out in a single layer.

5. Roast 10 minutes, and then stir carrots around sheet once. Return to oven and roast and stir once more, cooking another 20 minutes total. Carrots are done when tender and look glossy and caramelized.

6. Sprinkle dill over carrots and stir. Transfer to a serving bowl and serve immediately. Carrots also taste delicious cold.

Per Serving   Calories: 120 | Fat: 5g | Protein: 4g |
Sodium: 499mg | Fiber: 4g | Carbohydrates: 19g | Sugar: 11g

Hasselback Potatoes

Hasselback potatoes can be made with different ingredients, but the key is how you slice them and how marvelous you want them to be! No heavy cream here, just lactose-free milk and sour cream and cheese. Yum.

INGREDIENTS | SERVES 6

6 medium baking potatoes
4 tablespoons melted butter, divided
1 teaspoon paprika
⅛ teaspoon sea salt
1 teaspoon freshly ground black pepper
2 cups lactose-free milk
2 cups lactose-free sour cream
3 tablespoons finely grated fresh Pecorino-style cheese
1 cup gluten-free panko bread crumbs
1 teaspoon dried oregano

1. Preheat oven to 425°F.

2. Place potatoes on a cutting board and use a sharp knife to make slices across each potato, leaving about ¼" in between each slice and leaving about ⅛" of potato uncut from bottom, not cutting all the way through and keeping potato connected.

3. Place potatoes cut side up in a small roasting pan or a shallow baking dish. (A rimmed baking sheet works too, but other options are better to keep potatoes from moving too much.)

4. Drizzle potatoes with 2 tablespoons melted butter then sprinkle with paprika, salt, and pepper.

5. Whisk milk and sour cream in a bowl and pour over potatoes.

6. Stir to combine Pecorino cheese, bread crumbs, and oregano in a small bowl, and then sprinkle over top of potatoes. Drizzle remaining 2 tablespoons of butter over potatoes.

7. Place potatoes in oven 35–45 minutes. When done, potatoes should be cooked through, crispy, and golden brown. Serve hot.

Per Serving Calories: 357 | Fat: 15g | Protein: 11g | Sodium: 271mg | Fiber: 3g | Carbohydrates: 49g | Sugar: 6g

Lemon Pepper Green Beans

These fragrant and delicate green beans go nicely with meat or fish and are easy to make.

INGREDIENTS | SERVES 6

1 pound fresh green beans, trimmed

2 tablespoons butter

¼ cup sliced almonds

2 teaspoons lemon pepper

⅛ teaspoon salt

1. Place green beans in a large pot of boiling salted water. Cook about 4–5 minutes; drain.

2. Meanwhile, melt butter in a large skillet over medium heat. Add almonds and sauté until lightly browned. Sprinkle in lemon pepper and salt. Add green beans and toss to coat.

Per Serving   Calories: 82 | Fat: 6g | Protein: 2g | Sodium: 54mg | Fiber: 3g | Carbohydrates: 6g | Sugar: 3g

Sesame and Ginger Bok Choy

This dish is great when paired with Maple-Glazed Salmon (see recipe in Chapter 8). For vegans, this dish is great with the addition of brown rice and some protein such as Savory Baked Tofu (see recipe in Chapter 9).

INGREDIENTS | SERVES 2

1 tablespoon sesame oil

½ tablespoon minced fresh gingerroot

1 scallion, chopped, green part only

½ cup sliced water chestnuts

4 cups chopped fresh bok choy

1 tablespoon gluten-free soy sauce (tamari)

1. Heat oil in a large skillet over medium heat. Add ginger and scallion and cook 1 minute.

2. Add water chestnuts, bok choy, and soy sauce; cook 3–5 minutes or until bok choy greens are wilted. Bok choy stalks should be crisp-tender.

Per Serving   Calories: 115 | Fat: 7g | Protein: 3g | Sodium: 545mg | Fiber: 3g | Carbohydrates: 12g | Sugar: 4g

Spaghetti Squash with Goat Cheese

Very light and earthy, this dish fares well as a side with fish.

INGREDIENTS | SERVES 4

1 (5-pound) spaghetti squash

½ cup water

½ tablespoon extra-virgin olive oil

2 tablespoons pine nuts

⅛ teaspoon salt

½ teaspoon freshly ground black pepper

1 ounce crumbled goat cheese

1. Preheat oven to 400°F.

2. Carefully cut squash down middle, leaving two halves. Next, use a spoon to scoop out seeds. If desired, keep seeds to roast in oven, much like Roasted Pumpkin Seeds (see recipe in Chapter 14). Arrange squash cut side down in a 9" × 13" baking dish. Pour water into dish and bake 30–35 minutes.

3. Check to make sure squash is tender, then use a fork to rake the squash and pull up its fleshy strands.

4. Add squash to a large bowl and stir in olive oil, pine nuts, salt, and pepper. Finish by topping with goat cheese crumbles. Serve immediately.

Per Serving   Calories: 180 | Fat: 9g | Protein: 10g | Sodium: 114mg | Fiber: 7g | Carbohydrates: 20g | Sugar: 12g

Quinoa Tabbouleh

Quinoa soaks up the flavors of the herbs, lemon juice, and olive oil, and makes for an excellent base for tabbouleh.

INGREDIENTS | SERVES 2

½ cup quinoa

1 cup Vegetable Stock (see recipe in Chapter 4)

1 tablespoon extra-virgin olive oil

1 tablespoon fresh lemon juice

⅛ teaspoon sea salt

1 cup finely chopped parsley

¼ cup finely chopped mint leaves

6 cherry tomatoes, halved

¼ cup finely diced cucumber

½ cup crumbled feta cheese

1. Place quinoa in a sieve and rinse well with water. Combine quinoa with stock in a medium saucepan and bring to a boil. Cover, reduce heat to low, and simmer 12–15 minutes or until quinoa is tender. Drain thoroughly.

2. In a large salad bowl, whisk oil and lemon juice to combine. Add quinoa, salt, parsley, mint, tomatoes, and cucumber and toss. Garnish with feta. Serve at room temperature or chilled.

Per Serving   Calories: 435 | Fat: 21g | Protein: 18g | Sodium: 1514mg | Fiber: 6g | Carbohydrates: 45g | Sugar: 4g

CHAPTER 6

Sandwiches

Baba Ghanoush Sandwich
122

Cucumber Goat Cheese
Sandwich
122

Avocado, Goat Cheese, and
Spinach Panini
123

Turkey Pesto Wrap
123

Open-Faced Shrimp Salad
Sandwich with Cucumbers
124

Greek Salad Wrap
124

Brie and Orange Marmalade
Sandwich
125

Curry Chickpea and Vegetable
Spread Sandwich
125

Barbecue Chicken Wrap
126

Baba Ghanoush Sandwich

This vegetarian sandwich is so addictive that you'll want it every week!

INGREDIENTS | SERVES 4

8 tablespoons Baba Ghanoush (see recipe in Chapter 3)

8 pieces gluten-free bread

3 vine-ripe tomatoes, sliced thin

1 medium cucumber, sliced into thin rounds

4 large leaves romaine lettuce, trimmed and sliced in half

1 medium lemon

1. Spread 1 tablespoon Baba Ghanoush on each piece of bread.

2. For each sandwich, place 3 thin slices tomato, 3 thin slices cucumber, and 2 pieces romaine on 1 slice of bread.

3. Squeeze lemon juice on opposite slice of bread. Place pieces of bread together to form a sandwich.

Per Serving   Calories: 224 | Fat: 2g | Protein: 9g | Sodium: 425mg | Fiber: 4g | Carbohydrates: 45g | Sugar: 6g

Cucumber Goat Cheese Sandwich

This sandwich is great to have for lunch, at a picnic, or with afternoon tea.

INGREDIENTS | SERVES 4

¼ cup Basic Mayonnaise (see recipe in Chapter 13)

⅛ teaspoon wheat-free asafetida powder

⅛ teaspoon salt

1 teaspoon gluten-free Worcestershire sauce

8 slices gluten-free bread

½ cup goat cheese

1 medium cucumber, thinly sliced

1. In a small bowl, combine mayonnaise, asafetida, salt, and Worcestershire.

2. To assemble sandwiches, lay out pieces of bread and spread mayonnaise mixture across one side of bread and then spread goat cheese on other slice. Layer on the cucumber slices. Repeat process for second sandwich.

3. Cut sandwiches from corner to corner to make triangle slices.

Per Serving   Calories: 423 | Fat: 22g | Protein: 17g | Sodium: 680mg | Fiber: 2g | Carbohydrates: 40g | Sugar: 4g

Avocado, Goat Cheese, and Spinach Panini

Goat cheese is always delicious especially when warmed between bread and vegetables!

INGREDIENTS | SERVES 1

⅛ medium avocado, sliced

2 sun-dried tomatoes, chopped

¼ cup crumbled goat cheese

½ cup baby spinach

2 tablespoons sprouts

1 (4-ounce) gluten-free ciabatta roll, or other gluten-free bread

Where to Find Gluten-Free Ciabatta Rolls

You can find gluten-free ciabatta rolls in the freezer section in most natural foods stores, or you can buy them online.

1. Layer avocado, tomatoes, goat cheese, spinach, and sprouts on each side of a roll or bread. Close up sandwich.

2. Spray skillet or panini pan with cooking spray and heat sandwich over medium heat. Cook 4 minutes in a panini maker or place in a skillet and cook with a smaller skillet on top of the sandwich weighted with a heavy object (such as a large can) and cook 2 minutes; flip, place skillet on top again, and cook another 2 minutes.

Per Serving   Calories: 320 | Fat: 13g | Protein: 16g | Sodium: 512mg | Fiber: 3g | Carbohydrates: 36g | Sugar: 3g

Turkey Pesto Wrap

Make your own Pesto Sauce at home (see recipe in Chapter 13) and use for this recipe as a take-to-work/school sandwich. Use leftover pesto with your morning eggs, in potato salad, or spread on gluten-free bread, pizzas, and burgers.

INGREDIENTS | SERVES 1

1 tablespoon Pesto Sauce

1 (6") gluten-free tortilla

2 slices deli turkey meat

⅛ medium avocado, sliced

2 tablespoons sprouts

Spread pesto on tortilla. Layer turkey, avocado, and sprouts on top of pesto. Wrap and enjoy!

Per Serving   Calories: 241 | Fat: 14g | Protein: 10g | Sodium: 587mg | Fiber: 3g | Carbohydrates: 21g | Sugar: 2g

Open-Faced Shrimp Salad Sandwich with Cucumbers

Try this light and refreshing way to enjoy shrimp salad with these dainty open-faced sandwiches. You can also make an appetizer with this recipe by leaving out the bread and placing shrimp salad on top of cucumber slices on a rectangular serving plate.

INGREDIENTS | SERVES 4

1 pound cooked medium shrimp, peeled and deveined

1 medium stalk celery, diced

½ cup Basic Mayonnaise (see recipe in Chapter 13)

½ teaspoon ground red pepper

½ teaspoon paprika

½ teaspoon ground nutmeg

½ teaspoon ground allspice

½ teaspoon ground cardamom

2 teaspoons lemon juice

¼ teaspoon gluten-free Worcestershire sauce

¼ teaspoon freshly ground black pepper

8 slices gluten-free bread

1 large cucumber, cut into ¼" slices

2 scallions, chopped, green part only

1. Dice shrimp into small chunks and place in a medium bowl. Add celery, mayonnaise, red pepper, paprika, nutmeg, allspice, cardamom, lemon juice, Worcestershire, and black pepper. Stir well to combine.

2. Place 2 slices bread on each of 4 plates. Place 4 cucumber slices on each slice of bread, overlapping slices in middle. Top with shrimp salad and garnish with scallions.

Per Serving Calories: 512 | Fat: 25g | Protein: 32g | Sodium: 837mg | Fiber: 2g | Carbohydrates: 41g | Sugar: 3g

Greek Salad Wrap

If you're bringing this wrap to work, cut in half and roll up in tinfoil for easy transport.

INGREDIENTS | SERVES 1

½ tablespoon garlic-infused olive oil

1 (6") gluten-free wrap

⅛ teaspoon dried oregano

5 cherry tomatoes, halved

5 pitted black olives, cut into slices

1 large leaf romaine lettuce, or ½ cup spinach

4 slices cucumber, quartered

¼ cup crumbled feta cheese

3 basil leaves

⅛ teaspoon freshly ground black pepper

1. Using a spoon, spread oil onto wrap and add oregano. Place tomatoes, olives, romaine, cucumber, feta, basil, and pepper down middle of wrap.

2. Fold sides of tortilla halfway in. Fold bottom third up. Press down and pinch as you keep rolling. Tuck in fillings as you go. Press down to seal.

Per Serving Calories: 435 | Fat: 19g | Protein: 16g | Sodium: 1,039mg | Fiber: 6g | Carbohydrates: 55g | Sugar: 11g

Brie and Orange Marmalade Sandwich

Brie typically goes really well with high-FODMAP fruit such as pears and apples but it also tastes delicious with low-FODMAP orange marmalade, berries, or berry jams.

INGREDIENTS | SERVES 1

2 slices gluten-free bread, fresh or toasted

2 wedges brie cheese (about 1.5 ounces)

1½ tablespoons orange marmalade

Place bread on a plate and spread each slice with cheese and marmalade. Enjoy immediately or wrap in tinfoil and refrigerate to enjoy the next day.

Per Serving Calories: 263 | Fat: 6g | Protein: 7g | Sodium: 464mg | Fiber: 1g | Carbohydrates: 45g | Sugar: 20g

Make It a Panini

This sandwich also is excellent when the cheese is warmed as a panini! If you don't have a panini maker at home, you can always place the sandwich in a skillet and apply pressure by using a smaller, heavier skillet weighed down with a heavy object such as a large can.

Curry Chickpea and Vegetable Spread Sandwich

This spread is great on gluten-free bread or collard green wraps.

INGREDIENTS | SERVES 4

½ (15-ounce) can chickpeas, drained and rinsed

¼ cup peeled and grated carrots

½ teaspoon curry powder

¾ teaspoon chili powder

½ teaspoon ground cumin

1 teaspoon ground coriander

4 teaspoons lemon juice

1/16 teaspoon salt

1 tablespoon extra-virgin olive oil

8 slices gluten-free bread

4 slices tomato

12 large basil leaves, torn

1 cup spinach

1. Combine chickpeas with carrots, curry, chili powder, cumin, coriander, lemon juice, salt, and extra-virgin olive oil in a food processor and mix until a paste forms.

2. Spread mixture on 4 slices bread and top other slices with tomato, basil, and spinach. Press pieces of bread together and serve.

Per Serving Calories: 317 | Fat: 6g | Protein: 14g | Sodium: 819mg | Fiber: 8g | Carbohydrates: 54g | Sugar: 5g

Barbecue Chicken Wrap

Adults and kids alike love these wraps. To make low-FODMAP barbecue sauce see recipe in Chapter 13 or use a brand that does not contain high-FODMAP ingredients such as onions, garlic, onion powder, or garlic powder.

INGREDIENTS | SERVES 4

3 (4-ounce) boneless, skinless chicken breasts
¼ cup barbecue sauce
4 (6") gluten-free tortillas
½ cup shredded Cheddar cheese
2 large romaine lettuce leaves, halved

Make It Crunchy

Alternatively for a crunchier chicken wrap, you can dredge chicken tenders in flour, egg, and then gluten-free panko bread crumbs and cook in a pan with 1 tablespoon oil on medium heat, cooking each side for 6–7 minutes. You would then add the chicken tenders to the wrap and drizzle on the barbecue sauce.

1. Place chicken breasts in a medium pan and cover with water. Place pan over medium heat, bring to a boil, and simmer 10–12 minutes or until chicken meat is cooked through. Allow chicken to cool on a plate and then shred with forks.

2. In a small saucepan over low heat, add barbecue sauce and chicken and stir to combine. Keep warm while you begin making wraps.

3. Warm a small skillet over low heat and add a tortilla. Sprinkle on cheese and wait until cheese is melted. Remove from heat and place wrap on a wide plate or clean work surface.

4. Add ¼ of barbecue chicken and top with lettuce. Place wrap horizontally in front of you, fold bottom and top edges over, rotate wrap, and roll up from bottom. Repeat with remaining tortillas. Place any leftover barbecue chicken in an airtight container.

Per Serving   Calories: 378 | Fat: 12g | Protein: 44g | Sodium: 660mg | Fiber: 1g | Carbohydrates: 22g | Sugar: 5g

CHAPTER 7

Poultry, Pork, and Beef

Chicken Burgers
128

Pork and Fennel
Meatballs
128

Turkey Quinoa
Meatballs with
Mozzarella
129

Roast Beef Tenderloin
with Parmesan Crust
130

Citrus Flank Steak
131

Prosciutto-Stuffed
Chicken
132

Stuffed Peppers with
Ground Turkey
133

Orange Chicken and
Broccoli Stir-Fry
134

Beef with Spinach and
Sweet Potatoes
135

Pork Chops with
Carrots and Toasted
Buckwheat
136

Lemon Thyme Chicken
137

Spinach and Feta-
Stuffed Chicken Breast
137

Cumin Turkey with
Fennel
138

Victor's Chicken
Parmesan
139

Chicken Piccata
140

Easy Pan Chicken
141

Turkey Bolognese
with Pasta
142

Coq au Vin
143

Blueberry-Glazed
Chicken
144

Parmesan-Crusted
Chicken
144

Sweet and Savory
Brazilian Meat and
Cheese Tart
145

Zucchini Lasagna with
Meat Sauce
146

Pumpkin Maple Roast
Chicken
147

Barbecue Pork
Macaroni and Cheese
148

Sourdough Meatballs
149

Polenta-Crusted
Chicken
149

Aunt Bete's
Chicken Tart
150

Chicken, Sweet
Potato, and
Spinach Curry
151

Mustard and Thyme
Roasted Chicken
152

Crispy Baked Chicken
with Gravy
153

Turkey Pasta with Kale
154

Chicken Burgers

These burgers are great for garlic lovers as they have a nice hint of garlic from the asafetida powder. Serve these on gluten-free buns slathered with Aioli (see Chapter 13) and top with spinach and tomatoes.

INGREDIENTS | SERVES 4

1 pound ground chicken

⅛ teaspoon wheat-free asafetida powder

½ teaspoon salt

½ teaspoon white pepper

1 large egg, beaten

¼ cup grated Parmesan cheese

1 tablespoon olive oil

1. Mix all ingredients except oil together in a bowl with your hands until well blended.

2. Shape into 4 patties.

3. In a large skillet heat oil on medium-high and add burgers. Brown on one side until cooked throughout, about 5 minutes, then flip and cook other side.

Per Serving Calories: 283 | Fat: 20g | Protein: 23g | Sodium: 493mg | Fiber: 0g | Carbohydrates: 1g | Sugar: 0g

Pork and Fennel Meatballs

These meatballs can be described as earthy and definitely tasty. Serve either as appetizers or as a full meal with a sprinkle of chopped fresh parsley and pasta with Basic Marina Sauce from Chapter 13.

INGREDIENTS | MAKES 24

1 pound lean ground pork

2 tablespoons roughly chopped fresh flat-leaf parsley

3 tablespoons gluten-free panko bread crumbs

1 large egg

⅛ teaspoon wheat-free asafetida powder

¼ teaspoon salt

½ teaspoon freshly ground black pepper

1½ tablespoons olive oil

2 teaspoons fennel seeds

1. In a mixing bowl, combine pork, parsley, bread crumbs, egg, asafetida, salt, and pepper. Stir to combine or mix well with hands. Shape into 1" meatballs.

2. In a medium skillet, heat oil over medium heat and toast fennel seeds until fragrant, about 4 minutes. Add meatballs to pan.

3. Brown meatballs on all sides, cooking about 4–5 minutes per side, 20 minutes total. Meatballs are cooked through when no longer pink inside.

Per Serving (1 meatball) Calories: 64 | Fat: 5g | Protein: 4g | Sodium: 47mg | Fiber: 0g | Carbohydrates: 1g | Sugar: 0g

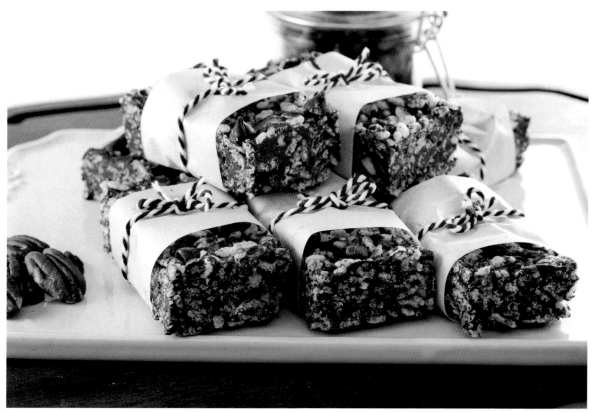

No-Bake Crispy Almond Pecan Bars (Chapter 11)

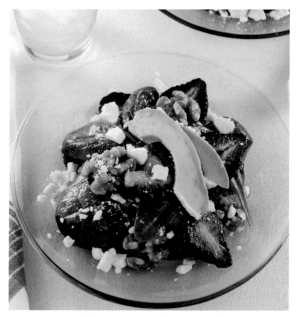

Glorious Strawberry Salad (Chapter 4)

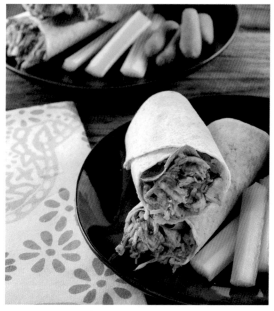

Barbecue Chicken Wrap (Chapter 6)

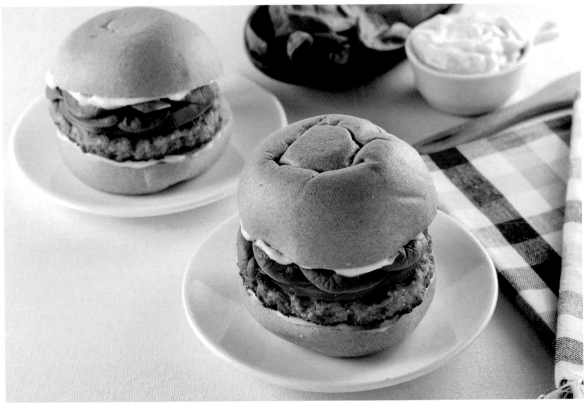

Chicken Burgers (Chapter 7) with Aioli (Chapter 13)

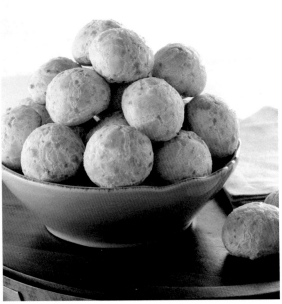

Pão de Queijo (Cheese Bread) (Chapter 3)

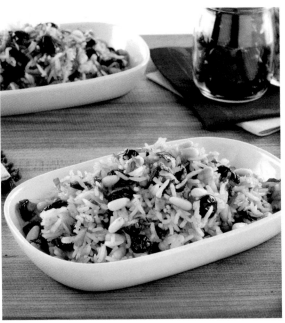

Turmeric Rice with Cranberries (Chapter 9)

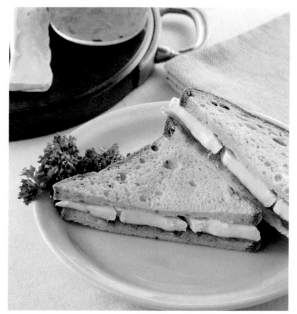

Brie and Orange Marmalade Sandwich (Chapter 6)

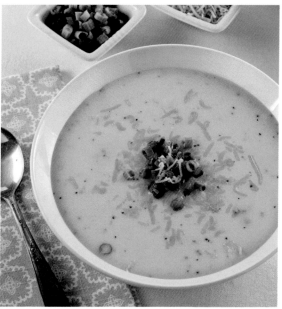

Potato Soup (Chapter 4)

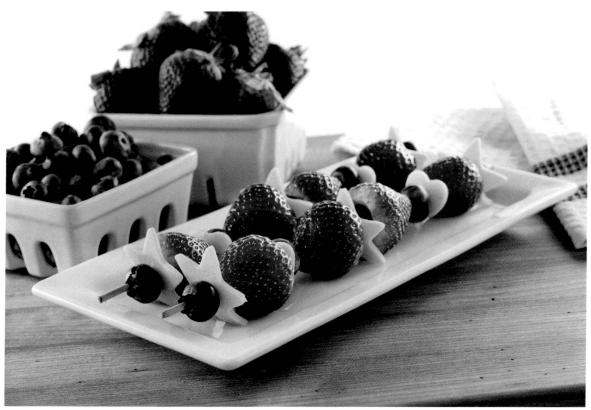

Fruit and Cheese Kebabs (Chapter 10)

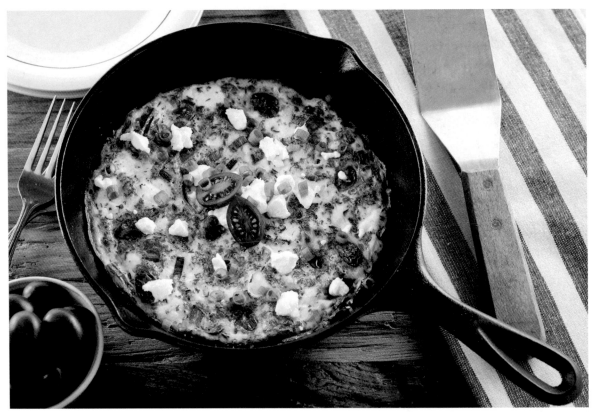

Tomato and Leek Frittata (Chapter 2)

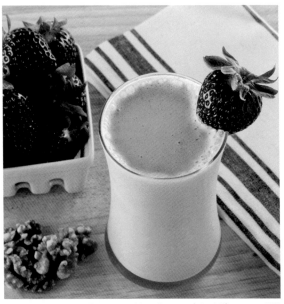

Banana-Nut Smoothie (Chapter 15)

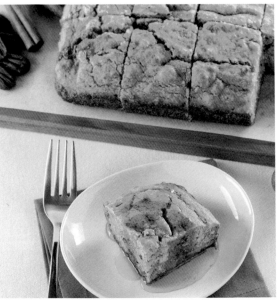

Pumpkin Spice Pecan Cornbread
(Chapter 12) with maple syrup

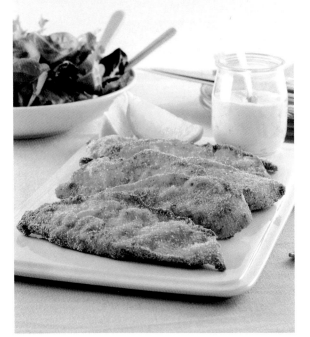

Cornmeal-Crusted Tilapia (Chapter 8)
with Tartar Sauce (Chapter 13)

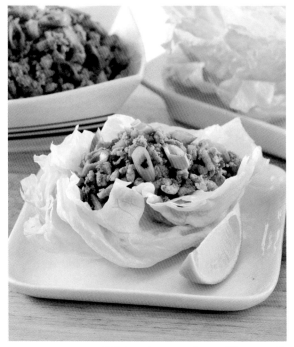

Chicken Lettuce Cups (Chapter 3)

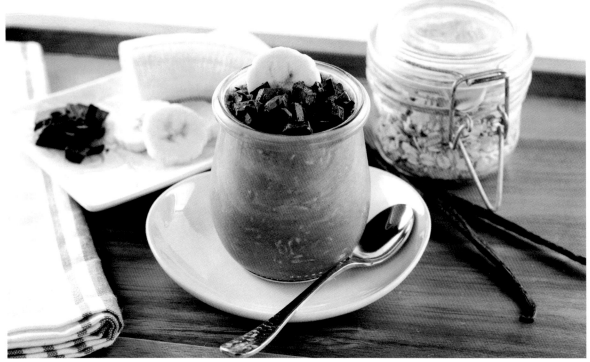

Overnight Banana Chocolate Oats (Chapter 2)

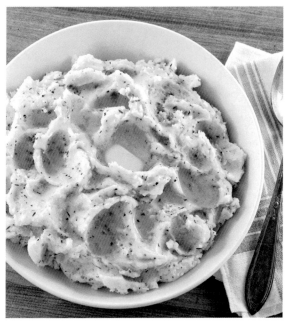
Herbed Mashed Potatoes (Chapter 5)

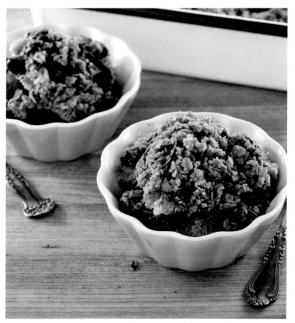
Mixed Berry Cobbler (Chapter 12)

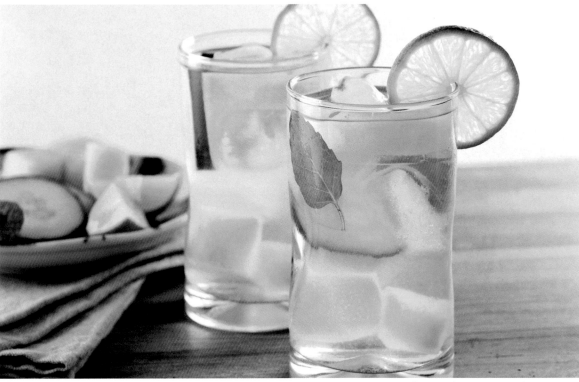
Cucumber Melon Water (Chapter 15)

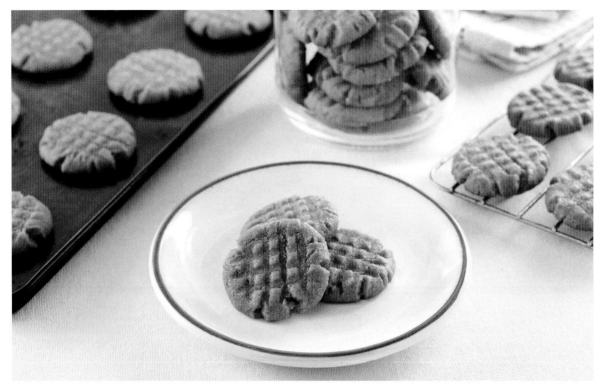

Peanut Butter Cookies (Chapter 11)

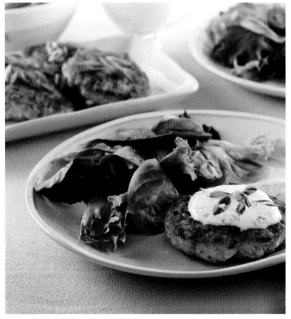

Salmon Cakes with Fresh Dill Sauce (Chapter 8)

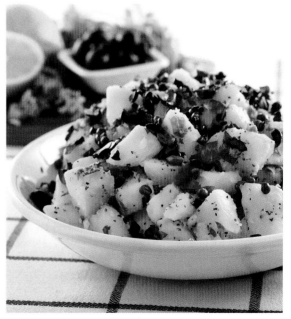

Vegan Potato Salad, Cypriot-Style (Chapter 9)

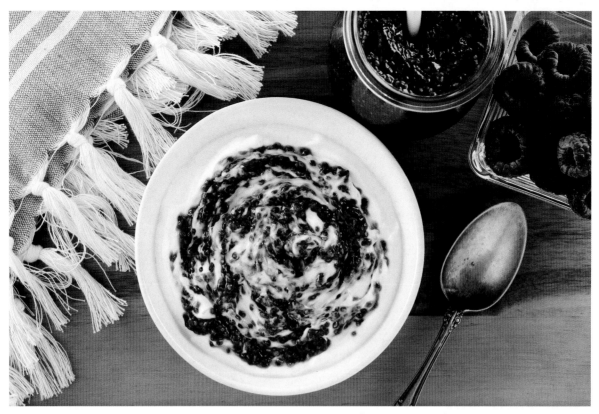

Raspberry Lemon Chia Seed Jam (Chapter 13)
stirred into lactose-free yogurt

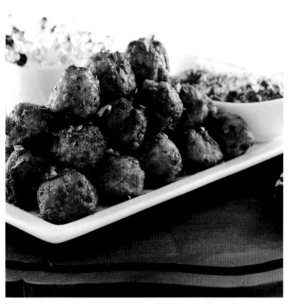

Pork and Fennel Meatballs (Chapter 7)
with Basic Marinara Sauce (Chapter 13)

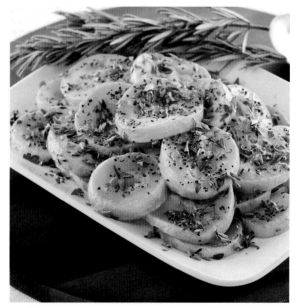

Herbed Yellow Squash (Chapter 5)

Turkey Quinoa Meatballs with Mozzarella

Easy and cozy for a Sunday night, try these meatballs topped on gluten-free pasta mixed with diced Roma tomatoes and Parmesan cheese or serve as appetizers.

INGREDIENTS | MAKES 15 MEATBALLS

1 cup cooked quinoa

1 pound ground lean turkey meat

2 large eggs

½ teaspoon freshly ground black pepper

½ teaspoon paprika

½ teaspoon dried oregano

½ teaspoon dried thyme

½ teaspoon dried parsley

8 ounces fresh mozzarella, cubed

2 tablespoons chopped fresh flat-leaf parsley

½ cup grated Parmesan cheese

1. Preheat oven to 350°F. Line a baking sheet with parchment paper.

2. Mix all ingredients together (except mozzarella, parsley, and Parmesan cheese) in a large bowl.

3. Divide meat mixture into 15 portions.

4. Place 1 small mozzarella cube in the center of each portion and shape into a ball.

5. Bake 30 minutes or until meatballs are not pink inside.

6. Garnish with fresh parsley and Parmesan cheese.

Per Serving Calories: 128 | Fat: 8g | Protein: 11g | Sodium: 183mg | Fiber: 0g | Carbohydrates: 3g | Sugar: 0g

Roast Beef Tenderloin with Parmesan Crust

If you like roast beef you'll love it even more when it's coated with a lovely Parmesan crust.

INGREDIENTS | SERVES 8

1 (4-pound) center-cut beef tenderloin, fat and silver skin trimmed

¼ teaspoon kosher salt

5 teaspoons freshly ground black pepper, divided

⅔ cup gluten-free fine bread crumbs

¾ cup finely grated Parmesan cheese

⅔ cup Basic Mayonnaise (see recipe in Chapter 13)

1 tablespoon Dijon mustard

1 tablespoon finely grated lemon zest

1 tablespoon gluten-free Worcestershire sauce

Tips on Buying Beef Tenderloin

If you want to purchase the roast completely trimmed and don't mind paying extra, just ask your butcher to prepare the roast "side muscle off and skinned."

1. Season tenderloin lightly with salt and 1 teaspoon pepper. Wrap in plastic wrap and refrigerate overnight.

2. Uncover tenderloin; let stand at room temperature for up to 2 hours.

3. Preheat oven to 400°F.

4. Set a rack inside a rimmed baking sheet. Transfer tenderloin to rack.

5. In a small food processor, pulse 4 teaspoons black pepper and remaining ingredients until well blended. Using your hands, pack Parmesan mixture around tenderloin.

6. Roast until crust is golden brown, about 30–40 minutes for medium-rare. An instant-read thermometer inserted into the thickest part of the tenderloin should register 120°F–125°F.

7. Transfer to a carving board; cover loosely with foil and let rest 10 minutes. Cut into ½"-thick slices, being careful to keep the delicate crust in place.

Per Serving   Calories: 401 | Fat: 24g | Protein: 37g | Sodium: 497mg | Fiber: 1g | Carbohydrates: 6g | Sugar: 1g

Citrus Flank Steak

Enjoy this dish on a warm day and pair with a light pasta salad or hearty green salad.

INGREDIENTS | SERVES 3

¼ cup toasted sesame oil

1 tablespoon fresh lime juice

1 tablespoon pineapple juice

1 tablespoon maple syrup

⅛ teaspoon wheat-free asafetida powder

1 (5") piece gingerroot, peeled and thinly sliced

¼ teaspoon kosher salt

¼ teaspoon freshly ground black pepper

1 (1½-pound) flank steak

2 teaspoons olive oil

1. In a food processor, mix oil, lime juice, pineapple juice, maple syrup, asafetida, ginger, salt, and pepper until smooth; pour into a large bowl.

2. Add steak to bowl and cover. Place in refrigerator and marinate 2–4 hours.

3. Heat olive oil in a large cast-iron skillet over medium-high heat or heat grill on medium-high.

4. Grill steak 6–8 minutes on each side for medium-rare. Transfer to a cutting board; cover loosely with foil and let rest about 10 minutes.

5. Slice steak against the grain and serve.

Per Serving Calories: 388 | Fat: 26g | Protein: 34g | Sodium: 283mg | Fiber: 1g | Carbohydrates: 6g | Sugar: 5g

Prosciutto-Stuffed Chicken

Have an Italian-inspired night and serve this dish with some gluten-free pasta.

INGREDIENTS | SERVES 4

4 boneless, skinless chicken breasts (2 pounds total)

$\frac{1}{16}$ teaspoon salt

$\frac{1}{4}$ teaspoon freshly ground black pepper

8 thin slices prosciutto

8 thin slices mozzarella cheese

20 fresh basil leaves

2 tablespoons unsalted butter, divided

1 tablespoon safflower oil

$\frac{1}{2}$ cup chicken broth

2 tablespoons Maple Mustard Dressing (see recipe in Chapter 13)

$\frac{1}{8}$ teaspoon wheat-free asafetida powder

$\frac{1}{4}$ cup thinly sliced basil leaves

1. Butterfly chicken breasts by carefully slicing them in half horizontally from the thick end to the thin end, keeping the edge intact; open the breasts like a book. Use a meat tenderizer to pound breasts to a $\frac{1}{4}$" thickness. Season with salt and pepper.

2. On a clean work surface, place a chicken breast cut side up. Leaving a $\frac{1}{2}$" border, place 2 slices prosciutto on top of chicken, then 2 slices mozzarella, and 5 basil leaves. Roll up chicken lengthwise and tie with kitchen twine. Repeat with remaining chicken breasts.

3. Preheat oven to 450°F.

4. Heat 1 tablespoon butter and oil in a 12" ovenproof skillet. Add chicken and cook until browned on all sides, about 8–10 minutes.

5. Transfer skillet to oven and bake 7–8 minutes. An instant-read thermometer inserted into center of chicken should register 165°F. Transfer chicken to plates.

6. Carefully wipe the skillet clean. Heat 1 tablespoon butter, broth, mustard dressing, and asafetida and bring to a boil over high heat; cook until slightly thickened, about 5 minutes. Stir in sliced basil.

7. Cut off and discard twine from chicken. Cut chicken into $\frac{1}{2}$" slices. Drizzle sauce over chicken.

Per Serving Calories: 593 | Fat: 32g | Protein: 68g | Sodium: 1,197mg | Fiber: 0g | Carbohydrates: 4g | Sugar: 2g

Stuffed Peppers with Ground Turkey

Enjoy these stuffed peppers as a side dish or main dish.
Alternatively, try ground chicken or different low-FODMAP cheeses.

INGREDIENTS | SERVES 3

1 tablespoon olive oil
1 pound ground turkey
1 tablespoon garlic-infused oil, divided
1 cup roasted corn kernels
2 Roma tomatoes, chopped
2 tablespoons pine nuts
1 cup cooked brown rice
½ tablespoon chili powder
½ teaspoon ground cumin
1 teaspoon smoked paprika
3 tablespoons chopped fresh cilantro
3 large bell peppers: orange, yellow, and green; halved and seeded
2 tablespoons coconut oil
6 slices goat cheese
3 tablespoons Fiesta Salsa (see recipe in Chapter 13)

How to Roast Corn in the Oven

To roast corn in your oven, first preheat oven to 450°F. Remove husks and silk threads from two ears of corn. Rub 1 tablespoon of butter on corn cobs and wrap cobs in foil. Place on cookie sheet and roast for 20–25 minutes.

1. Preheat oven to 375°F.

2. Heat 1 tablespoon olive oil in a large skillet over medium-high heat and cook ground turkey until browned.

3. Add ½ tablespoon garlic-infused oil to skillet along with corn, tomatoes, and pine nuts; stir and heat through.

4. Add brown rice and stir to combine. Stir in remaining ½ tablespoon oil, chili powder, cumin, paprika, and cilantro. Remove from heat.

5. Stuff halved peppers with brown rice mixture and brush outside of peppers with coconut oil. Place peppers in an 8" × 8" shallow baking dish.

6. Top each pepper with a slice of goat cheese. Loosely cover dish with foil.

7. Bake 30–40 minutes until peppers are tender. Garnish with salsa.

Per Serving Calories: 700 | Fat: 43g | Protein: 41g | Sodium: 364mg | Fiber: 8g | Carbohydrates: 41g | Sugar: 6g

Orange Chicken and Broccoli Stir-Fry

Create your own flavorful Asian dish without ordering take-out. Serve this dish over brown rice.

INGREDIENTS | SERVES 4

2 tablespoons fresh orange juice

2 tablespoons fresh lemon juice

2 tablespoons gluten-free soy sauce (tamari)

2 tablespoons orange marmalade (without high-fructose corn syrup)

2 teaspoons cornstarch

2 tablespoons safflower oil

2 pounds chicken tenders, cut into 1" pieces

1½ pounds broccoli, cut into florets

1 medium red bell pepper, seeded and chopped

1 green onion, chopped, green part only

2 teaspoons chopped fresh gingerroot

1 teaspoon chili powder

1. In a small bowl, combine orange juice, lemon juice, soy sauce, marmalade, and cornstarch. Set aside.

2. Heat oil over medium-high heat in a wok or 9" non-stick skillet. Add chicken and stir until cooked through, 2–3 minutes. Transfer chicken to a plate.

3. Add broccoli to wok and cook 3 minutes. Increase heat to high, add bell pepper and cook 2 minutes, stirring frequently. Transfer vegetables to plate with chicken.

4. Reduce heat to medium-high and add onion, ginger, and chili powder. Cook until fragrant, about 30 seconds.

5. Add orange sauce to pan and cook until slightly thickened, about 30 seconds. Add chicken and vegetables to wok and toss to coat.

Per Serving   Calories: 424 | Fat: 13g | Protein: 53g | Sodium: 780mg | Fiber: 5g | Carbohydrates: 23g | Sugar: 11g

Beef with Spinach and Sweet Potatoes

This dish does not need to be paired with anything else. It's filling and delicious as is.

INGREDIENTS | SERVES 4

1 pound organic or grass-fed beef tenderloin, cut into 4 medallions

¼ teaspoon salt

¼ teaspoon freshly ground black pepper

3 teaspoons olive oil, divided

½ pound sweet potatoes, peeled and cut into ½" cubes

½ teaspoon ground turmeric

¼ teaspoon chili powder

2 tablespoons rice wine vinegar

3 tablespoons maple syrup

10 ounces baby spinach

⅓ cup toasted pumpkin seeds

1. Season beef with salt and black pepper. Heat 2 teaspoons oil in a 9" cast-iron skillet over medium-high heat. Add beef to skillet and cook about 3 minutes for medium-rare, browning all sides. Transfer to plate and cover with foil.

2. Add remaining oil to skillet along with sweet potatoes. Cook until browned, about 10–15 minutes. Stir in turmeric and chili powder and cook 1 minute.

3. Add vinegar and maple syrup. If potatoes start to stick, add more vinegar. Add a few ounces spinach at a time and cook 2 minutes, stirring.

4. Slice beef into four medallions. Transfer spinach and sweet potatoes to plates and top with beef, then pumpkin seeds.

Per Serving   Calories: 373 | Fat: 17g | Protein: 30g | Sodium: 298mg | Fiber: 4g | Carbohydrates: 26g | Sugar: 12g

Pork Chops with Carrots and Toasted Buckwheat

The sweetness of the carrots and salt from the pork along with the earthy buckwheat makes this an all-around beautiful and pleasing dish.

INGREDIENTS | SERVES 4

1½ pound carrots, peeled, halved lengthwise and cut into 2" pieces

⅛ teaspoon wheat-free asafetida powder

4 teaspoons fresh lemon juice

¼ cup dill sprigs

2 tablespoons olive oil, divided

½ teaspoon kosher salt, divided

1 medium orange, cut in half

¾ cup buckwheat groats

1 tablespoon safflower oil

2 (1"-thick) bone-in pork shoulder chops (about 8–10 ounces each)

2 tablespoons unsalted butter, divided

1. Preheat oven to 450°F.

2. Place carrots, asafetida, lemon juice, dill, and 2 table-spoons olive oil in a medium bowl. Toss well to coat. Place on a rimmed baking sheet and season with ¼ teaspoon salt. Roast carrots until tender and browned, tossing once, about 20 minutes.

3. Remove carrots from oven. Squeeze juice from ½ orange over carrots. Set aside.

4. Meanwhile, in a large saucepan of boiling salted water, cook buckwheat until tender, 10–15 minutes. Drain and rinse well under cold water, rinsing away any pinkish-red film (or mucilage). Spread out on a baking sheet and allow to dry.

5. Heat safflower oil on high in a 10" heavy or cast-iron skillet. Season pork with ¼ teaspoon salt and cook until browned and slightly pink in the center, about 5–6 minutes per side. Transfer to a cutting board.

6. Add buckwheat and 1 tablespoon butter to the same skillet. Cook 5 minutes, stirring frequently. Remove from heat. Divide buckwheat onto 4 plates.

7. Add 1 tablespoon butter and squeeze in juice from remaining orange half into skillet; heat until butter has melted.

8. Slice pork into thin slices. Top buckwheat with pork slices and carrots. Drizzle with orange-butter mixture.

Per Serving   Calories: 471 | Fat: 27g | Protein: 17g | Sodium: 460mg | Fiber: 9g | Carbohydrates: 44g | Sugar: 11g

Lemon Thyme Chicken

Thyme is one of many beautiful herbs that you can use on the low-FODMAP diet and it dresses chicken perfectly. Serve this dish with Lemon Kale Salad (see recipe in Chapter 4).

INGREDIENTS | SERVES 3

4 chicken thighs and 4 drumsticks (about 2½ pounds)
3 medium lemons
Zest of 1 medium lemon
1 tablespoon butter
¼ teaspoon sea salt
½ teaspoon freshly ground black pepper
2 tablespoons fresh thyme leaves
6 basil leaves, torn

1. Preheat oven to 375°F.

2. Add chicken to a large bowl. Slice lemons in half and juice into bowl.

3. Add lemon zest, butter, salt, pepper, and thyme; toss well with your hands. Place chicken in a 9" × 13" baking dish.

4. Bake 35–40 minutes, basting every 10 minutes. Skin should get crispy and meat should be cooked through.

5. Garnish with basil leaves.

Per Serving   Calories: 90 | Fat: 5g | Protein: 6g | Sodium: 219mg | Fiber: 3g | Carbohydrates: 9g | Sugar: 2g

Spinach and Feta-Stuffed Chicken Breast

This recipe is relatively easy to make and only needs a few ingredients, including low-FODMAP ingredients that you may already have.

INGREDIENTS | SERVES 2

1 tablespoon garlic-infused oil
8 ounces spinach
½ cup crumbled feta cheese
2 boneless, skinless chicken breasts, pounded to a ¼" thickness
1 large egg, lightly beaten
1 cup gluten-free bread crumbs

1. Preheat oven to 350°F.

2. Heat oil in a medium skillet over low heat; cook spinach until soft, about 2–3 minutes. Add feta, stir a few times, and remove from heat.

3. Lay spinach mixture onto each chicken breast. Wrap chicken around mixture and secure with toothpicks.

4. Place egg in a shallow bowl. Place bread crumbs in a separate shallow bowl. Roll each breast in egg, tap off any excess, then roll in bread crumbs until well coated.

5. Place in an 8" × 8" casserole dish. Bake 30 minutes and serve.

Per Serving   Calories: 468 | Fat: 17g | Protein: 46g | Sodium: 807mg | Fiber: 3g | Carbohydrates: 30g | Sugar: 4g

Cumin Turkey with Fennel

A nice one-pot appetizing meal that's quick to prepare and clean up.

INGREDIENTS | SERVES 4

1 tablespoon brown sugar

¼ teaspoon ground cinnamon

½ tablespoon ground cumin

¼ teaspoon kosher salt

½ teaspoon freshly ground black pepper

¼ teaspoon cayenne pepper

1 cup cubed celeriac

1 cup halved seedless red grapes

1 fennel bulb (about ½ pound), cut into 1" chunks

1 tablespoon olive oil

2 pounds lean turkey fillets

1. Preheat oven to 425°F. Position rack in upper third of oven.

2. Mix brown sugar, cinnamon, cumin, salt, pepper, and cayenne in a small bowl.

3. In a medium bowl, combine celeriac, grapes, and fennel with oil and half of spice mixture. Spread out evenly in a single layer in an 18" × 13" rimmed baking sheet.

4. Rub remaining spice mixture on both sides of turkey fillets and place on top of grapes and vegetables.

5. Bake 40 minutes; check at 30 minutes to be sure food is not burning—if so, move pan to a lower rack.

Per Serving Calories: 354 | Fat: 7g | Protein: 52g | Sodium: 357mg | Fiber: 3g | Carbohydrates: 19g | Sugar: 10g

Victor's Chicken Parmesan

A healthier spin on a classic, inspired by the author's brother. This dish will always be a crowd pleaser!

INGREDIENTS | SERVES 4

3 large eggs

3 cups gluten-free panko bread crumbs

1/16 teaspoon salt

1/2 teaspoon freshly ground black pepper

1 teaspoon dried oregano

4 (6-ounce) boneless, skinless chicken breasts, pounded to a 1/2" thickness

1 tablespoon safflower oil

2 cups Basic Marinara Sauce (see recipe in Chapter 13)

2 cups baby spinach

2 cups shredded mozzarella cheese

1/4 cup grated Parmesan cheese

6 whole basil leaves

1. Preheat oven to 400°F. Grease a 9" × 13" casserole dish.

2. Whisk eggs in shallow bowl and set aside. Place bread crumbs, salt, pepper, and oregano on a plate. Stir to combine. Dredge chicken in egg, tapping off any excess; dredge in bread crumb mixture and place on a clean plate.

3. Heat oil in a medium skillet over medium-high heat. Add chicken and cook 2–3 minutes per side, or until golden brown.

4. Spoon a thin layer of marinara sauce in casserole dish. Lay down each piece of chicken. Then layer more marinara and half of the spinach, mozzarella, and 2 tablespoons Parmesan cheese. Repeat again with another layer of the same ingredients.

5. Bake until chicken is cooked through and cheese is melted, about 5–7 minutes. Remove from oven. Garnish with basil.

Per Serving Calories: 777 | Fat: 28g | Protein: 65g | Sodium: 1,633mg | Fiber: 6g | Carbohydrates: 63g | Sugar: 14g

Chicken Piccata

This is a delicious, quick, and flourless chicken piccata recipe. It's also wheat-free, soy-free, and nut-free. If your capers are salt-packed, rinse them before using, and if they're brine-packed, drain them.

INGREDIENTS | SERVES 4

4 (6–8 ounce, ½–¾"-thick) chicken breasts

2 teaspoons sea salt

4 tablespoons unsalted butter, divided

⅛ cup dry white wine

¼ cup capers

½ cup halved cherry tomatoes

2 teaspoons finely chopped fresh flat-leaf parsley

2 large lemons, pitted

Make a Seafood Piccata

Fish is another nice option for this recipe instead of chicken. Choose a light fish such as flounder, red snapper, tilapia, or rainbow trout. Cook the fish until it easily flakes apart with a fork.

1. Sprinkle all sides of chicken breasts with salt.

2. Melt 2 tablespoons butter in a 10" skillet over medium-high heat.

3. Add chicken and cook until opaque halfway through, 4–5 minutes.

4. Add wine and 1 tablespoon butter to skillet; as soon as butter is melted, flip chicken and finish cooking through, 3–4 minutes.

5. Transfer chicken to plates.

6. Add capers to hot skillet and let sizzle 30 seconds. Add tomatoes and parsley and 1 tablespoon butter. Squeeze juice from lemons over capers and stir everything to combine.

7. Cook another 30 seconds, then drizzle mixture over chicken. Serve immediately.

Per Serving Calories: 202 | Fat: 14g | Protein: 16g | Sodium: 1,519mg | Fiber: 2g | Carbohydrates: 4g | Sugar: 1g

Easy Pan Chicken

This makes for a comforting home-cooked meal that's easy to assemble and ready in less than 45 minutes.

INGREDIENTS | SERVES 4

3 tablespoons whole-grain mustard

2 teaspoons dried oregano

1 teaspoon dried thyme

1 tablespoon unsalted butter, softened

2 teaspoons Dijon mustard

3 pounds bone-in chicken thighs and drumsticks, patted dry

½ teaspoon salt

1 teaspoon freshly ground black pepper

⅔ cup plain gluten-free bread crumbs

4 medium carrots, peeled and halved lengthwise

1 tablespoon garlic-infused olive oil

1. Heat oven to 425°F.

2. In a small bowl, combine whole-grain mustard, oregano, thyme, butter, and Dijon mustard.

3. Season chicken with salt and pepper. Rub mustard-butter mixture all over chicken.

4. Place bread crumbs in a wide bowl and coat chicken evenly with bread crumbs.

5. Place carrots (cut side down) with chicken on a baking sheet and drizzle with olive oil.

6. Bake until chicken is golden and no longer pink, 35–40 minutes.

Per Serving   Calories: 564 | Fat: 21g | Protein: 70g | Sodium: 733mg | Fiber: 3g | Carbohydrates: 20g | Sugar: 4g

Turkey Bolognese with Pasta

*Bolognese sauce is a favorite for many and this low-FODMAP version
will soothe the soul just as well as the traditional version.*

INGREDIENTS | SERVES 4

1 tablespoon olive oil

1 large carrot, peeled and diced small

⅛ teaspoon wheat-free asafetida powder

1 teaspoon salt, divided

½ teaspoon dried oregano

4 ounces pancetta, visible fat discarded and pancetta minced

1 pound ground turkey

2 tablespoons Tomato Paste (see recipe in Chapter 13)

½ cup Lambrusco wine

1 (14-ounce) can San Marzano tomatoes

1 tablespoon balsamic vinegar

1 pound gluten-free angel hair pasta

¼ cup shaved Parmesan cheese

Choosing the Perfect Wine for Bolognese Sauce

The wine that hails from Bologna, Italy, is Lambrusco. It's a sparkling wine that ranges from light pink to dark and tannic. Choose a Lambrusco somewhere in the middle, with bright red fruit.

1. Heat oil in a wide, deep skillet or saucepan over medium heat. Add carrots, asafetida, ½ teaspoon salt, and oregano and cook for 6 minutes. Add pancetta and continue cooking everything until carrots are softened, 8–10 minutes.

2. Add ground turkey and remaining ½ teaspoon salt. Cook until meat is lightly browned. Add tomato paste and cook 2–3 minutes.

3. Add wine. Cook until wine has reduced by half, 4–5 minutes.

4. Add tomatoes and stir. Cook 5 minutes. Stir balsamic vinegar into sauce. Set heat to low and simmer.

5. Meanwhile, cook pasta according to package directions. Drain. Stir Parmesan into pasta and top with Bolognese sauce.

Per Serving Calories: 528 | Fat: 18g | Protein: 40g | Sodium: 1,010mg | Fiber: 6g | Carbohydrates: 93g | Sugar: 8g

Coq au Vin

Coq au vin is said to date back to King Henry IV of France but it's Julia Child who really made it famous. While several versions exist for this recipe, most include high FODMAPs such as onions, mushroom, and brandy. This recipe is free of high FODMAPs and will still win over foodies!

INGREDIENTS | SERVES 4

1 (2-pound) whole free-range chicken, cut into 8 serving pieces

¼ teaspoon salt

½ teaspoon freshly ground black pepper

2 tablespoons gluten-free all-purpose flour

1 tablespoon garlic-infused olive oil

¼ cup butter

¼ pound bacon (preferably smoked), cut into short strips

1 large carrot, peeled and diced

1 medium stalk celery, diced

3 cups Beaujolais wine

1¾ cups Easy Onion- and Garlic-Free Chicken Stock (see recipe in Chapter 4)

2 bay leaves

1 cup finely chopped fresh flat-leaf parsley

1. Place chicken pieces in a large bowl and toss with salt, pepper, and flour until well coated.

2. Heat oil and butter in a large, wide ovenproof pan over medium heat and brown chicken on all sides; work in batches if necessary to avoid overcrowding the pan. Remove and set aside.

3. Add bacon to pan and cook until lightly browned, 3–4 minutes. Remove with a slotted spoon and set aside with chicken. Add carrot and celery and cook 5 minutes or until softened and lightly browned. Set aside.

4. Add wine to pan and stir well; add stock and bay leaves, and return vegetables, chicken, and bacon to pan. Heat until just about boiling, reduce heat to low, and simmer uncovered for 30 minutes or until chicken is cooked through.

5. Remove chicken pieces, increase heat, and simmer sauce until reduced, thickened, and glossy, about 25 minutes.

6. Return chicken to pan and serve immediately. Garnish with parsley.

Per Serving   Calories: 592 | Fat: 29g | Protein: 44g | Sodium: 594mg | Fiber: 1g | Carbohydrates: 12g | Sugar: 3g

Blueberry-Glazed Chicken

Enjoy this savory sauce and delectable chicken with mashed potatoes or jasmine rice. A great wine to pair with this dish is a Pinot Noir, especially from New Zealand!

INGREDIENTS | SERVES 4

2 tablespoons balsamic vinegar

2 tablespoons olive oil

2 tablespoons lemon juice

2 teaspoons Dijon mustard

⅓ cup Blueberry Chia Seed Jam (see recipe in Chapter 13)

1 tablespoon pure maple syrup

½ teaspoon salt

2 tablespoons coconut oil

4 (4-ounce) boneless, skinless chicken breasts

1. In a medium bowl, combine vinegar, olive oil, lemon juice, mustard, blueberry jam, maple syrup, and salt.

2. Heat coconut oil in a large skillet over medium heat. Add chicken breasts and brown on both sides.

3. Turn heat to low and add blueberry sauce.

4. Cover and simmer until cooked through, about 20 minutes.

5. Spoon extra sauce over chicken to serve.

Per Serving   Calories: 486 | Fat: 20g | Protein: 50g | Sodium: 611mg | Fiber: 0g | Carbohydrates: 24g | Sugar: 17g

Parmesan-Crusted Chicken

This tasty chicken is ready in less than 30 minutes and pairs well with gluten-free pasta or green beans.

INGREDIENTS | SERVES 2

2 boneless, skinless chicken breast halves (about 1 pound)

¼ cup Basic Mayonnaise (see recipe in Chapter 13)

2 tablespoons grated Parmesan cheese

1 tablespoon gluten-free bread crumbs

1 teaspoon dried oregano

1 teaspoon dried parsley

1. Preheat oven to 425°F. Arrange chicken on a baking sheet.

2. Combine mayonnaise with cheese in a medium bowl.

3. In a small bowl, mix bread crumbs with oregano and parsley.

4. Evenly top chicken with mayonnaise mixture, then sprinkle with bread crumbs.

5. Bake until chicken is thoroughly cooked, about 20 minutes.

Per Serving   Calories: 508 | Fat: 30g | Protein: 53g | Sodium: 551mg | Fiber: 0g | Carbohydrates: 4g | Sugar: 0g

Sweet and Savory Brazilian Meat and Cheese Tart

Try this savory comfort food—an ode to traditional Brazilian tarts.

INGREDIENTS | SERVES 6

2½ cups gluten-free all-purpose flour

½ cup butter

½ cup vegetable shortening

1 teaspoon salt, divided

1 teaspoon turbinado sugar

4–6 tablespoons ice water, for blending

1 tablespoon coconut oil, divided

2 pounds ground beef

⅛ teaspoon wheat-free asafetida powder

2 bunches spinach, finely chopped (stems removed)

½ teaspoon freshly ground black pepper

¼ teaspoon cayenne pepper

½ cup grated Parmesan cheese

6 large eggs

1 egg beaten with 1 tablespoon water (egg wash)

4 medium limes, cut in quarters

1. For the pie crust: In a bowl of a stand mixer fitted with a paddle attachment (or using a pastry cutter or two knives), combine flour, butter, vegetable shortening, ½ teaspoon salt, and sugar; work dough until mixture resembles oatmeal. Slowly add ice water and mix until pliable but not very wet. Wrap in plastic wrap and refrigerate 30 minutes. Dough can be kept in refrigerator up to 3 days or frozen up to 3 months.

2. Preheat oven to 375°F.

3. For the filling: In a medium saucepan on medium-high heat, warm half of coconut oil and add ground beef, breaking up into pieces and cooking until browned. Add remaining oil, asafetida, spinach, remaining salt, pepper, and cayenne pepper. Cook 2–3 minutes or until spinach is wilted. Remove from heat and mix in Parmesan. If there is any extra juice, drain first before putting filling into pie.

4. Take half of dough out of refrigerator. Cover your work surface with flour and sprinkle more flour onto rolling pin and dough.

Working quickly, roll dough until it's about 18", a little larger than size of 9" pie dish. Dust dough with flour occasionally to ensure it does not stick to surface or rolling pin. Transfer dough to pie dish. Gently tuck dough inside dish and allow remaining dough to drape over sides of dish. Prick pie crust all over with a fork.

5. Pour filling into 9" pie dish and spread out evenly. Make 6 small holes in filling, evenly around dish, and slowly drop 1 egg into each hole. Roll out remaining dough with flour and drape it on top of filling and eggs. Using your fingers, seal crust around edges. Cut 2–3 slits on top to vent during baking.

6. Brush egg wash all over top and place into middle rack of oven. Bake 50–55 minutes or until crust is golden brown. Let cool 15 minutes before slicing and serving with lime wedges.

Per Serving Calories: 927 | Fat: 59g | Protein: 50g | Sodium: 795mg | Fiber: 5g | Carbohydrates: 51g | Sugar: 3g

Zucchini Lasagna with Meat Sauce

Get your fill of Italian food and more green vegetables at the same time with this super-easy and healthy recipe!

INGREDIENTS | SERVES 5

2 cups Roasted Tomato Sauce (see recipe in Chapter 13)

1½ large zucchini, cut lengthwise into thin slices

1 tablespoon olive oil

10 ounces ground beef

1 small green bell pepper, seeded and diced

1 tablespoon dried oregano

½ cup plus 2 tablespoons tomato paste

2 tablespoons chopped fresh basil

¼ cup red wine (like Cabernet Sauvignon)

4 cups baby spinach

2 cups grated mozzarella cheese

½ cup grated Parmesan cheese

A Very Resourceful Tool for Healthy Eating

Investing in a mandoline can be rather helpful to get the perfect slice of zucchini. A mandoline offers several creative options for the kitchen and it might encourage you to eat more vegetables!

1. Preheat oven to 325°F.

2. Grease a 9" × 13" casserole dish. Pour in enough tomato sauce to lightly coat bottom of dish, a little less than ½ cup. Layer a few zucchini slices side by side in bottom of dish.

3. Heat oil in a large skillet over medium-high heat. Add beef, stir, and cook 5 minutes. Add green pepper and oregano. Once meat is no longer pink, stir in tomato paste, remaining tomato sauce, basil, and wine. Bring to a boil; reduce heat and simmer sauce 20 minutes, stirring frequently.

4. Spoon a layer of meat sauce over the zucchini in casserole dish. Add a layer of spinach and then mozzarella. Repeat same process one more time—layer zucchini, meat sauce, spinach, and mozzarella. Finish by topping with Parmesan cheese.

5. Cover dish with foil and bake 45 minutes. Remove foil; increase temperature to 350°F and bake an additional 12–15 minutes. Lasagna will be very hot; let stand 5 minutes before serving.

Per Serving   Calories: 387 | Fat: 22g | Protein: 30g | Sodium: 1,270mg | Fiber: 5g | Carbohydrates: 18g | Sugar: 12g

Pumpkin Maple Roast Chicken

Once in the oven, this simple roast chicken with pumpkin, maple syrup, cinnamon, and thyme will cast a fragrant spell over your kitchen. After carving, be sure to drizzle each serving with Pumpkin Maple Glaze (see recipe in Chapter 13).

INGREDIENTS | SERVES 4

1½ tablespoons butter
1 tablespoon canned pumpkin
1 tablespoon pure maple syrup
1 teaspoon ground cinnamon
1 teaspoon dried thyme
½ teaspoon sea salt
¼ teaspoon freshly ground black pepper
1 (4-pound) whole chicken

Canned Pumpkin

You need to be cautious when purchasing canned pumpkin, because there is a very similar-looking canned product known as pumpkin pie filling. Pumpkin pie filling contains ingredients that may not be appropriate for a low-FODMAP diet. Pure canned pumpkin should be nothing but pumpkin and so can be enjoyed for its nutrition without worry.

1. Preheat oven to 375°F.

2. Melt butter in a small saucepan. Stir in pumpkin, maple syrup, cinnamon, thyme, salt, and pepper. Refrigerate 10 minutes.

3. Cut small slit under skin on both sides of chicken breast and under legs. Once the pumpkin mixture is cool, generously rub it under skin and all over the top of skin. Place chicken, breast side up, on the rack of a roasting pan. Roast 50–60 minutes or until a meat thermometer registers 165°F at thickest part of thigh.

4. Tent with foil and let rest 5 minutes before carving.

Per Serving   Calories: 588 | Fat: 18g | Protein: 96g | Sodium: 641mg | Fiber: 1g | Carbohydrates: 4g | Sugar: 3g

Barbecue Pork Macaroni and Cheese

This sweet and savory blend of flavors is a real crowd pleaser. Remove the meats and substitute low-FODMAP vegetable stock for the chicken stock and this recipe makes a wonderful vegetarian main dish.

INGREDIENTS | SERVES 8

1 pound gluten-free macaroni

1½ cups peeled and cubed butternut squash

1 teaspoon extra-virgin olive oil

1 teaspoon sea salt, divided

½ teaspoon freshly ground black pepper, divided

¼ teaspoon ground nutmeg

¼ teaspoon ground ginger

½ pound boneless pork loin, cut into ½" cubes

¼ cup Sweet Barbecue Sauce (see recipe in Chapter 13)

¾ cup chicken stock

¾ cup canned coconut milk

1½ cups shredded Cheddar cheese, divided

1 loosely packed cup thinly sliced kale leaves

2 slices bacon, cooked, cooled, and crumbled

½ cup freshly grated Parmesan cheese

1. Cook macaroni al dente according to package directions. Drain and pour macaroni into a 9" × 13" baking dish. Set aside.

2. Heat oven to 375°F. On a parchment-lined baking sheet, toss squash with olive oil. Sprinkle with ½ teaspoon salt, ¼ teaspoon pepper, nutmeg, and ginger. Bake 25 minutes. Remove from oven and set aside to cool.

3. In a medium skillet over medium heat, brown all sides of pork. Add barbecue sauce; toss to coat. Simmer uncovered 1–2 minutes, remove from heat, and set aside to cool.

4. Transfer squash to the bowl of a food processor. Add stock, coconut milk, and remaining salt and pepper and process to combine. Add 1 cup Cheddar and pulse until combined.

5. Pour squash mixture over macaroni and stir to combine.

6. Tuck kale here and there between the noodles. Dot top of casserole evenly with the barbecue pork cubes and bacon.

7. Sprinkle top of casserole evenly with remaining ½ cup Cheddar and Parmesan. Bake 20 minutes or until cheese is melted and bubbling. Let sit 5 minutes, then serve.

Per Serving Calories: 487 | Fat: 20g | Protein: 26g | Sodium: 843mg | Fiber: 3g | Carbohydrates: 51g | Sugar: 5g

Sourdough Meatballs

You can still enjoy meatballs on the low-FODMAP diet if you don't use gluten-containing bread crumbs. The toasted sourdough bread crumbs add a zest to these classic savory meatballs.

INGREDIENTS | SERVES 4

1 slice gluten-free sourdough bread, toasted

1 large egg

¼ cup freshly grated Parmesan cheese

1 teaspoon sea salt

½ teaspoon freshly ground black pepper

½ pound ground meat (mix of beef, pork, and veal)

1. Pulse bread in a food processor to create coarse crumbs.

2. In a large bowl, whisk egg, cheese, salt, and pepper. Add bread crumbs and meat. Hand mix just until combined.

3. Preheat broiler. Form mixture into 16 equally sized balls and place on a foil-lined baking sheet. Broil 8–10 minutes, or until tops are evenly browned. Remove sheet, carefully turn meatballs over, and broil 8–10 minutes more or until fully cooked. Serve.

Per Serving Calories: 212 | Fat: 14g | Protein: 19g | Sodium: 913mg | Fiber: 0g | Carbohydrates: 5g | Sugar: 0g

Polenta-Crusted Chicken

Polenta crust makes for a deliciously crunchy and very fulfilling chicken dinner night. Serve with spinach, green beans, or a generous salad.

INGREDIENTS | SERVES 2

1 large egg

½ teaspoon salt, divided

½ teaspoon freshly ground black pepper, divided

¼ cup gluten-free all-purpose flour

¼ cup quick-cooking polenta

1 teaspoon dried oregano

1 teaspoon dried thyme

¾ pound boneless, skinless chicken breasts

¼ cup safflower oil

¼ cup olive oil

1. In a shallow bowl, beat egg with ¼ teaspoon each of salt and pepper. In another shallow bowl, whisk together flour, polenta, oregano, thyme, and ¼ teaspoon each of salt and pepper.

2. Dip chicken in egg, tapping off any excess, then dredge in polenta mixture.

3. Heat safflower oil and olive oil in a 6" nonstick skillet over medium heat.

4. Cook chicken in batches until golden brown, 4–6 minutes on one side and 2 minutes on other side.

Per Serving Calories: 383 | Fat: 31g | Protein: 20g | Sodium: 410mg | Fiber: 0g | Carbohydrates: 7g | Sugar: 0g

Aunt Bete's Chicken Tart

This recipe was inspired by one very similar, made by a loving, happy, and upbeat Aunt Bete living in southern Brazil.

INGREDIENTS | SERVES 6

2 (4-ounce) boneless, skinless chicken breasts
1 (.25-ounce) packet instant yeast
1 cup lactose-free milk, warmed
½ cup butter, room temperature
3 cups gluten-free all-purpose flour
½ teaspoon salt, divided
1 tablespoon coconut oil
⅛ teaspoon wheat-free asafetida powder
½ cup corn kernels
1 cup peeled and grated carrots
1½ cups broccoli florets
1 teaspoon dried tarragon
1 teaspoon dried thyme
1 teaspoon lemon juice
½ teaspoon freshly ground black pepper, divided
1 tablespoon cornstarch
½ cup Parmesan cheese
1 large egg, beaten

1. Place chicken breasts in a medium saucepan and cover with water. Place saucepan over medium heat, bring to a boil covered, and then simmer uncovered 10–12 minutes or until chicken meat is cooked through. Reserve 1 cup cooking water. Allow chicken to cool on a plate and then shred with forks.

2. Dissolve yeast in warm milk within bowl of a stand mixer. Add in butter, flour and ¼ teaspoon salt. Use a paddle attachment and mix just until a ball forms. Transfer dough to a lightly floured surface, and knead a few times. Divide dough in half, pat each half into a disc, and wrap in plastic. Refrigerate for 1 hour.

3. Preheat oven to 350°F.

4. Heat oil in a medium saucepan over medium heat. Sauté shredded chicken with asafetida. Add corn, carrots, broccoli, tarragon, thyme, lemon juice, ¼ teaspoon salt, and ¼ teaspoon pepper.

5. Dissolve 1 tablespoon cornstarch in cup of reserved cooking water. Add to saucepan, stir and continue cooking for another 2–3 minutes. Remove pan from heat.

6. Remove dough from refrigerator and lightly flour surface again and top of dough. Cover dough with plastic wrap or wax paper and use rolling pin to start gently rolling out dough, turning 90° with each roll and removing plastic wrap or wax paper to flour dough if it begins to stick, also flouring surface below if dough sticks there as well. Gradually roll out dough to a 13" circle.

7. Transfer dough to a 9" glass pie plate, allowing excess dough to hang over edge of plate. Trim dough off edges. Add chicken mixture evenly into pie plate. Top with cheese and ¼ teaspoon pepper.

8. On a lightly floured surface, roll out second disc of dough to a 13" circle. Transfer to top of tart. Fold top crust over bottom, and crimp edges together with your fingers. Cut a few small vents around in a circle and in middle. Beat egg with a few drops of water, and brush over surface of dough. Bake 40 minutes.

Per Serving Calories: 484 | Fat: 21g | Protein: 18g | Sodium: 685mg | Fiber: 3g | Carbohydrates: 56g | Sugar: 4g

Chicken, Sweet Potato, and Spinach Curry

Try this comforting, earthy, and creamy curry dish! You can easily use other meats or fish instead of chicken and it's also perfectly satisfying without any meat at all.

INGREDIENTS | SERVES 3

2 medium sweet potatoes, peeled

½ teaspoon salt, divided

½ tablespoon safflower oil

6 chicken thighs with bone and skin, about 2¼ pounds

1 tablespoon freshly grated gingerroot

1 (13.5-ounce) can coconut milk, chilled overnight in refrigerator

½ teaspoon ground cinnamon

½ teaspoon ground cumin

½ teaspoon ground coriander

½ teaspoon ground turmeric

½ teaspoon chili powder

2 tablespoons butter or vegan substitute

1 cup canned chickpeas, drained and rinsed

1 (13.5-ounce) can crushed tomatoes

4 cups spinach

2 tablespoons chopped fresh cilantro

1. Place sweet potatoes in a pot. Fill pot with just enough water to cover sweet potatoes. Add ⅛ teaspoon salt. Bring to a boil. Cover and cook 8–10 minutes or until just tender on outside but not completely tender throughout whole potato. Remove from pot and let cool. When cool enough to handle, cut into chunks and set aside.

2. Heat oil in medium saucepan over medium-high heat. Add chicken thighs and sear on both sides. Insides should still be slightly pink. Remove chicken from pan and place on a plate. Wipe pan clean with a paper towel.

3. Return pan to stove and add ginger. Cook 2 minutes. Open coconut milk can and spoon out coconut cream from top (save coconut liquid for another use). Add coconut cream, cinnamon, cumin, coriander, turmeric, chili powder, butter, and remaining salt. Stir until well combined. Mixture should go from white to golden orange.

4. Add chickpeas, tomatoes, and chicken. Make sure chicken is sitting in middle of pan.

5. Reduce heat to simmer and occasionally scoop up sauce from sides and baste chicken. About 5 minutes in, add spinach and sweet potatoes to outer edges of pan and gently stir to combine.

6. Once chicken is cooked through, serve immediately with curry sauce and garnish with cilantro.

Per Serving   Calories: 520 | Fat: 38g | Protein: 11g | Sodium: 928mg | Fiber: 10g | Carbohydrates: 41g | Sugar: 8g

Mustard and Thyme Roasted Chicken

Delicate thyme and slightly spicy Dijon mustard blend with flour to make a delectable sauce.

INGREDIENTS | SERVES 2

1 tablespoon olive oil

¼ teaspoon salt, divided

½ teaspoon freshly ground black pepper, divided

4 bone-in skinless chicken thighs (about 1¼ pounds)

1 cup chicken stock

4 teaspoons gluten-free all-purpose flour

1 tablespoon butter

2 teaspoons chopped fresh thyme

1 teaspoon Dijon mustard

½ tablespoon chopped fresh flat-leaf parsley

1. Preheat oven to 425°.

2. Heat oil in a medium nonstick skillet over medium-high heat. Sprinkle ⅛ teaspoon salt and ¼ teaspoon pepper on both sides of chicken. Add chicken to skillet and cook 4–6 minutes on first side and 2 minutes on other or until both sides are golden browned.

3. Place chicken in a 11" × 7" glass baking dish and bake uncovered for 16 minutes or until an instant-read thermometer registers 165°F.

4. Meanwhile, combine ¼ cup stock and flour in a small bowl and whisk until smooth. Coat surface of skillet with butter.

5. Once chicken is done, transfer chicken to a plate and keep warm, covering with aluminum foil. Reserve drippings from chicken and add to skillet over medium-high heat. Add thyme and flour mixture and remaining stock. Bring to a boil and cook 2–4 minutes or until sauce is somewhat thickened.

6. Remove sauce from heat and whisk in mustard and remaining salt and pepper. Spoon sauce over chicken, garnish with parsley, and serve immediately.

Per Serving Calories: 341 | Fat: 20g | Protein: 31g | Sodium: 666mg | Fiber: 1g | Carbohydrates: 9g | Sugar: 2g

Crispy Baked Chicken with Gravy

When you're in the mood for a cozy dish, this chicken will hit the spot.

INGREDIENTS | SERVES 4

2 cups brown rice

4 cups water

2½ pounds boneless, skinless chicken breasts

1 cup gluten-free panko bread crumbs

4 tablespoons olive oil, divided

2 tablespoons minced fresh flat-leaf parsley

¼ cup Dijon mustard

2 tablespoons water

¼ teaspoon salt, divided

½ teaspoon freshly ground black pepper, divided

6 tablespoons butter

½ cup plus 6 tablespoons gluten-free all-purpose flour

1 cup lactose-free milk

1 cup chicken stock

¼ teaspoon dried thyme

1. Place rice in a medium saucepan with water. Bring to a boil, reduce heat to low, and cover; simmer 20 minutes. Rice should be tender. Remove from heat, stir, and keep covered. Set aside.

2. Preheat oven to 400°F. Line a baking sheet with aluminum foil. Place a rack over pan and spray rack with nonstick cooking spray.

3. Using a meat tenderizer, pound each chicken breast to a ¼" thickness. Set aside.

4. In a shallow dish, combine bread crumbs, 2 tablespoons olive oil, and parsley. In a separate shallow dish, combine mustard, water, ⅛ teaspoon salt, and ¼ teaspoon pepper, and remaining olive oil.

5. Coat each breast with mustard mixture; dredge each in bread crumb mixture. Place on prepared rack in pan.

6. Bake 25–30 minutes or until chicken is golden brown. About 15–20 minutes into baking chicken, prepare gravy.

7. For gravy: Over medium heat, melt butter in a medium saucepan and whisk in flour to make a roux (a mixture of fat and flour used in making sauces). Whisk constantly until bubbling and flour turns light brown in color. Gradually whisk in milk, stock, and thyme, and continue to stir. Add ⅛ teaspoon salt and ¼ teaspoon pepper. Mixture should thicken after about 5 minutes.

8. Divide rice onto 4 plates. Place chicken breasts on rice and spoon gravy on top. Serve immediately.

Per Serving   Calories: 765 | Fat: 30g | Protein: 51g | Sodium: 573mg | Fiber: 3g | Carbohydrates: 69g | Sugar: 3g

Turkey Pasta with Kale

This one-pot, one-pan meal is quick and easy to make and other low-FODMAP ingredients can be added effortlessly for other tasty variations.

INGREDIENTS | SERVES 2

½ pound gluten-free pasta

2 cups chopped kale (thick ribs and stems removed)

1 tablespoon extra-virgin olive oil

1/16 teaspoon salt

1 tablespoon olive oil

1 large carrot, peeled and thinly sliced

½ medium stalk celery, thinly sliced

1 tablespoon dried oregano

½ teaspoon freshly ground black pepper

1 pound ground lean turkey meat

½ cup chicken stock

1 (13.5-ounce) can diced tomatoes

3 tablespoons chopped fresh flat-leaf parsley

6 black olives

¾ cup grated mozzarella cheese

1. Cook pasta according to package directions.

2. Meanwhile, add kale to a small bowl with extra-virgin olive oil and salt. Massage until leaves are soft. Set aside.

3. Heat a large saucepan with olive oil over medium-high heat. Add carrot, celery, oregano, and pepper; sauté until carrots are tender, about 8–10 minutes.

4. Add turkey and break up into bite-sized pieces with spatula. Cook until browned. Add stock, tomatoes, and parsley and reduce heat to low; cook covered 5 minutes.

5. Once pasta is cooked and drained, add to saucepan. Stir in kale, olives, and mozzarella and toss to combine. Remove from heat and cover 2 minutes, then serve.

Per Serving Calories: 1,104 | Fat: 46g | Protein: 68g | Sodium: 867mg | Fiber: 8g | Carbohydrates: 103g | Sugar: 8g

CHAPTER 8

Fish and Shellfish

Seafood Risotto
156

Shrimp and Cheese Casserole
157

Grilled Swordfish with
Pineapple Salsa
157

Seared Sesame Tuna
158

Salmon with Herbs
158

Poached Salmon with
Tarragon Sauce
159

Light Tuna Casserole
160

Mediterranean Flaky Fish with
Vegetables
161

Coconut-Crusted Fish with
Pineapple Relish
162

Salmon Cakes with Fresh
Dill Sauce
162

Sole Meunière
163

Rita's Linguine with Clam Sauce
163

Basic Baked Scallops
164

Creamy Halibut
164

Cornmeal-Crusted Tilapia
165

Fish and Chips
166

Bacon-Wrapped Maple Scallops
167

Citrusy Swordfish Skewers
167

Atlantic Cod with Basil
Walnut Sauce
168

Shrimp Puttanesca with Linguine
168

Maple-Glazed Salmon
169

Baked Moroccan-Style Halibut
170

Seafood Risotto

Creamy risotto helps set the stage for plump clams, shrimp, and scallops.
This dish is best paired with something light such as a basic green salad.

INGREDIENTS | SERVES 6

2½ cups water

2 (8-ounce) bottles clam juice

6 tablespoons olive oil, divided

1½ cups arborio rice

½ cup dry white wine

¾ pound uncooked large shrimp, peeled, deveined, coarsely chopped

¾ pound bay scallops

⅛ teaspoon wheat-free asafetida powder

1 tablespoon butter

½ cup grated Parmesan cheese

2 tablespoons finely chopped fresh Italian parsley

1. Combine water and clam juice in a medium saucepan. Bring to simmer. Keep warm over low heat.

2. Heat 3 tablespoons oil in heavy, large saucepan over medium heat. Add rice; sauté 2 minutes.

3. Add wine; stir until liquid is absorbed, about 2 minutes. Add 1 cup clam juice mixture to rice. Simmer until liquid is absorbed, stirring often. Continue adding clam juice mixture ½ cup at a time, stirring often and simmering until liquid is absorbed before each addition. Simmer until rice is tender but still slightly firm in center and mixture is creamy, about 25 minutes.

4. Heat remaining 3 tablespoons oil in a separate heavy, large skillet over medium-high heat. Add shrimp, scallops, and asafetida. Sauté until shrimp and scallops are opaque in center, about 6 minutes.

5. Add seafood to rice. Stir and add butter; cook 4 minutes longer. Remove from heat and stir in Parmesan cheese. Transfer to serving bowl.

6. Garnish with chopped parsley and serve.

Per Serving   Calories: 514 | Fat: 22g | Protein: 30g | Sodium: 478mg | Fiber: 2g | Carbohydrates: 43g | Sugar: 0g

Shrimp and Cheese Casserole

This Greek-inspired dish is delicious paired with mashed potatoes and a green salad.

INGREDIENTS | SERVES 4

3 tablespoons butter

⅛ teaspoon salt

⅛ teaspoon freshly ground black pepper

⅛ teaspoon wheat-free asafetida powder

¼ cup dry white wine

10 ounces fresh spinach, chopped

1 (14.5-ounce) can diced tomatoes, drained

10 ounces medium shrimp, peeled and deveined

2 tablespoons olive oil

¼ pound crumbled feta cheese

¼ pound shredded mozzarella cheese

1. Preheat oven to 350°F. Grease a 9" × 13" casserole dish.

2. In a large skillet, melt butter over medium-high heat; add salt, pepper, and asafetida and stir.

3. Add wine and spinach and cook 2–3 minutes.

4. Put spinach mixture into prepared casserole dish and layer in diced tomatoes. Place shrimp on top, drizzle with olive oil. Sprinkle with feta and mozzarella.

5. Bake 25 minutes or until cheese is bubbly and slightly brown.

Per Serving Calories: 346 | Fat: 22g | Protein: 27g | Sodium: 790mg | Fiber: 2g | Carbohydrates: 8g | Sugar: 3g

Grilled Swordfish with Pineapple Salsa

Perfect for a summer day. Get your grill fired up and enjoy this recipe with a crisp green salad.

INGREDIENTS | SERVES 4

2 tablespoons finely chopped cilantro

2 medium limes, juiced and zested

1 medium orange, juiced and zested

½ whole pineapple, cut into small chunks

¼ teaspoon kosher salt

½ teaspoon freshly ground black pepper

4 (3.5-ounce) swordfish steaks, 1" thick

2 tablespoons olive oil

1. In a medium bowl, combine cilantro, lime and orange juice and zest, and pineapple; set aside.

2. Set a gas grill to medium-high or heat a cast-iron skillet over medium-high heat. Mix salt and pepper together in a small bowl.

3. Brush swordfish with oil and sprinkle with salt and pepper.

4. Cook fish 5 minutes on one side and 3 minutes on other side.

5. Transfer swordfish to plates; top with pineapple salsa.

Per Serving Calories: 267 | Fat: 11g | Protein: 20g | Sodium: 238mg | Fiber: 4g | Carbohydrates: 24g | Sugar: 16g

Seared Sesame Tuna

*Just 3 ingredients and ready in less than 15 minutes, this recipe is a
beautiful and delicious way to enjoy fish at home.*

INGREDIENTS | SERVES 2

¾ pound tuna steak

¼ cup sesame seeds

1 tablespoon garlic-infused olive oil

1. Prepare fish by discarding veiny stub from the tuna, then slice into 1" pieces.

2. Place sesame seeds on a plate and add tuna pieces, tossing to coat all sides with seeds.

3. Heat oil in a 10" nonstick frying pan over medium heat. Add tuna and sear on one side 15–20 seconds. Use tongs to turn tuna and continue searing all sides of fish. Transfer to a plate.

Per Serving   Calories: 269 | Fat: 16g | Protein: 28g | Sodium: 45mg | Fiber: 1g | Carbohydrates: 3g | Sugar: 1g

Salmon with Herbs

*The low-FODMAP diet includes many fresh herbs for you to enjoy, and this recipe utilizes a few of them.
This lovely fish is ready in less than 30 minutes. Serve with a green salad and rice or quinoa.*

INGREDIENTS | SERVES 2

1 pound salmon fillets

¼ teaspoon salt

½ teaspoon freshly ground black pepper

¼ cup plus 2 tablespoons olive oil

¼ cup chopped fresh dill

2 tablespoons roughly chopped fresh rosemary

¼ cup fresh flat-leaf parsley leaves

2 tablespoons fresh thyme leaves

2 tablespoons lemon juice

1. Preheat oven to 250°F.

2. Coat a 9" × 13" casserole dish with cooking spray. Lay salmon skin-side down and sprinkle with salt and pepper.

3. Blend ¼ cup plus 2 tablespoons olive oil with dill, rosemary, parsley, thyme, and lemon juice in a small food processor. Use a spatula or your hands to pat the herb paste over the salmon.

4. Bake 22–28 minutes depending on thickness of salmon. Insert tines of a fork into thickest part of fillet and gently pull. If fish flakes easily, it is done.

5. Slide a spatula under fish and set on a cutting board. Cut into equal pieces and serve.

Per Serving   Calories: 588 | Fat: 44g | Protein: 45g | Sodium: 403mg | Fiber: 1g | Carbohydrates: 3g | Sugar: 1g

Poached Salmon with Tarragon Sauce

This recipe makes for a delicate and flavorful fish, which pairs nicely with green beans or brown rice.

INGREDIENTS | SERVES 4

½ cup Basic Mayonnaise (see recipe in Chapter 13)

½ cup lactose-free sour cream

2 teaspoons chopped fresh tarragon

1 tablespoon chopped green onion, green part only

1 tablespoon lemon juice

⅛ teaspoon sea salt, divided

1 teaspoon freshly ground black pepper, divided

1¾ cups dry white wine

2 cups water

2-pound salmon fillet with skin

Tips for Poached Salmon

When poaching salmon, the key is to not overcook. Gently simmer and if you're not sure if the salmon is done, use a fork to check. If the fish flakes easily, it's done. The USDA recommends a minimum internal temperature of 145°F, which should be measured at the thickest part of the filet with an instant-read thermometer. Poached salmon may be cooked 1 day ahead and chilled, covered.

1. In a food processor combine mayonnaise, sour cream, tarragon, onion, lemon juice, ¹⁄₁₆ teaspoon salt, and ½ teaspoon pepper; purée until smooth. (Make 1 day ahead if desired; chill and cover.) If making sauce ahead of time, allow sauce to cool to room temperature before serving.

2. In a deep 12" skillet bring water and wine to a simmer, covered.

3. Cut salmon into 4 pieces and season with ¹⁄₁₆ teaspoon salt and ½ teaspoon pepper. Submerge salmon skin-side down in pot. Make sure there is enough water to cover salmon. Simmer about 8 minutes or until just cooked through. Do not overcook fish.

4. Using a slotted spatula to drain any excess water, transfer salmon to a platter or dish to cool. Once salmon is cool, remove skin. Let salmon cool to room temperature before serving. Spoon tarragon sauce over salmon.

Per Serving Calories: 516 | Fat: 25g | Protein: 45g | Sodium: 380mg | Fiber: 0g | Carbohydrates: 11g | Sugar: 3g

Light Tuna Casserole

This is not your mama's tuna casserole! It's on the lighter side and low in FODMAPs. Kids will love it too.

INGREDIENTS | SERVES 8

1 tablespoon butter

2 large carrots, peeled and diced

¼ cup gluten-free all-purpose flour

1½ cups chicken stock

1½ cups lactose-free milk

1 cup frozen green beans, thawed

1 teaspoon dried oregano

1 teaspoon dried marjoram

1 teaspoon dried rosemary

1 teaspoon dried thyme

½ teaspoon salt

¼ teaspoon freshly ground black pepper

3 (5-ounce) cans tuna in water, drained

8 ounces gluten-free egg noodles, cooked al dente

½ cup shredded sharp Cheddar cheese

½ cup shredded Colby cheese

2 tablespoons gluten-free panko bread crumbs

1. Preheat oven to 400°F.

2. Melt butter in a large saucepan over medium-high heat. Add carrots, and sauté 5–7 minutes, or until soft. Stir in flour and cook 1 minute.

3. Whisk in stock, then stir in milk, green beans, oregano, marjoram, rosemary, thyme, salt, pepper, and tuna. Continue cooking, stirring occasionally, about 5 minutes.

4. Add sauce mixture to noodles and toss to combine. Stir in Cheddar and Colby cheese.

5. Pour noodles into a greased 9" × 13" baking pan. Sprinkle bread crumbs on top. Bake 18–20 minutes or until top is crispy and golden and filling is bubbling. Serve immediately.

Per Serving Calories: 339 | Fat: 11g | Protein: 23g | Sodium: 650mg | Fiber: 2g | Carbohydrates: 35g | Sugar: 4g

Mediterranean Flaky Fish with Vegetables

Lovely flavors of the Mediterranean paired with flaky fish make for a healthy and tasty dinner. Pair with a salad and potatoes.

INGREDIENTS | SERVES 4

4 (3.5-ounce) skinless Atlantic cod fillets

1 cup grated zucchini

¼ cup thinly sliced fresh basil, plus 4 whole basil leaves

20 cherry tomatoes, halved

10 black olives, sliced

¼ teaspoon kosher salt

½ teaspoon freshly ground black pepper

4 tablespoons dry white wine, divided

4 tablespoons extra-virgin olive oil, divided

What Are Other Fish Options?

Other great options for this recipe are halibut, flounder, red snapper, and tilapia.

1. Preheat oven to 400°F.

2. Make parchment pockets: Pull out a 17" × 11" piece of parchment paper. With one longer edge closest to you, fold in half from left to right. Using scissors, cut out a large heart shape. On a large cutting board or clean work surface, lay down parchment heart and place fish on one half of heart, leaving at least a 1½" border around fillet. Repeat with remaining fish fillets. Lay parchment hearts in a 9" × 13" baking dish.

3. In a medium bowl, combine zucchini, sliced basil, tomatoes, olives, salt, and pepper. Stir to combine.

4. Evenly distribute the vegetables over each fish fillet in the parchment hearts.

5. Take opposite side of each parchment heart and fold over, making both edges of heart line up. Starting at rounded end, crimp edges together tightly. Leave a few inches at pointed end unfolded. Grab pointed edge and tilt heart to pour in 1 tablespoon each of wine and oil. Finish by crimping edges and twisting pointed end around and under packet.

6. Bake until just cooked through, about 10–12 minutes. Poke a toothpick through parchment paper. Fish should be done if toothpick easily slides through fish. Carefully cut open packets (steam will escape). Garnish with whole basil leaves.

Per Serving Calories: 246 | Fat: 16g | Protein: 19g | Sodium: 304mg | Fiber: 2g | Carbohydrates: 6g | Sugar: 3g

Coconut-Crusted Fish with Pineapple Relish

Love tropical flavors? You'll love this pairing of tropical coconut and pineapple flavor. Pair with brown rice or a basic side salad.

INGREDIENTS | SERVES 2

½ cup shredded unsweetened coconut

½ cup gluten-free panko bread crumbs

½ teaspoon paprika

1 large egg

1 pound cod fillets

2 cups chopped pineapple

¼ cup finely chopped red bell pepper

1 tablespoon fresh lemon juice

2 teaspoons palm sugar

1 finely chopped seeded jalapeño pepper

⅛ teaspoon salt

1. Preheat oven to 400°F.

2. In a medium bowl, mix together coconut, bread crumbs, and paprika. In a separate small bowl whisk egg. Dredge fish fillets in egg, then coconut-panko mixture.

3. Place in a baking pan and bake 12–15 minutes or until firm.

4. Make pineapple relish by combining pineapple, bell pepper, lemon juice, sugar, and jalapeño pepper and then stirring in salt. Top fish with relish and serve.

Per Serving Calories: 423 | Fat: 11g | Protein: 46g | Sodium: 224mg | Fiber: 5g | Carbohydrates: 36g | Sugar: 24g

Salmon Cakes with Fresh Dill Sauce

Paired with a fresh dill sauce, these salmon cakes are a great way to get your omega-3 fatty acids, which are vital to your health. You can serve these salmon cakes alone or with a side salad.

INGREDIENTS | SERVES 8

1 pound skinless wild-caught salmon fillet

3 scallions, chopped, green part only, divided

2 tablespoons lemon juice, divided

2 tablespoons Dijon mustard

1 teaspoon salt, divided

¼ teaspoon freshly ground black pepper

¼ cup gluten-free panko bread crumbs

1 tablespoon coconut oil

2 tablespoons fresh dill

7 ounces lactose-free sour cream

1. In a food processor, pulse salmon, 2 scallions, 1 tablespoon lemon juice, mustard, ½ teaspoon salt, and pepper until coarsely chopped.

2. Mix in the bread crumbs and form into 8 patties.

3. Heat oil in a large nonstick skillet over medium heat. Cook patties until opaque throughout, about 2 minutes per side.

4. Dill sauce: In your food processor combine dill, sour cream, 1 tablespoon lemon juice, and ½ teaspoon salt. Pulse until blended. Dollop onto salmon cakes. Sprinkle on remaining scallions.

Per Serving Calories: 160 | Fat: 11g | Protein: 12g | Sodium: 409mg | Fiber: 0g | Carbohydrates: 4g | Sugar: 1g

Sole Meunière

This low-FODMAP version of the classic French dish pays homage to the late Julia Child, who famously said, "You don't have to cook fancy or complicated masterpieces—just good food from fresh ingredients."

INGREDIENTS | SERVES 2

2 (4-ounce) boneless, skinless sole fillets
¼ teaspoon kosher salt
¼ teaspoon freshly ground black pepper
¼ cup gluten-free all-purpose flour
4 tablespoons unsalted butter, divided
1½ tablespoons finely chopped fresh flat-leaf parsley
½ teaspoon grated lemon zest
Pulp ½ large lemon, seeds removed

1. Season fillets on both sides with salt and pepper and lay on a plate. Place flour in a shallow bowl. Dredge fillets in flour, shaking off any excess.

2. Heat 2 tablespoons butter in a 12" skillet over medium-high heat. Place fillets in skillet and cook until browned on both sides and just cooked through, about 6 minutes.

3. Transfer fillets to plates; sprinkle with parsley.

4. Using a paper towel, carefully wipe skillet clean and return to heat. Add remaining butter, stir, and cook until it starts to brown. Add lemon zest and pulp; cook 3–4 minutes, then pour over fillets. Serve immediately.

Per Serving Calories: 364 | Fat: 25g | Protein: 23g | Sodium: 390mg | Fiber: 1g | Carbohydrates: 12g | Sugar: 1g

Rita's Linguine with Clam Sauce

This recipe is dedicated to Rita, a sweet lady from New York who loved linguine with clam sauce!

INGREDIENTS | SERVES 4

12 ounces gluten-free linguine
1 tablespoon olive oil
1 tablespoon garlic-infused olive oil
⅛ teaspoon wheat-free asafetida powder
2 tablespoons unsalted butter, divided
½ cup dry white wine
1 teaspoon dried oregano
2 dozen cherrystone clams, rinsed and scrubbed
¼ cup coarsely chopped fresh flat-leaf parsley
½ teaspoon freshly ground black pepper

1. Cook pasta until al dente according to package directions. Reserve ½ cup pasta water; drain pasta. Set aside.

2. While pasta cooks, heat oils over medium heat in a 5-quart saucepan. Add asafetida, 1 tablespoon butter, wine, and oregano and bring to a boil; cook 2 minutes.

3. Add clams; cover and simmer until clams open, about 10 minutes. If any clams have not opened, discard.

4. Add pasta to clams and stir 1 minute. Remove from heat and stir in 1 tablespoon butter, parsley, black pepper, and reserved pasta water; stir to combine. Serve immediately.

Per Serving Calories: 456 | Fat: 14g | Protein: 12g | Sodium: 14mg | Fiber: 3g | Carbohydrates: 65g | Sugar: 3g

Basic Baked Scallops

This recipe will take less than 30 minutes and pairs well with green beans or a side salad.

INGREDIENTS | SERVES 2

¾ pound sea scallops

2 tablespoons lemon juice

2½ tablespoons unsalted butter, melted

¼ teaspoon sea salt

½ teaspoon freshly ground black pepper

2 tablespoons chopped fresh flat-leaf parsley

½ cup gluten-free bread crumbs

½ teaspoon smoked paprika

2 tablespoons olive oil

1. Preheat oven to 425°F.

2. Toss together scallops, lemon juice, melted butter, salt, and pepper in a 2-quart baking dish.

3. In a medium bowl, combine parsley, bread crumbs, paprika, and olive oil. Sprinkle on top of scallops.

4. Bake 12–14 minutes or until scallops are heated through and bread crumbs are golden. Serve immediately.

Per Serving Calories: 426 | Fat: 30g | Protein: 17g | Sodium: 621mg | Fiber: 2g | Carbohydrates: 23g | Sugar: 2g

Creamy Halibut

This recipe might be creamy, but it's lower in fat than other creamy sauces. Enjoy!

INGREDIENTS | SERVES 4

2 teaspoons sunflower oil

1½ pounds halibut, cut into 4 portions

⅓ cup Basic Mayonnaise (see recipe in Chapter 13)

2½ tablespoons lemon juice

2¼ tablespoons grated Parmesan cheese

⅛ teaspoon wheat-free asafetida powder

1 teaspoon Dijon mustard

½ teaspoon crushed red pepper flakes

2 tablespoons chopped fresh flat-leaf parsley

1. Preheat oven to 400°F.

2. Heat oil in a large nonstick skillet over medium-high heat. Brown halibut on both sides, about 3 minutes each side.

3. Remove fish from skillet and place in a 9" × 13" oven-proof casserole dish. Bake 7 minutes.

4. While fish is baking, mix together remaining ingredients except parsley in a medium bowl.

5. Once fish is done baking, spoon mixture over fish and broil in oven 2 minutes. Garnish with parsley.

Per Serving Calories: 358 | Fat: 22g | Protein: 37g | Sodium: 267mg | Fiber: 0g | Carbohydrates: 2g | Sugar: 0g

Cornmeal-Crusted Tilapia

If you miss fried fish, try this crunchy and flaky fish, using cornmeal made from whole-grain corn. Serve this dish with some lemon wedges and the Tartar Sauce from Chapter 13.

INGREDIENTS | SERVES 2

1 pound tilapia

¼ cup gluten-free bread crumbs

¾ cup coarse cornmeal

2 tablespoons gluten-free all-purpose flour

½ teaspoon salt

1 teaspoon freshly ground black pepper

⅛ teaspoon wheat-free asafetida powder

1 large egg

1 tablespoon lactose-free milk

1 tablespoon sunflower oil

1. Rinse and pat fish dry. Slice into 2 pieces.

2. In a large bowl, combine bread crumbs, cornmeal, flour, salt, pepper, and asafetida. In a small bowl, whisk together egg and milk.

3. Dip tilapia in egg mixture, tapping off any excess. Then dip both sides of fish in cornmeal mixture.

4. Heat oil in a 9" frying pan on medium-high heat. Pan-fry fish 3–5 minutes each side; fish should be opaque throughout and flaky.

Per Serving Calories: 561 | Fat: 13g | Protein: 50g | Sodium: 882mg | Fiber: 3g | Carbohydrates: 58g | Sugar: 2g

Uses for Cornmeal on the Low-FODMAP Diet

On the low-FODMAP diet, cornmeal is a grain that can be used not only to coat fish, but it can also be turned into creamy polenta and used as a side or for pizza crust (see recipe in Chapter 16).

Fish and Chips

*This recipe favors good health by baking the fish and potatoes rather than frying them—
but the millet coating adds the familiar crunch of fried fish.*

INGREDIENTS | SERVES 4

¼ cup millet

¼ cup chopped pecans

2 tablespoons coarse cornmeal

1½ teaspoons sea salt, divided

⅛ teaspoon ground red pepper

4 small red potatoes, thinly sliced

1 tablespoon extra-virgin olive oil

½ cup lactose-free milk

2 tablespoons lactose-free sour cream

12 ounces tilapia fillets

Corn and the Low-FODMAP Diet

On the low-FODMAP diet, sweet corn is limited to half of a cob, as eating the whole cob would expose you to high levels of GOS and sorbitol. However, products such as cornmeal, cornstarch, and popcorn are permitted because they are made from a different variety of corn.

1. In a medium bowl, cover millet with boiling water and soak 30 minutes.

2. Preheat oven to 400°F. Line 2 baking sheets with parchment paper.

3. Drain millet completely and spread on baking sheet. Add pecans to second baking sheet. Roast millet and pecans 10 minutes, tossing halfway through.

4. Process pecans in a food processor until finely ground. Transfer to a medium shallow dish; toss with millet, cornmeal, ½ teaspoon salt, and red pepper.

5. Toss potato slices in oil and 1 teaspoon salt. Reline a baking sheet with parchment paper and scatter it with potatoes. Roast in oven 30 minutes or until brown and crisp.

6. In a separate shallow dish, whisk together milk and sour cream.

7. Reline the second baking sheet and coat with cooking spray. Working with 1 piece at a time, dip tilapia in milk mixture and then carefully coat both sides in millet mixture. Transfer to baking sheet.

8. Bake 15 minutes or until fish is cooked through. Serve with the potato chips.

Per Serving Calories: 351 | Fat: 11g | Protein: 22g | Sodium: 957mg | Fiber: 5g | Carbohydrates: 42g | Sugar: 4g

Bacon-Wrapped Maple Scallops

Easy to make, these scallops can make for elegant dinner fare or talk-of-the-party hors d'oeuvres.

INGREDIENTS | SERVES 10

20 sea scallops
10 slices bacon, halved
1 recipe Pumpkin Maple Glaze (see recipe in Chapter 13)

1. Preheat broiler and line a baking sheet with foil.

2. Wrap each scallop with bacon; secure with a toothpick and transfer to baking sheet.

3. Broil 10–12 minutes, turning once, until bacon is fully cooked on all sides.

4. Drizzle glaze evenly over scallops and serve immediately.

Per Serving   Calories: 97 | Fat: 6g | Protein: 2g | Sodium: 187mg | Fiber: 0g | Carbohydrates: 8g | Sugar: 6g

Citrusy Swordfish Skewers

This sweet and savory marinade works just as well with tuna steak. Serve these skewers with a glass of Sauvignon Blanc (please see note on alcohol in Appendix B).

INGREDIENTS | SERVES 4

2 tablespoons garlic-infused olive oil
1 tablespoon orange juice
1 teaspoon dried oregano
½ teaspoon sea salt
4 (4-ounce) swordfish steaks, cut into 2" cubes
2 medium oranges, peeled and cut into 6 portions each

1. Combine oil, orange juice, oregano, and salt in a medium bowl. Whisk to combine.

2. Add fish and orange pieces to marinade. Toss to coat. Marinate 60 minutes, tossing occasionally.

3. Skewer the swordfish and orange pieces in an alternating fish/fruit pattern.

4. Heat grill or broiler to medium. Grill or broil skewers 15 minutes, turning once, until fish is cooked through. Serve immediately.

Per Serving   Calories: 228 | Fat: 11g | Protein: 23g | Sodium: 396mg | Fiber: 2g | Carbohydrates: 8g | Sugar: 6g

Atlantic Cod with Basil Walnut Sauce

This sauce is a lovely complement to cod or other fish such as haddock, tilapia, pollock, or striped bass.

INGREDIENTS | SERVES 4

2 (6-ounce) Atlantic cod fillets

¼ teaspoon kosher salt, divided

½ teaspoon freshly ground black pepper, divided

Zest of 1 large lemon

3 tablespoons extra-virgin olive oil, divided

¼ packed cup fresh basil leaves

1 tablespoon small walnut pieces

1. Preheat oven to 400°F.

2. Place fish fillets in a 9" × 13" baking dish and sprinkle ⅛ teaspoon salt, ¼ teaspoon pepper, and lemon zest over both sides of fish. Brush with 1 tablespoon olive oil.

3. Using a food processor, combine basil, walnuts, ⅛ teaspoon salt, and ¼ teaspoon pepper. Process until it becomes a paste. With processor running, gradually add 2 tablespoons olive oil. Pat mixture evenly over fish.

4. Place baking dish in oven and bake for 13–17 minutes or until flesh is opaque in color. Serve with rice, spooning the juices from the pan over the fish and rice.

Per Serving   Calories: 176 | Fat: 12g | Protein: 16g | Sodium: 194mg | Fiber: 1g | Carbohydrates:2g | Sugar: 1g

Shrimp Puttanesca with Linguine

A more traditional puttanesca sauce calls for onions and garlic, but this version replaces them with ingredients just as tasty.

INGREDIENTS | SERVES 4

1 pound gluten-free linguine

2 tablespoons olive oil

1 (24-ounce) can diced tomatoes

2 cups shredded kale

½ cup black olives

½ cup green olives

2 tablespoons capers, rinsed and drained

1 teaspoon red pepper flakes

1 pound large shrimp

½ cup crumbled feta cheese

1. Cook pasta according to package directions. Drain and set aside.

2. Heat oil in a large skillet over medium heat. Stir in tomatoes, kale, black and green olives, capers, and red pepper flakes. Bring to a boil, then reduce heat to a simmer and cook 15 minutes.

3. Add pasta, shrimp, and cheese to sauce. Cook 3–5 minutes or until shrimp is cooked through.

Per Serving   Calories: 529 | Fat: 18g | Protein: 42g | Sodium: 1,130mg | Fiber: 7g | Carbohydrates: 98g | Sugar: 8g

Maple-Glazed Salmon

There are so many uses for maple syrup. Like this salmon for example. This recipe is flavorful, healthy, and delicious with Sesame and Ginger Bok Choy (see recipe in Chapter 5) and brown rice.

INGREDIENTS | SERVES 2

2 tablespoons toasted sesame seeds

3 tablespoons maple syrup

3 tablespoons sesame oil

¼ cup gluten-free soy sauce (tamari)

⅛ teaspoon freshly ground black pepper

⅛ teaspoon wheat-free asafetida powder

2 (6-ounce) wild salmon fillets

1 tablespoon thinly sliced fresh gingerroot

2 scallions, chopped, green part only

1. To toast sesame seeds, use a small dry skillet and place over medium heat. Toast 3–5 minutes or until lightly browned, stirring occasionally. Set aside on a plate.

2. In a large, shallow dish, whisk maple syrup, sesame oil, tamari, pepper, and asafetida. Once evenly combined, add salmon to mixture and using tongs, turn fish to evenly coat every side. Place ginger slices on top of salmon. Cover and refrigerate at least 2 hours. If possible, refrigerate up to 24 hours so more of the flavors marinate throughout the fish.

3. Preheat oven to 450°F.

4. Remove salmon from refrigerator and using tongs, coat both sides of fish with toasted sesame seeds. Place salmon in a 9" × 13" baking dish and cook 10–12 minutes or until salmon is opaque in center. An instant-read thermometer should register 145°F in thickest part of fillet.

5. Transfer to plates and garnish with scallions.

Per Serving   Calories: 573 | Fat: 35g | Protein: 37g | Sodium: 1,876mg | Fiber: 2g | Carbohydrates: 26g | Sugar: 19g

Baked Moroccan-Style Halibut

This recipe was created with a combination of ingredients and spices you may find the next time you eat a Moroccan dish!

INGREDIENTS | SERVES 4

1 pint cherry tomatoes
¼ cup pitted black olives
⅛ teaspoon wheat-free asafetida powder
½ teaspoon ground cumin
¼ teaspoon ground cinnamon
¼ teaspoon freshly ground black pepper
4 (6-ounce) fresh halibut fillets
2 tablespoons olive oil

1. Preheat oven 450°F.

2. In a medium mixing bowl, stir together tomatoes, olives, asafetida, cumin, cinnamon, and black pepper.

3. Add halibut to a large baking dish. Sprinkle tomato mixture evenly over fish. Drizzle oil over fish.

4. Bake 10–15 minutes or until an instant-read thermometer inserted into the thickest fillet reads 145°F. Serve immediately.

Per Serving Calories: 269 | Fat: 12g | Protein: 36g | Sodium: 168mg | Fiber: 1g | Carbohydrates: 4g | Sugar: 2g

CHAPTER 9

Vegan and Vegetarian Main Dishes

Tempeh Coconut Curry Bowls
172

Mexican Risotto
173

Lentil Pie
174

Vegan Potato Salad, Cypriot-Style
175

Lemon and Mozzarella Polenta Pizza
176

Summer Vegetable Pasta
177

Latin Quinoa-Stuffed Peppers
178

Mixed Grains, Seeds, and Vegetable Bowl
179

Vegetable Nori Roll
179

Broccoli Greenballs
180

Orange Tempeh and Rice Salad
181

Goat Cheese and Potato Tacos with Red Chili Cream Sauce
182

Baked Tofu and Vegetables
183

Vegetable and Rice Noodle Bowl
184

Mediterranean Noodles
185

Turmeric Rice with Cranberries
185

Savory Baked Tofu
186

Swiss Chard with Lentils, Pine Nuts, and Feta Cheese
186

Vegetable Fried Rice
187

Vegan Pad Thai
188

Mac 'n' Cheeze
189

Tempeh Tacos
190

Collard Green Wraps with Thai Peanut Dressing
191

Tempeh Coconut Curry Bowls

Tempeh lovers will enjoy this hearty and flavorful bowl with a cool undertone of coconut.

INGREDIENTS | SERVES 2

1 tablespoon canola oil

½ teaspoon ground turmeric

½ teaspoon ground coriander

1 teaspoon mustard seeds

½ teaspoon cayenne pepper

1 tablespoon minced fresh gingerroot

2 tablespoons fresh minced lemongrass

2 tablespoons red curry paste

1/16 teaspoon salt

1 pound Yukon Gold potatoes, peeled and cut into small cubes (about 3 cups)

1 cup water

1 (13.5-ounce) can light coconut milk

8 ounces tempeh, cut into ¾" cubes

2 teaspoons gluten-free soy sauce (tamari)

½ tablespoon fresh lime juice

½ tablespoon fresh lemon juice

1 cup uncooked basmati rice

¼ cup shredded unsweetened coconut

1. Heat oil in a large nonstick skillet over medium-high heat. Add turmeric, coriander, mustard seeds, cayenne pepper, ginger, lemongrass, and curry paste; cook 4 minutes, stirring frequently.

2. Add salt, potatoes, water, coconut milk, and tempeh; bring to a boil. Cover, reduce heat, and simmer 15 minutes or until potatoes are tender.

3. Stir in soy sauce and lemon and lime juices. Simmer uncovered 5 minutes.

4. Cook rice according to package instructions. Once rice is done, add coconut shreds. Serve with curry in bowls.

Per Serving   Calories: 648 | Fat: 42g | Protein: 21g | Sodium: 631mg | Fiber: 5g | Carbohydrates: 54g | Sugar: 2g

All Curry Pastes Are Not Alike!

Oftentimes curry pastes are made with high FODMAPs such as garlic and onions. If you cannot find a curry paste that is free of FODMAPs, you can always make your own! See Chapter 13 for a recipe.

Mexican Risotto

Kick things up a notch and try this comforting Mexican version of risotto.

INGREDIENTS | SERVES 6

½ each large red, green, yellow, and orange bell peppers, seeded and chopped

1 cup frozen corn

¼ teaspoon salt, divided

¼ teaspoon freshly ground black pepper, divided

2 tablespoons butter

1 cup arborio rice

3 cups vegetable stock

1 cup white cooking wine

½ tablespoon ground cumin

2 teaspoons chili powder

1 teaspoon dried oregano

1 teaspoon ground coriander

Juice of 1 large lime

1 cup shredded Cheddar cheese

⅓ cup chopped fresh cilantro

1 medium avocado, cut into sixths

1. Coat a small saucepan with cooking spray and sauté peppers over medium-high heat. After about 5 minutes, add corn and season with ⅛ teaspoon salt and ⅛ teaspoon pepper. Cook peppers until slightly charred, about 8 minutes. Set aside.

2. Meanwhile, in a medium skillet over medium-high heat, melt butter and add rice; fry until translucent, stirring for about 2 minutes.

3. Slowly add ½ cup stock and continuously stir until rice has absorbed all liquid. Follow this process again in ½-cup increments until stock is gone and then move on to two ½-cup increments of wine. Rice should be creamy and tender after 25–35 minutes. If rice is not completely cooked through, add more stock or wine. When cooked through, stir in peppers.

4. In a small bowl, stir together cumin, chili powder, oregano, coriander, lime juice, ⅛ teaspoon salt, and ⅛ teaspoon pepper. Stir into cooked rice along with cheese.

5. Top each serving with some cilantro and 1 slice of avocado. Serve immediately.

Per Serving Calories: 385 | Fat: 12g | Protein: 12g | Sodium: 758mg | Fiber: 6g | Carbohydrates: 48g | Sugar: 3g

Lentil Pie

Lentils, Swiss chard, Parmesan cheese, and potatoes make this dish perfect for a chilly day, or you can bring it to your next fall or winter holiday gathering!

INGREDIENTS | SERVES 4

1 small sweet potato, peeled and grated

1 small white potato, peeled and grated

2 tablespoons olive oil, divided

4 ounces Parmesan cheese, grated

1 medium leek, finely sliced, leaves only

1 large carrot, peeled and cut into rounds

1 medium celeriac, peeled and sliced

⅓ cup dry white wine

8 ounces Swiss chard, cut into thin ribbons (ribs and stems removed)

2 cups Vegetable Stock (see recipe in Chapter 4)

1 (15-ounce) can red lentils, thoroughly rinsed and drained

1 medium tomato, diced

½ teaspoon sea salt

1 teaspoon freshly ground black pepper

1. Preheat oven to 350°F. Grease an 8" × 8" ovenproof casserole dish.

2. Stir together sweet potato, white potato, 1 tablespoon olive oil, and Parmesan in a medium bowl. Set aside.

3. Heat 1 tablespoon olive oil in a medium nonstick pan over medium-high heat. Add leek, carrot, celeriac, and white wine. Cook covered 8–10 minutes, stirring occasionally. Vegetables should be soft. Add Swiss chard and stock; stir occasionally and bring to a boil.

4. Add lentils, tomato, salt, and black pepper. Stir and cook 5 minutes.

5. Transfer vegetable filling to casserole dish and top evenly with potato mixture. Bake 20 minutes. Filling should be steaming hot and potato topping should be golden and cooked through.

Per Serving   Calories: 473 | Fat: 19g | Protein: 26g | Sodium: 1,894mg | Fiber: 4g | Carbohydrates: 54g | Sugar: 4g

Vegan Potato Salad, Cypriot-Style

This low-FODMAP version of traditional Greek Cypriot-style potato salad is a delightful taste of the Mediterranean. For a vegetarian version, toss in ¼ cup feta cheese in the last step.

INGREDIENTS | SERVES 6

2½ pounds Cyprus or Yukon Gold potatoes, peeled

Juice of 1 medium lemon

2 tablespoons extra-virgin olive oil

½ teaspoon sea salt

1 teaspoon freshly ground black pepper

1 tablespoon dried oregano

1 bunch fresh cilantro, roughly chopped

¼ cup chopped fresh flat-leaf parsley

3 scallions, chopped, green part only

1 tablespoon olive oil

¼ cup roughly chopped black olives

2 tablespoons capers, rinsed and drained

1. In a shallow pan of salted boiling water, cook potatoes 25 minutes. Drain and set aside until cool, then slice into small chunks.

2. Place potatoes in a large bowl with lemon juice and extra-virgin olive oil. Add salt, pepper, and oregano. Toss to coat evenly.

3. Add cilantro, parsley, and scallions. Toss to mix.

4. Heat olive oil in a small skillet over medium heat. Add olives and capers and fry 3 minutes. Sprinkle over potatoes in bowl. Tastes best when served immediately, but can be stored in refrigerator in an airtight container up to 2 days.

Per Serving Calories: 203 | Fat: 8g | Protein: 4g | Sodium: 345mg | Fiber: 6g | Carbohydrates: 32g | Sugar: 3g

Lemon and Mozzarella Polenta Pizza

Taste the warm polenta crust with lemon, mozzarella, basil, and truffle salt, and you have found your new Friday night date.

INGREDIENTS | SERVES 4

For the crust:

1 tablespoon extra-virgin olive oil

2½ cups vegetable stock (or use water)

1¼ teaspoons salt, divided

1 cup coarse cornmeal

1 tablespoon garlic-infused olive oil

2 teaspoons freshly ground black pepper

For the pizza topping:

½ pound mozzarella, cut into small cubes

1 small lemon, cut into thin slices

5 large leaves fresh basil, chopped

1 teaspoon truffle salt

1 teaspoon freshly ground black pepper

Where Can I Buy Truffle Salt?

If you have trouble finding truffle salt at your local store, plenty of specialty gourmet stores sell it online. Amazon.com has a wide variety of truffle salts to choose from.

1. Preheat oven to 450°F. Brush olive oil on a pizza pan or baking sheet.

2. In a medium saucepan over medium-high heat, add stock or water and ¼ teaspoon salt. Bring just about to a boil, reduce heat to medium, and add cornmeal. Turn heat to low and simmer, whisking frequently for about 10–15 minutes. Polenta needs to be thick, so add more water only if needed.

3. Stir garlic-infused oil into polenta. Quickly spread polenta out onto prepared pan, into a thickness of about ½". Sprinkle with 1 teaspoon salt and pepper. Cover baking sheet with plastic wrap and place in refrigerator until firm, about 1 hour. Can be refrigerated overnight.

4. Place polenta in oven and bake 25–30 minutes or until brown and crisp on edges.

5. Take polenta out of oven, sprinkle with mozzarella cheese, then spread lemon and basil on top. Sprinkle with truffle salt and pepper. Put pizza back in oven 2–4 minutes or until cheese has melted. Cut into square or triangle slices and serve hot or at room temperature.

Per Serving   Calories: 364 | Fat: 20g | Protein: 15g | Sodium: 1,685mg | Fiber: 2g | Carbohydrates: 31g | Sugar: 2g

Summer Vegetable Pasta

This dish tastes like a warm summer day at the farmers' market. Switch it up with other low-FODMAP vegetables from the fall, winter, and spring. Can be served hot, warm, or cold.

INGREDIENTS | SERVES 4

1 pound gluten-free penne pasta, cooked and drained

2½ tablespoons extra-virgin olive oil, divided

1 medium eggplant, diced into ½" cubes

1 medium zucchini, sliced lengthwise into ¼"-thick planks

1 cup halved grape tomatoes

1 tablespoon garlic-infused olive oil

2 tablespoons lemon juice

1 tablespoon rice wine vinegar

1 teaspoon fresh dill

1 medium cucumber, peeled and cut into quarters

2 tablespoons chopped fresh basil leaves

1 tablespoon chopped fresh cilantro leaves

1 teaspoon salt

1 teaspoon freshly ground black pepper

1. Place penne in a large salad bowl and add ½ tablespoon extra-virgin olive oil. Toss noodles gently to coat.

2. Heat a wok or large frying pan to medium heat. Add eggplant, zucchini, and tomatoes. Sauté until slightly tender. Transfer to salad bowl with pasta.

3. Make the dressing: Combine remaining olive oil, garlic-infused oil, lemon juice, vinegar, and dill in a food processor and blend until smooth. Set aside.

4. Toss cucumber, basil, cilantro, salt, and black pepper into salad bowl. Add dressing. Toss until all ingredients are evenly distributed.

Per Serving   Calories: 577 | Fat: 14g | Protein: 17g | Sodium: 608mg | Fiber: 9g | Carbohydrates: 97g | Sugar: 9g

Latin Quinoa-Stuffed Peppers

The spices and macadamia nuts really make these quinoa-stuffed peppers super tasty and filling.

INGREDIENTS | SERVES 4

½ cup quinoa

1 cup Vegetable Stock (see recipe in Chapter 4)

3 tablespoons nutritional yeast

2 cups spinach

2 teaspoons ground cumin

1 tablespoon chili powder

1 cup whole-kernel corn, drained

2 tablespoons macadamia nuts

4 large red, yellow, green, or orange bell peppers, tops cut off, seeds removed, halved

2 tablespoons coconut oil

½ ripe medium avocado, sliced into eighths

1 tablespoon fresh lime juice

1. Preheat oven to 375°F and lightly grease a 9" × 13" baking dish or rimmed baking sheet with cooking spray.

2. Combine quinoa with stock in a medium saucepan. Bring to a boil. Cover, reduce heat to low, and simmer 15 minutes or until quinoa is tender.

3. Add cooked quinoa to a large mixing bowl and thoroughly mix together with yeast, spinach, cumin, chili powder, corn, and macadamia nuts.

4. Place peppers in baking dish and brush with coconut oil. Stuff peppers with quinoa mixture. Make sure none of the spinach is showing. Cover dish with foil.

5. Bake 30 minutes, then remove foil and increase heat to 400°F; bake another 30 minutes.

6. Top with avocado, then lime juice. Serve immediately.

Per Serving   Calories: 418 | Fat: 22g | Protein: 14g | Sodium: 1,188mg | Fiber: 11g | Carbohydrates: 46g | Sugar: 9g

Mixed Grains, Seeds, and Vegetable Bowl

This bowl is very nutritious and comes with a nice dose of healthy fats, magnesium, and iron, as well as vitamins A, B$_6$, and C—all helpful for digestion.

INGREDIENTS | SERVES 4

2 medium sweet potatoes, peeled and cut into 2" chunks

2 tablespoons olive oil

1½ tablespoons balsamic vinegar

½ teaspoon dried rosemary

½ teaspoon dried thyme

½ teaspoon dried oregano

2 tablespoons pumpkin seeds

1⅓ of a whole fennel bulb, halved lengthwise and cut into quarters

½ cup brown rice, cooked

¾ cup red quinoa, rinsed and cooked

1 cup buckwheat, rinsed and cooked

½ tablespoon coconut oil

3 cups baby spinach

1. Preheat oven to 375°F.

2. Place sweet potatoes in a medium bowl. Add oil, vinegar, rosemary, thyme, and oregano. Toss with hands to coat. Place on rimmed baking sheet and roast 1 hour, flipping halfway through cooking and adding pumpkin seeds and fennel.

3. Add rice, quinoa, and buckwheat to same bowl used to prepare sweet potatoes. Stir in coconut oil.

4. Once sweet potatoes have finished baking and are tender, immediately add to bowl. Add spinach and toss. Serve immediately.

Per Serving Calories: 411 | Fat: 14g | Protein: 12g | Sodium: 72mg | Fiber: 9g | Carbohydrates: 63g | Sugar: 5g

Vegetable Nori Roll

Rich and nutty tahini, lemon, and creamy avocado steal the show for these vegan nori rolls. These rolls are great for dinner, as appetizers, or they can be made the night before and enjoyed for lunch.

INGREDIENTS | SERVES 1

1 perforated half cut (0.08-ounce) nori sheet

½ tablespoon tahini

1 ounce medium tofu, drained, patted dry

⅛ cup peeled and shredded carrot

1 small cucumber, peeled and cut into thin slices

⅛ medium avocado, thinly sliced

Pulp of 1 small lemon slice, cut into thirds

1. Use a bamboo mat to arrange nori sheet horizontally in front of you, rough side facing up.

2. Spread tahini horizontally in a line across nori sheet.

3. Spread tofu, carrots, cucumber, avocado, and lemon across bottom center of nori sheet.

4. Gently but firmly roll together like a sushi-like roll.

5. With a sharp knife, carefully slice your roll and serve immediately.

Per Serving Calories: 153 | Fat: 9g | Protein: 6g | Sodium: 36mg | Fiber: 4g | Carbohydrates: 17g | Sugar: 6g

Broccoli Greenballs

Italian grandmothers everywhere are aghast! No need for meat in this recipe! Pair with vegetable pasta for an entrée, or serve as an appetizer, in sliders, or in lettuce wraps.

INGREDIENTS | MAKES 24 GREENBALLS

2¼ teaspoons salt, divided
4 cups broccoli florets
1 cup raw almonds
¼ cup finely grated Parmesan cheese
¼ teaspoon dried oregano
¼ cup finely chopped fresh basil
¼ cup finely chopped fresh flat-leaf parsley
1⁄16 teaspoon wheat-free asafetida powder
¼ teaspoon freshly ground black pepper
2 large eggs

1. Preheat oven to 350°F. Line a baking sheet with parchment paper or spray a nonstick baking sheet with cooking spray.

2. Bring a medium pot of water to a rolling boil. Add 2 teaspoons salt. Add broccoli florets and cook until crisp-tender, about 1½ minutes. Remove with a slotted spoon.

3. Using a food processor, pulse almonds into a fine powder. Transfer to a large mixing bowl.

4. Add steamed broccoli to food processor and pulse until coarsely chopped. Transfer to bowl with ground almonds. Add Parmesan, oregano, basil, parsley, asafetida, remaining salt, and pepper.

5. In a small bowl, whisk eggs until fluffy and stir into broccoli mixture.

6. With your hands, shape mixture into 24 small balls, pressing firmly. The mixture will be very wet. Place on baking sheet. Bake 25–30 minutes or until golden brown. (Three Greenballs is equal to 1 low-FODMAP serving.)

Per Serving   Calories: 264 | Fat: 18g | Protein: 16g | Sodium: 1,618mg | Fiber: 6g | Carbohydrates: 13g | Sugar: 3g

Orange Tempeh and Rice Salad

*Satisfying and easy to make, this salad is very healthy and
can also be used as a side to pair with an entrée.*

INGREDIENTS | SERVES 2

For the salad:

4 tablespoons coconut oil, divided

¾ cup tempeh, diced into small cubes

1½ cups cooked basmati rice

1 cup common (green) cabbage, shredded

1 cup broccoli florets

1 cup peeled and shredded carrots

1 cup diced red bell pepper

1 teaspoon ground ginger

1 teaspoon ground cumin

1 teaspoon curry powder

⅛ teaspoon wheat-free asafetida powder

⅛ teaspoon salt

1 teaspoon freshly ground black pepper

1 medium orange, halved, seeds removed

For the vinaigrette:

Juice of ½ medium orange

2 tablespoons extra-virgin olive oil

2 tablespoons rice wine vinegar

1 tablespoon maple syrup

2 teaspoons ground ginger

1 teaspoon salt

1 teaspoon pepper

1. In a large nonstick skillet, heat 1 tablespoon coconut oil over medium-high heat. Add tempeh and sear 1–2 minutes each side. Add tempeh to a large mixing bowl. Set aside.

2. Add 1 tablespoon coconut oil to skillet and add rice, stirring 2 minutes. Add rice to mixing bowl. Set aside.

3. Add 2 tablespoons coconut oil to skillet along with all vegetables; stir and add ginger, cumin, curry powder, asafetida, ⅛ teaspoon salt, and 1 teaspoon pepper. Stir to evenly coat vegetables. Cook 5 minutes or until softened. Add to mixing bowl with rice and tempeh.

4. Slice half orange into small pieces. Add to mixing bowl.

5. To make vinaigrette: In a medium bowl, squeeze juice from other orange half; add remaining dressing ingredients. Whisk to combine.

6. Pour dressing into mixing bowl; toss gently to combine.

Per Serving   Calories: 1,153 | Fat: 50g | Protein: 26g | Sodium: 1,389mg | Fiber: 11g | Carbohydrates: 154g | Sugar: 23g

What Else Can I Do with Tempeh?

Tempeh is a versatile vegan protein. You can use it in salads, sandwiches, curry dishes, stir-fries, tacos, and pizza.

Goat Cheese and Potato Tacos with Red Chili Cream Sauce

*Comforting potato tacos with mild goat cheese and spicy
red chili cream sauce are sure to please foodies who love tacos.*

INGREDIENTS | SERVES 4

2 white potatoes, peeled

1 teaspoon salt, divided

1 small red chili, seeded and sliced

1 (6-ounce) container lactose-free plain yogurt

1 teaspoon light brown sugar

1 tablespoon lemon juice

1½ teaspoons chili powder

1 teaspoon ground cumin

¼ teaspoon freshly ground black pepper

1 tablespoon coconut oil

1 (10-ounce) package frozen corn, thawed

8 (6") corn tortillas, warmed

¾ cup crumbled goat cheese

¼ cup finely chopped fresh cilantro

½ medium avocado, cut into 4 slices

1. Preheat oven to 400°F.

2. In a medium saucepot, cover potatoes with cold water. Add ½ teaspoon salt and bring to a boil. Cook at a rolling boil about 20–30 minutes or until a fork can be inserted fully into potatoes. Drain and set aside to cool.

3. For the chili sauce: Blend chili, yogurt, brown sugar, and lemon juice in a small blender or food processor. Sauce should be pinkish-red in color. Set aside.

4. Cut potatoes into ¾" chunks and add to a medium bowl. Add chili powder, cumin, remaining salt, and pepper. Toss to combine.

5. Add coconut oil to a medium skillet over medium-high heat. Add potatoes and toss until golden brown, turning occasionally, about 10 minutes. Set aside in bowl.

6. Add corn to skillet and cook 2 minutes.

7. Fill tortillas with potatoes, corn, goat cheese, and cilantro.

8. Serve with avocado and red chili cream sauce.

Per Serving   Calories: 538 | Fat: 26g | Protein: 22g |
Sodium: 799mg | Fiber: 10g | Carbohydrates: 61g | Sugar: 6g

Baked Tofu and Vegetables

Delicious sesame, sweet bok choy, and tofu make for a healthy dish and a happy tummy.

INGREDIENTS | SERVES 4

2 (14-ounce) packages extra-firm tofu, pressed between paper towels and patted dry

2 tablespoons toasted sesame oil, divided

2 teaspoons sesame seeds

2½ tablespoons gluten-free soy sauce (tamari), divided

7–8 cups chopped bok choy (about 8 stalks)

1 bunch scallions, diced, green part only

1 medium red bell pepper, seeded and diced

¼ cup slivered almonds

2 tablespoons rice wine vinegar

1. Preheat oven to 400°F. Grease a large rimmed baking sheet with cooking spray.

2. Cut tofu into 1" pieces and toss in a large bowl with 1 tablespoon sesame oil, sesame seeds, and 2 tablespoons soy sauce.

3. Spread in a single layer on the prepared baking sheet. Bake tofu on lower rack of oven. Bake until browned, 25–30 minutes, flipping once.

4. While tofu is baking, heat a large skillet on medium-high and coat with 1 tablespoon sesame oil.

5. Add bok choy, scallions, bell pepper, almonds, remaining ½ tablespoon soy sauce, and vinegar. Cook until bok choy is slightly tender, stirring frequently. Place in same bowl used to prepare tofu.

6. Once tofu is ready, add to vegetables in bowl and stir until combined. Divide into 4 bowls and serve.

Per Serving   Calories: 267 | Fat: 16g | Protein: 18g | Sodium: 725mg | Fiber: 3g | Carbohydrates: 12g | Sugar: 6g

Vegetable and Rice Noodle Bowl

This Asian-inspired dish has the taste of garlic without the unsettling effects of the fructans. It's perfect to make on a busy weeknight.

INGREDIENTS | SERVES 2

For the teriyaki sauce:

¼ cup rice wine vinegar

1 tablespoon sesame oil

1 tablespoon light brown sugar

1/16 teaspoon wheat-free asafetida powder

1½ teaspoons minced fresh gingerroot

¼ teaspoon red pepper flakes

1 teaspoon freshly ground black pepper

For the noodles:

1 tablespoon coconut oil

2 cups finely chopped broccoli florets

1 small stalk celery, chopped

2 medium carrots, peeled and shredded

3 ounces rice noodles, cooked and drained

1 scallion, chopped, green part only

2 teaspoons toasted sesame seeds

1. In a medium bowl, whisk together all sauce ingredients until combined. Set aside.

2. Preheat a wok over medium-high heat. Add oil to coat pan. Add broccoli, celery, carrots, and 2 tablespoons of teriyaki sauce. Sauté about 8 minutes.

3. Stir drained noodles into wok along with remaining teriyaki sauce. Cook 2–3 minutes and serve immediately garnished with scallions and sesame seeds.

Per Serving Calories: 281 | Fat: 16g | Protein: 4g | Sodium: 92mg | Fiber: 6g | Carbohydrates: 32g | Sugar: 12g

Some Like It Hot!

Red pepper flakes have not been formally analyzed for FODMAPs; however, ¼ teaspoon divided by 2 servings may not cause symptoms. If you think it may, leave it out of the recipe.

Mediterranean Noodles

This fresh pasta recipe is like a walk through an Italian garden in the countryside.

INGREDIENTS | SERVES 4

1 medium eggplant

½ cup garlic-infused olive oil

½ teaspoon sea salt

2 teaspoons freshly ground black pepper

1 (12-ounce) package gluten-free fusilli, cooked, drained, and rinsed under cold water

20 grape tomatoes, halved

½ cup sliced black olives

20 fresh basil leaves, torn

1 teaspoon dried oregano

Juice of 2 medium lemons

½ cup grated Parmesan cheese

1. Preheat oven to 475°F.

2. Cut eggplant into chunks and place in a large bowl. Using your hands, toss eggplant with oil, salt, and black pepper.

3. Place eggplant in a single layer on a baking sheet. Bake 20 minutes, flipping halfway through baking. When done, remove from oven and cool. Eggplant should be soft. Transfer back to large bowl along with cooked noodles.

4. Stir in tomatoes, olives, basil, oregano, lemon juice, and Parmesan and serve.

Per Serving Calories: 470 | Fat: 33g | Protein: 11g | Sodium: 680mg | Fiber: 8g | Carbohydrates: 36g | Sugar: 7g

Turmeric Rice with Cranberries

This Persian-style dish is a tad sweet and nutty, and beautifully paired with fluffy basmati rice. Finish this dish with a sprinkle of parsley.

INGREDIENTS | SERVES 2

½ cup no-sugar-added dried cranberries

2 cups lukewarm water

1 tablespoon coconut oil

2 tablespoons pine nuts

½ teaspoon ground turmeric

1/16 teaspoon wheat-free asafetida powder

½ teaspoon saffron dissolved in ¼ cup hot water

2 tablespoons light brown sugar

¼ teaspoon sea salt

1 cup cooked basmati rice

1. Soak cranberries in lukewarm water for about 10 minutes to plump. Drain.

2. In a wok or medium skillet on medium-high, heat coconut oil and stir in cranberries and pine nuts. Add turmeric, asafetida, saffron, sugar, and salt and reduce heat to low; cook 7 minutes.

3. Add rice and stir until evenly coated; serve immediately.

Per Serving Calories: 396 | Fat: 16g | Protein: 4g | Sodium: 307mg | Fiber: 4g | Carbohydrates: 63g | Sugar: 32g

Savory Baked Tofu

Savory Baked Tofu makes a great addition when served on vegetable quinoa or Vegetable Fried Rice (see recipe in this chapter).

INGREDIENTS | SERVES 4

1 (14-ounce) package firm tofu, drained and patted dry

2 teaspoons paprika

1/16 teaspoon wheat-free asafetida powder

2 teaspoons curry powder

2 tablespoons extra-virgin olive oil

1. Preheat oven to 400°F.

2. Cut tofu widthwise into ½" slices.

3. Lay tofu in a lightly greased 9" × 13" casserole dish. Sprinkle on paprika, asafetida, and curry powder, and drizzle with olive oil. Bake 30 minutes.

Per Serving Calories: 677 | Fat: 33g | Protein: 68g | Sodium: 355mg | Fiber: 2g | Carbohydrates: 26g | Sugar: 13g

Swiss Chard with Lentils, Pine Nuts, and Feta Cheese

This dish is super easy and healthy. It can also be served as a small side.

INGREDIENTS | SERVES 4

1 tablespoon garlic-infused olive oil

¼ cup pine nuts

1 (15-ounce) can lentils, drained and thoroughly washed

¼ teaspoon kosher salt

1 teaspoon freshly ground black pepper

12 ounces Swiss chard (about 1 bunch), cut into thin ribbons (ribs and stems removed)

¼ cup rice wine vinegar

½ cup crumbled feta cheese

1. Heat 1 tablespoon oil in a large skillet over high heat. Add pine nuts, lentils, salt, and pepper and cook about 8 minutes, stirring occasionally. Reduce heat to medium.

2. Add Swiss chard and cook, stirring occasionally, until wilted, about 2 minutes.

3. Add vinegar and stir 2 minutes. Remove from heat. Place in large bowl.

4. Fold in feta and stir to combine. Serve immediately.

Per Serving Calories: 321 | Fat: 20g | Protein: 15g | Sodium: 556mg | Fiber: 3g | Carbohydrates: 29g | Sugar: 2g

Vegetable Fried Rice

This flavorful and healthy dish is especially enjoyable when topped with Savory Baked Tofu (see recipe in this chapter)!

INGREDIENTS | SERVES 2

2 large eggs

1 tablespoon sesame oil

½ medium carrot, peeled and thinly sliced

½ medium red bell pepper, seeded and diced

1 teaspoon palm sugar

1/16 teaspoon wheat-free asafetida powder

1 tablespoon gluten-free soy sauce (tamari)

1 teaspoon gluten-free fish sauce

1 tablespoon rice wine vinegar

1 large green onion, chopped, green part only

1 tablespoon freshly grated gingerroot

1 cup cooked brown rice

2 cups baby spinach

Make It Vegan with Vegan Fish Sauce

To make this dish totally vegan, use vegan fish sauce. You can make your own at home by trying this recipe at *http://veganmiam.com/recipes/vegan-fish-sauce* (it says "vegetarian" but it is vegan) and *make sure* to swap out the garlic for an ⅛ teaspoon asafetida powder.

1. Whisk eggs in a small bowl. Heat a wok or medium skillet on medium-high; spray with cooking spray and add eggs to pan. Cook 4–5 minutes or until eggs are cooked but still slightly moist. Set eggs aside on cutting board.

2. Add sesame oil to pan, then add carrot and bell pepper. Cook about 3 minutes, stirring occasionally.

3. Meanwhile, in a small bowl, stir together sugar, asafetida, soy sauce, fish sauce, and vinegar until sugar is dissolved.

4. Add green onion to pan and stir 1 minute; add ginger and cook 1 more minute.

5. Add rice and cook 2 minutes, stirring. Add soy sauce mixture and continue stirring until absorbed into rice, about 2 minutes.

6. Add spinach and cook until wilted, about 3 minutes. Coarsely chop egg and stir into rice.

Per Serving Calories: 296 | Fat: 13g | Protein: 11g | Sodium: 790mg | Fiber: 4g | Carbohydrates: 35g | Sugar: 5g

Vegan Pad Thai

This vegan version of pad thai is full of flavor and will win over your vegan foodie friends.

INGREDIENTS | SERVES 2

2½ cups water, divided

1 (10-ounce) package rice noodles or ramen-style noodles

2 tablespoons peanut butter

Juice of 2 medium limes

3 tablespoons palm sugar

1 chili (about 4" long), chopped and seeded

4 tablespoons gluten-free soy sauce (tamari), divided

2 tablespoons garlic-infused olive oil

½ (12-ounce package) extra-firm tofu, drained and cut into cubes

1 medium head broccoli, florets chopped small

2 cups bean sprouts

1 large scallion, green part only

2 tablespoons chopped unsalted peanuts

1. Bring 1½ cups water to boil in a medium pot and submerge noodles to soak. Turn off heat.

2. In a small bowl, whisk together peanut butter, lime juice, sugar, chili, 3 tablespoons soy sauce, and 1 cup water.

3. In a large frying pan, heat oil on medium and add tofu. Drizzle 1 tablespoon soy sauce over tofu and sauté until golden brown. Add broccoli and bean sprouts. Cook 4–5 minutes.

4. Drain noodles. Add peanut butter mixture and stir well. Add to tofu and cook through, about 5 minutes.

5. Garnish with scallions and peanuts. Serve immediately.

Per Serving Calories: 454 | Fat: 13g | Protein: 16g | Sodium: 920mg | Fiber: 6g | Carbohydrates: 73g | Sugar: 12g

Mac 'n' Cheeze

This dish is so creamy, non-vegans wouldn't know it wasn't made with real cheese!

INGREDIENTS | SERVES 4

1 pound brown rice pasta noodles

3 tablespoons nutritional yeast

½ teaspoon sea salt, divided

¼ cup coconut oil

¼ cup sweet rice flour

2¾ cups unsweetened almond milk

1 teaspoon rice wine vinegar

½ cup dairy-free cheese shreds

¼ teaspoon freshly ground black pepper

1 teaspoon paprika

Read the Label

When buying any brand of almond milk, read labels carefully. Many contain carrageenan, which is said to trigger gastrointestinal discomfort. Also, when buying dairy-free cheese be sure to read the labels carefully. Pea protein is sometimes included. As of the publishing of this book, pea protein has not been analyzed for FODMAPs, so it is unclear whether it could trigger symptoms. Pea protein is included in many vegan foods. Consider trying a small amount of dairy-free cheese or other products made with pea protein to test your tolerance.

1. Bring a large pot of salted water to a rolling boil and cook pasta until al dente according to package directions. Drain and set aside.

2. In a small bowl, combine yeast and ¼ teaspoon sea salt. Set aside.

3. In a large skillet, heat coconut oil over medium-low heat. Whisk in flour and continue whisking constantly 3–5 minutes or until flour smells toasty but hasn't browned.

4. In a steady stream, whisk in almond milk, stirring constantly. Add yeast mixture and vinegar. Cook 3 minutes or until slightly thickened.

5. Add cheese shreds and mix until well incorporated.

6. Add pasta and toss with sauce, black pepper, and remaining salt. Cook 1–2 minutes more to reheat pasta. Sprinkle on paprika. Serve immediately.

Per Serving Calories: 574 | Fat: 16g | Protein: 13g | Sodium: 646mg | Fiber: 3g | Carbohydrates: 91g | Sugar: 5g

Tempeh Tacos

The new "taco meat" in town is tempeh!

INGREDIENTS | SERVES 4

1 (8-ounce) package tempeh

2 small vine-ripe tomatoes, chopped

1 teaspoon chili powder

½ teaspoon ground cumin

3 tablespoons lime juice, divided

2–4 tablespoons water

1½ tablespoons coconut oil, divided

½ medium green bell pepper, seeded and diced

2 cups common (green) cabbage, diced

8 (6") soft corn tortillas, warmed

1½ cups Fiesta Salsa (see recipe in Chapter 13)

½ medium avocado, cut into eighths

How Do You Like Your Cabbage?

Though common (green) cabbage is low in FODMAPs at 1 cup per serving, it still might be troublesome for some people with IBS. Cooking the cabbage helps to "predigest" it, making it easier for some to break it down in the gut. Cabbage as well as other cruciferous vegetables (raw or cooked) can trigger unpleasant gas and bloating so be sure to stick to recommended servings!

1. Crumble tempeh into a large mixing bowl. Add tomatoes, chili powder, cumin, and 1 tablespoon lime juice. Stir in 1 tablespoon water and mix again. If tempeh mixture seems a little dry, add more water. Set aside.

2. Heat 1 tablespoon oil in large skillet over medium-high heat. Add bell pepper and cabbage. Cook for 10–12 minutes, stirring occasionally.

3. Add tempeh mixture and cook 8–10 minutes, stirring frequently. Halfway through cooking, add 1 tablespoon lime juice, 1 tablespoon water, and ½ tablespoon coconut oil. Add 2 more tablespoons of water and 1 tablespoon lime juice toward end of cooking. Stir again. Remove from heat. Mixture should be moist. Add more water if necessary.

4. Fill tortillas with tempeh mixture, salsa, and cabbage, and top with avocado.

Per Serving   Calories: 472 | Fat: 24g | Protein: 19g | Sodium: 992mg | Fiber: 9g | Carbohydrates: 52g | Sugar: 7g

Collard Green Wraps with Thai Peanut Dressing

*These wraps are bursting with healthy ingredients, and along with the dressing,
they will make taste buds sing!*

INGREDIENTS | SERVES 3

¼ teaspoon salt

2 teaspoons lemon juice

6 large collard green leaves

9 ounces semi-firm tofu

⅔ cup bean sprouts

2 medium carrots, peeled and julienned

1 medium cucumber, peeled and julienned

2 tablespoons chopped fresh cilantro leaves

½ small avocado

Thai Peanut Dressing (see recipe in Chapter 13)

Why Are Collard Greens So Awesome?

Collard greens are packed with soluble fiber, vitamins C, K, and A, as well as folate, manganese, calcium, and tryptophan.

1. Set a wide saucepan over high heat. Fill with 3" of water. Add salt and lemon juice. Bring water to a simmer and reduce heat to medium. Place 1 collard green leaf at a time in water 35–45 seconds. When leaves are done, they should turn a bright-colored green. When done with each leaf, remove from water and place on a plate with paper towels to cool.

2. Place 1½ ounces tofu toward top of each collard green leaf. Top each with an equal amount sprouts, carrots, cucumber, and cilantro. Cut out three (⅛) portions of avocado and place over vegetables. Drizzle Thai peanut dressing over vegetables.

3. Roll up wraps like you would a burrito, tucking in sides as you roll. Slice rolls in half and serve.

Per Serving   Calories: 255 | Fat: 13g | Protein: 14g | Sodium: 713mg | Fiber: 8g | Carbohydrates: 27g | Sugar: 5g

CHAPTER 10

Snacks and Main Dishes for Kids

Pumpkin Parfait
194

Strawberry Toast
194

SunButter and Jelly Crepes
195

Ants on a Trunk
195

Baked Cornflake-Crusted
Chicken Tenders with Maple
Mustard
196

Cornflake-Crusted
Chicken Wraps
197

Grilled S'mores Sandwich
197

Fiesta Nachos
198

Vegetable and Cream Cheese
Sandwich
199

Chicken, Ham, and
Blueberry Melt
199

Turkey Sloppy Joes
200

Panko-Coconut Fish Sticks
201

Spaghetti and Meatballs
202

Peanut Butter Banana
Quesadilla
202

Meatloaf Muffins
203

Mac 'n' Cheese Taco Bake
204

Barbecue Chicken Pizza
205

Chicken Potpie
206

Chicken Pizza Quesadilla
207

Broccoli and Cheddar Quesadilla
208

Collard Green Eggs and Ham
Breakfast Wrap
209

Quinoa Pizza Muffins
210

Fruit and Cheese Kebabs
211

PB and J Kebabs
211

Maple Almond Strawberry
Banana Rice Cake
212

Pumpkin Parfait

Whether your kids are in the mood for something that reminds them of the fall or they just love pumpkin, this sweet and spicy parfait may have them dreaming of pumpkin patches and autumn leaves (and hopefully schoolwork)!

INGREDIENTS | SERVES 2

12 ounces lactose-free vanilla yogurt

1 tablespoon maple syrup

½ cup pumpkin purée

¼ teaspoon pumpkin pie spice

1 cup Cinnamon Spice Granola (see recipe in Chapter 2)

¼ teaspoon ground nutmeg

1. In a small bowl, mix together yogurt and maple syrup.

2. In a separate small bowl, combine purée and pumpkin pie spice.

3. Using two parfait glasses, tall glasses, or canning jars, layer in ingredients in each: half purée mixture, half yogurt, half granola, then remaining purée mixture, yogurt, and finally top with granola. Sprinkle nutmeg on top and serve or refrigerate up to 1 day.

Per Serving   Calories: 476 | Fat: 17g | Protein: 17g | Sodium: 127mg | Fiber: 6g | Carbohydrates: 64g | Sugar: 42g

Strawberry Toast

This sandwich has a nice amount of fiber and protein to keep your little one satisfied.

INGREDIENTS | SERVES 1

2 slices gluten-free bread

1½ tablespoons lactose-free cream cheese

1 tablespoon finely ground walnuts

10 strawberries, thinly sliced

1 tablespoon maple syrup

Buying Bread for the Low-FODMAP Diet

When buying bread for the low-FODMAP diet you should always carefully read the label.

1. Place bread on a plate and spread both slices with cheese. Sprinkle walnuts on one slice and apply a little bit of pressure so they stick to cream cheese.

2. Layer strawberries on other slice of bread and apply pressure so they stick.

3. Drizzle both sides with maple syrup. Enjoy immediately or wrap in foil and refrigerate to enjoy the next day.

Per Serving   Calories: 390 | Fat: 13g | Protein: 11g | Sodium: 488mg | Fiber: 4g | Carbohydrates: 61g | Sugar: 20g

SunButter and Jelly Crepes

Make your own crepes at home (see Chapter 2) and spread on some SunButter or other low-FODMAP butter and jelly for breakfast or lunch with the kiddos.

INGREDIENTS | SERVES 4

4 crepes

¼ cup SunButter or other sunflower seed butter

¾ cup Raspberry Lemon Chia Seed Jam (see recipe in Chapter 13)

½ tablespoon confectioners' sugar

1. Spread equal amounts of sunflower seed butter on each crepe and top with jam.

2. Roll up and place on plates.

3. Lightly dust crepes with confectioners' sugar and serve.

Per Serving Calories: 179 | Fat: 9g | Protein: 5g | Sodium: 131mg | Fiber: 1g | Carbohydrates: 22g | Sugar: 14g

SunButter Is Allergen-Friendly

SunButter is a great brand of sunflower seed butter, free of peanuts, tree nuts, gluten, dairy, egg, or sesame. You can also make your own sunflower seed butter at home.

Ants on a Trunk

Celery and raisins (like Ants on a Log) get swapped out for a more modern twist for this fun snack.

INGREDIENTS | SERVES 1

1 tablespoon almond butter

1 medium banana, cut in half lengthwise

1 tablespoon pumpkin seeds

Spread almond butter on banana halves. Sprinkle with seeds.

Per Serving Calories: 248 | Fat: 13g | Protein: 8g | Sodium: 76mg | Fiber: 5g | Carbohydrates: 31g | Sugar: 16g

Get Creative with Seeds

Having seeds on hand is great for adults and kids for a snack. Try also topping Ants on a Trunk with Roasted Pumpkin Seeds with Cinnamon and Sugar (see recipe in Chapter 14)

Baked Cornflake-Crusted Chicken Tenders with Maple Mustard

Pull the cornflakes out of the pantry and try them with chicken.
You'll definitely be a superhero in your house!

INGREDIENTS | SERVES 2

For the chicken:

2 cups gluten-free cornflakes
¼ cup gluten-free all-purpose flour
½ teaspoon salt, divided
¼ teaspoon freshly ground black pepper
¼ teaspoon smoked paprika
2 large eggs
2 tablespoons lactose-free milk
1 teaspoon dried parsley
¾ pound boneless, skinless chicken tenders

For the dipping sauce:

¼ cup plus 1 tablespoon Dijon mustard
¼ cup maple syrup
¼ cup rice wine vinegar
1½ teaspoons kosher salt
¼ cup plus 2 tablespoons oil, such as soy, peanut, or corn

1. Preheat oven to 400°F. Grease a baking sheet with cooking spray.

2. Place cornflakes in a zip-top plastic bag, close bag, and use a rolling pin to roll over and crush flakes. Set aside.

3. In a shallow dish, combine flour with a ¼ teaspoon salt, pepper, and paprika.

4. In another shallow dish, whisk together eggs and milk.

5. In a third shallow dish, combine cornflakes, parsley, and remaining ¼ teaspoon salt.

6. Set up your bowls from left to right with flour, eggs, and then cornflakes. Dredge chicken in flour, then dip in egg, tapping off any excess and then firmly pressing both sides of chicken into cornflake mixture. Place on baking sheet.

7. Bake 12–15 minutes or until golden brown and cooked through. Flip tenders about halfway through baking.

8. Meanwhile, for dipping sauce, place mustard, maple syrup, vinegar, and salt in a blender. Pulse to combine, then with motor running, add in oil slowly. Place sauce in a small bowl. Serve with tenders.

Per Serving Calories: 475 | Fat: 26g | Protein: 23g |
Sodium: 1,671mg | Fiber: 2g | Carbohydrates: 38g | Sugar: 19g

Cornflake-Crusted Chicken Wraps

See recipe in this chapter to make Baked Cornflake-Crusted Chicken Tenders and add to wraps for a fun lunch or dinner.

INGREDIENTS | SERVES 2

2 servings Baked Cornflake-Crusted Chicken Tenders (see recipe in this chapter)

2 (8") gluten-free tortillas or wraps

2 tablespoons Basic Mayonnaise (see recipe in Chapter 13)

2 tablespoons Dijon mustard

½ cup shredded Cheddar cheese, divided

2 large leaves romaine lettuce, halved

1. Make cornflake-crusted chicken tenders and set aside.

2. Place 1 tortilla on a plate and spread 1 tablespoon mayonnaise and 1 tablespoon mustard, then add half chicken tenders, and top with ¼ cup cheese and 1 lettuce leaf. Roll up and repeat with other tortilla.

Per Serving Calories: 570 | Fat: 40g | Protein: 24g | Sodium: 1,092mg | Fiber: 4g | Carbohydrates: 30g | Sugar: 1g

Grilled S'mores Sandwich

Once you've spread chocolate onto these sandwiches you can always sprinkle on some cinnamon, coconut flakes, slivered almonds, or other low-FODMAP additions.

INGREDIENTS | SERVES 2

1 tablespoon butter or vegan substitute

4 pieces gluten-free bread

2 tablespoons lactose-free or vegan cream cheese

2 ounces dark chocolate chips

1. Heat a small skillet on medium heat. Butter outsides of 2 slices bread and smear cream cheese on other side of 1 slice. Place both slices butter side down in skillet.

2. Once cream cheese is slightly melted but not bubbling hot, use a spatula to transfer bread slices to a plate.

3. Set your microwave to low and heat 1 ounce dark chocolate chips 1 minute or until melted (microwave ovens vary). Once done, immediately spread chocolate on unbuttered side of 1 slice bread. Place sandwich together and finish making other sandwich.

Per Serving Calories: 380 | Fat: 15g | Protein:9g | Sodium: 439mg | Fiber: 3g | Carbohydrates: 56g | Sugar: 17g

Fiesta Nachos

Planning a fun night in? Try these fun nachos with all the low-FODMAP fixings.

INGREDIENTS | SERVES 4

½ pound ground lean beef

¼ teaspoon chili powder

¼ teaspoon dried oregano

¼ teaspoon paprika

¼ teaspoon ground cumin

⅛ teaspoon salt

⅛ teaspoon freshly ground black pepper

1 tablespoon safflower oil

35 tortilla chips

½ cup Fiesta Salsa (see recipe in Chapter 13)

¼ cup sliced black olives

1½ cups shredded Cheddar cheese

2 scallions, chopped, green part only

½ cup lactose-free sour cream

1. Preheat oven to 350°F. Spray a 9" × 13" baking dish with cooking spray.

2. In a medium bowl, add beef, chili powder, oregano, paprika, cumin, salt, and pepper and mix together with hands.

3. Set a large skillet to medium-high heat and add beef mixture and oil; cook 5 minutes, chopping up beef with a spatula into bite-sized pieces as you cook. Set aside.

4. Line baking dish with tortilla chips. Sprinkle on beef, salsa, olives, cheese, and scallions.

5. Bake 10 minutes or until cheese is melted. Top with sour cream. Serve immediately.

Per Serving Calories: 494 | Fat: 30g | Protein: 27g | Sodium: 895mg | Fiber: 3g | Carbohydrates: 30g | Sugar: 3g

Vegetable and Cream Cheese Sandwich

Kids will love the creamy cream cheese, and they may forget it's a vegetable sandwich!

INGREDIENTS | SERVES 1

½ tablespoon lactose-free cream cheese

1 gluten-free hamburger bun

⅛ medium avocado

3 slices cucumber

¼ cup peeled and shredded carrot

1 large leaf romaine lettuce, cut in half (stem removed)

1. Spread cream cheese on both sides of hamburger bun and place avocado on one side.

2. Top one side with cucumber slices and top other with carrots and romaine. Put sandwich together and serve.

Per Serving   Calories: 216 | Fat: 7g | Protein: 7g | Sodium: 64mg | Fiber: 8g | Carbohydrates: 39g | Sugar: 17g

Chicken, Ham, and Blueberry Melt

These yummy sandwiches will melt your little one's heart!

INGREDIENTS | SERVES 2

2 pieces gluten-free bread

¼ cup Blueberry Chia Seed Jam (see recipe in Chapter 13)

2 slices thin-sliced deli ham (about 2 ounces)

4 ounces shredded rotisserie chicken

2 slices Havarti cheese

1. Heat a broiler with rack set 4" from heat. Line a rimmed baking sheet with aluminum foil.

2. Place bread on baking sheet and spread with blueberry jam; layer each slice with 1 slice ham, about 2 ounces chicken, and 1 slice cheese.

3. Broil until cheese is melted, 4–6 minutes. Serve immediately, as open-faced sandwiches.

Per Serving   Calories: 378 | Fat: 10g | Protein: 28g | Sodium: 876mg | Fiber: 2g | Carbohydrates: 43g | Sugar: 14g

Turkey Sloppy Joes

Yes, kids can enjoy Sloppy Joes, especially when they're made with lean turkey meat and some spinach is sneaked in!

INGREDIENTS | SERVES 4

1 tablespoon olive oil

2 cups peeled and shredded carrots

¼ medium green pepper, seeded and chopped

¼ medium red pepper, seeded and chopped

¼ teaspoon dried parsley

¼ teaspoon paprika

⅛ teaspoon salt

¼ teaspoon freshly ground black pepper

3 tablespoons tomato paste

¾ pound lean ground turkey

3 tablespoons gluten-free Worcestershire sauce

¼ cup Sweet Barbecue Sauce (see recipe in Chapter 13)

¼ cup Artisanal Ketchup (see recipe in Chapter 13)

2 tablespoons gluten-free soy sauce (tamari)

3 cups baby spinach

4 gluten-free hamburger buns

1. In a large saucepan, heat oil over medium heat; add carrots, peppers, parsley, paprika, salt, and pepper. Cook, stirring occasionally, until peppers and carrots are softened, 5–6 minutes.

2. Add tomato paste and stir until combined; cook 1 minute.

3. Add turkey; cook 4–5 minutes and chop up meat with a spatula.

4. Add Worcestershire, barbecue sauce, ketchup, and soy sauce.

5. Stir occasionally 12–15 minutes, adding spinach about halfway through cooking. Sauce should become thickened. Serve on hamburger buns.

Per Serving   Calories: 247 | Fat: 11g | Protein: 17g | Sodium: 1,223mg | Fiber: 3g | Carbohydrates: 22g | Sugar: 13g

Panko-Coconut Fish Sticks

Never buy frozen fish sticks again and always make them fresh and healthy with this recipe!
Serve these fish sticks with Tartar Sauce (see recipe in Chapter 13).

INGREDIENTS | SERVES 8

1 cup gluten-free all-purpose flour

2 large eggs, beaten

⅛ teaspoon salt

1¼ teaspoon freshly ground black pepper, divided

3 cups gluten-free panko bread crumbs

1 cup shredded unsweetened coconut

1 teaspoon ground bay leaves

¼ teaspoon celery salt

1 teaspoon dry mustard

⅛ teaspoon ground nutmeg

⅛ teaspoon ground ginger

⅛ teaspoon paprika

⅛ teaspoon chili powder

3 pounds fresh tilapia fillets, cut into 1–2" strips

2 medium lemons, cut into quarters

1. Preheat oven to 475°F. Position racks on top and bottom third. Line 2 baking sheets with aluminum foil; set aside.

2. Place flour in a shallow bowl.

3. In another shallow bowl, whisk eggs with salt and ¼ teaspoon pepper. Whisk until fluffy.

4. In a third shallow bowl, combine panko, coconut, bay leaves, celery salt, mustard, 1 teaspoon pepper, nutmeg, ginger, paprika, and chili powder.

5. Dip tilapia into flour and then egg, tapping off any excess; roll in panko mixture, pressing to adhere on all sides of fish. Place on prepared baking sheets.

6. Bake until lightly golden brown, 12–15 minutes, rotating sheets from top to bottom rack halfway through.

7. Serve fish sticks with lemon wedges.

Per Serving   Calories: 411 | Fat: 8g | Protein: 39g | Sodium: 525mg | Fiber: 4g | Carbohydrates: 44g | Sugar: 3g

Spaghetti and Meatballs

If you don't have much time, skip making the marinara sauce and heat up 1 (14.5-ounce) can crushed tomatoes, 1 teaspoon dried oregano, ⅛ teaspoon salt, and 1 tablespoon unsalted butter.

INGREDIENTS | SERVES 4

¾ pound gluten-free spaghetti

Turkey Quinoa Meatballs with Mozzarella (see recipe in Chapter 7)

¼ cup plus 3 tablespoons finely grated Parmesan, divided

¼ teaspoon freshly ground black pepper

Basic Marinara Sauce (see recipe in Chapter 13)

2 tablespoons chopped fresh flat-leaf parsley

1. Cook spaghetti according to package directions.

2. Make recipe for turkey quinoa meatballs with mozzarella. (Note that you will have about 3 meatballs left over which can be used to make a sandwich for lunch next day! You will make medium slices of meatballs and place in between two pieces of gluten-free bread with 1 slice mozzarella cheese, and you can also use leftover marinara sauce.)

3. Drain spaghetti when done and add to a large serving bowl. Stir in ¼ cup Parmesan cheese and pepper.

4. Top with marinara sauce, meatballs, 3 tablespoons Parmesan, and parsley.

Per Serving Calories: 248 | Fat: 8g | Protein: 20g | Sodium: 674mg | Fiber: 3g | Carbohydrates: 24g | Sugar: 6g

Peanut Butter Banana Quesadilla

When your little one needs fuel to burn with a long day ahead, this makes for a great breakfast or snack. You can easily substitute the chocolate chips for other fun low-FODMAP ingredients.

INGREDIENTS | SERVES 1

2 tablespoons natural peanut butter

1 (8") gluten-free tortilla

½ medium banana, thinly sliced

1 tablespoon dark chocolate chips

1. Spread peanut butter over tortilla.

2. Lay banana slices over one half of tortilla. Sprinkle chocolate chips over banana slices and fold tortilla in half.

3. Spray a small skillet with cooking spray. Set heat to medium-low and place tortilla on skillet. Heat until golden brown on both sides. Cut into thirds and serve.

Per Serving Calories: 386 | Fat: 22g | Protein: 12g | Sodium: 341mg | Fiber: 5g | Carbohydrates: 42g | Sugar: 16g

Meatloaf Muffins

Meatloaf muffins are the new "thing" when it comes to fun at the dinner table! Serve these with salad, green beans, or sautéed spinach with Parmesan cheese.

INGREDIENTS | SERVES 6 (2 MUFFINS PER SERVING)

1 pound lean ground turkey

1 pound lean ground beef

¼ cup finely chopped red bell pepper

¼ cup chopped water chestnuts

2 large eggs

1 cup gluten-free bread crumbs

1 tablespoon gluten-free Worcestershire sauce

1 cup Artisanal Ketchup, divided (see recipe in Chapter 13)

½ teaspoon salt

1 teaspoon freshly ground black pepper

3 tablespoons light brown sugar

2 teaspoons yellow mustard

1. Preheat oven to 350°F. Lightly spray a 12-cup muffin pan with cooking spray.

2. In a large bowl, add ground turkey, ground beef, bell pepper, water chestnuts, eggs, bread crumbs, Worcestershire sauce, ½ cup ketchup, salt, and pepper. Mix with your hands.

3. Generously pack each muffin tin with meatloaf mixture. Place meatloaf in oven and bake 25 minutes. Remove from oven.

4. In a small bowl, mix together ½ cup ketchup, brown sugar, and mustard. Spread on top of each muffin.

5. Bake 10 minutes. Once done, remove from oven and allow to rest 10–15 minutes.

Per Serving Calories: 384 | Fat: 13g | Protein: 34g | Sodium: 935mg | Fiber: 1g | Carbohydrates: 32g | Sugar: 18g

Mac 'n' Cheese Taco Bake

Let the fiesta begin with this zesty take on taco night!

INGREDIENTS | SERVES 2

1 cup gluten-free penne pasta
8 ounces lean ground beef
¼ cup diced red bell pepper
¼ cup diced green bell pepper
¼ teaspoon chili powder
¼ teaspoon dried oregano
¼ teaspoon paprika
¼ teaspoon ground cumin
⅛ teaspoon salt
⅛ teaspoon freshly ground black pepper
1 tablespoon olive oil
¾ cup lactose-free cream cheese
1 cup grated Cheddar cheese
1 cup crushed tortilla chips (optional)
1 scallion, chopped, green part only

1. Preheat oven to 350°F.

2. Cook pasta according to package directions, more al dente than soft; set aside.

3. In a medium bowl, combine beef, bell peppers, chili powder, oregano, paprika, cumin, salt, and pepper. Mix together with hands.

4. Heat oil in a wide, deep skillet over medium-high heat; add beef mixture and cook 5 minutes. Remove from heat.

5. Add pasta and cream cheese; stir to combine. Transfer to a 9" × 13" casserole dish. Top with Cheddar and tortilla chips.

6. Bake 20–25 minutes or until cheese has melted. Top with scallions. Serve immediately.

Per Serving Calories: 624 | Fat: 28g | Protein: 27g | Sodium: 602mg | Fiber: 3g | Carbohydrates: 42g | Sugar: 4g

Barbecue Chicken Pizza

The Barbecue Chicken Pizza made by California Pizza Kitchen inspired this recipe and it's got all the delicious flavor without all the FODMAPs.

INGREDIENTS | MAKES 12" PIZZA (SERVES 8)

1 recipe Gluten-Free Pizza Dough (see recipe in Chapter 16)

1 tablespoon olive oil

½ cup Sweet Barbecue Sauce (see recipe in Chapter 13)

1 cup shredded cooked chicken

¼ cup shredded mozzarella cheese

¼ cup shredded Cheddar cheese

2 tablespoons chopped fresh cilantro

Choosing Barbecue Sauce

If you don't have time to make your own low-FODMAP barbecue sauce, look for brands that do not contain high-FODMAP ingredients such as cider vinegar, garlic, garlic salt, onions, and onion powder.

1. Make pizza dough according to directions.

2. Preheat oven to 350°F.

3. Coat pizza dough lightly with olive oil. Bake dough 30 minutes.

4. Remove from oven and spread half amount of barbecue sauce over crust. Top with chicken, remaining barbecue sauce, mozzarella, then Cheddar. Bake 25–35 minutes or until cheese is melted and crust is cooked through.

5. When pizza is done sprinkle with cilantro. Serve immediately.

Per Serving Calories: 209 | Fat: 12g | Protein: 9g | Sodium: 348mg | Fiber: 1g | Carbohydrates: 16g | Sugar: 4g

Chicken Potpie

Chicken potpie warms the heart and soul, especially this low-FODMAP version made with broccoli, coconut cream, and gluten-free flour.

INGREDIENTS | SERVES 8

1 Pie Crust (see recipe in Chapter 16)

¼ cup extra-virgin olive oil

4 medium carrots, peeled and chopped

1 medium stalk celery, diced

2 cups frozen broccoli florets

⅛ teaspoon salt

⅛ teaspoon freshly ground black pepper

2 cups shredded cooked chicken

1¾ cups chicken broth

¼ cup lactose-free milk

1 (13.5-ounce) can coconut cream

¼ cup gluten-free all-purpose flour

Time Saver

To save time, make more than 2 cups of shredded chicken the night before and use the extra for sandwiches, wraps, salads, or soups!

1. Make pie crust and lightly grease a 9" pie pan with cooking spray. Lay bottom portion of pie crust into pie pan.

2. Preheat oven to 350°F.

3. In a large skillet, heat olive oil over medium heat. Add carrots, celery, broccoli, salt, and pepper. Cook, stirring occasionally, about 5 minutes.

4. Add chicken, broth, milk, coconut cream, and flour to skillet. Mix well and cook over medium heat 3–4 minutes. Remove from heat and pour on top of dough in prepared pie tin. Cover with top of pie crust, crimp edges and using a sharp knife, cut 5–6 slits into dough.

5. Place baking dish on a baking sheet and bake 40 minutes or until crust is lightly browned. Allow to cool 10–12 minutes. Serve immediately.

Per Serving   Calories: 331 | Fat: 17g | Protein: 15g | Sodium: 350mg | Fiber: 3g | Carbohydrates: 32g | Sugar: 22g

Chicken Pizza Quesadilla

These are especially easy to put together if you've made the sauce and chicken ahead of time.

INGREDIENTS | SERVES 3

½ cup marinara or tomato sauce

2 (3-ounce) boneless, skinless chicken breasts

2 (8") gluten-free tortillas

½ cup shredded mozzarella cheese

1. Heat marinara or tomato sauce in a small saucepan over low heat.

2. To make shredded chicken, place chicken breasts into a saucepan and cover with water. Place saucepan over medium heat, bring to a boil, and simmer 10–12 minutes or until chicken is cooked through. Allow chicken to cool on a plate and then shred with forks.

3. Place sauce over half of 1 tortilla. Sprinkle ¼ cup cheese over sauce, add half the shredded chicken, and fold tortilla in half. Repeat with remaining tortilla.

4. Spray a skillet with cooking spray. Set heat to medium-low and place tortillas on skillet. Heat until golden brown on both sides. Cut into thirds and serve.

Per Serving   Calories: 248 | Fat: 8g | Protein: 20g | Sodium: 674mg | Fiber: 3g | Carbohydrates: 24g | Sugar: 6g

Broccoli and Cheddar Quesadilla

This is almost like the microwave version of snack foods we grew up with, but much healthier!

INGREDIENTS | SERVES 1

¼ cup broccoli florets
⅛ teaspoon salt
1 tablespoon water
¼ cup shredded Cheddar cheese
1 (8") gluten-free tortilla

Low-FODMAP Servings for Broccoli

Stick to a low-FODMAP serving of ¼ cup to ½ cup broccoli. A ⅔-cup serving contains moderate amounts of the polyol sorbitol, so intake should be limited.

1. Place broccoli in a small microwave-safe bowl and add salt and water.

2. Cover and microwave 2–3 minutes or until broccoli is tender and crunchy.

3. Drain any remaining water and set broccoli aside.

4. Sprinkle cheese over tortilla, add broccoli and fold tortilla in half.

5. Spray a small skillet with cooking spray. Set heat to medium-low and place tortilla on skillet. Heat until golden brown on both sides. Cut into thirds and serve.

Per Serving Calories: 215 | Fat: 12g | Protein: 10g | Sodium: 668mg | Fiber: 2g | Carbohydrates: 17g | Sugar: 1g

Collard Green Eggs and Ham Breakfast Wrap

The brightly-hued collard green wrap doesn't make this recipe sneaky when it comes to getting your kids to eat vegetables, but the taste of sweet potatoes, maple syrup, and ham will win them over!

INGREDIENTS | SERVES 1

⅛ teaspoon salt, divided

2 teaspoons lemon juice

1 large collard green leaf

1 large egg

1 tablespoon lactose-free milk (optional)

⅛ teaspoon freshly ground black pepper

6 slices (2-ounces) deli ham, sliced thinly

1 ounce grated Parmesan cheese

½ cup cooked mashed sweet potatoes

½ tablespoon maple syrup

1. Set a small, wide saucepan over high heat. Fill with 3" of water. Add ¹⁄₁₆ teaspoon salt and lemon juice. Bring water to a simmer and reduce heat to medium. Place collard green leaf in water 35–45 seconds. When done, leaf should turn a bright-colored green. Remove from water and place on a plate with paper towels to cool.

2. Beat egg in a small bowl with milk (if using), ¹⁄₁₆ teaspoon salt, and pepper. Heat a small skillet and lightly coat with cooking spray. Scramble egg to your desired level of doneness and add ham slices and Parmesan cheese.

3. Lay collard green on a plate with vein running horizontally. Place egg mixture slightly below vein and add sweet potatoes with a fork. Drizzle on maple syrup. Take bottom half of collard green leaf (closest to you) and roll up and tuck under egg mixture, continuing to roll tightly like a burrito. Tuck in sides and serve.

Per Serving   Calories: 363 | Fat: 15g | Protein: 24g | Sodium: 939mg | Fiber: 5g | Carbohydrates: 33g | Sugar: 14g

Quinoa Pizza Muffins

These are mini pizzas that you can hold in your hands! Great for dinner, kids' parties, or for adults.

INGREDIENTS | MAKES 12 MUFFINS

1½ cups Basic Marinara Sauce (see recipe in Chapter 13)

1 cup uncooked quinoa

2 cups water, divided

2 large eggs

1½ cups shredded mozzarella cheese

½ cup chopped fresh spinach

¼ cup chopped fresh basil

1 teaspoon dried oregano

½ teaspoon salt

½ teaspoon freshly ground black pepper

1. Make marinara sauce and keep warm on stove over low heat.

2. Rinse quinoa thoroughly in a sieve. In a medium saucepan, combine 1 cup quinoa with water. Bring to a boil. Reduce heat to low, cover, and simmer until quinoa is tender, about 12–15 minutes.

3. Preheat oven to 350°F. Grease a 12-cup muffin tin with cooking spray.

4. In saucepan, combine quinoa, eggs, cheese, spinach, basil, oregano, salt, and pepper.

5. Add ¼ cup mixture to each muffin well. Press down gently on mixture with back of a spoon or with your fingers.

6. Bake 15–20 minutes. Allow to cool and serve with marinara sauce.

Per Serving (1 muffin)   Calories: 88 | Fat: 4g | Protein: 4g | Sodium: 195mg | Fiber: 1g | Carbohydrates: 9g | Sugar: 2g

Fruit and Cheese Kebabs

This is a fun way to serve your child a healthy dose of fruit, protein, and carbohydrates, making for a balanced snack. Serve with rice crackers or other gluten-free crackers.

INGREDIENTS | SERVES 2

4 slices Cheddar cheese
10 medium strawberries
10 blueberries

1. Cut Cheddar into fun shapes like stars or hearts with 1" cookie cutters. You will use 2 pieces cheese for each skewer.

2. Thread fruit and cheese onto wooden skewers: a strawberry, a blueberry, then a piece of cheese—alternate to create a pattern. (For safety, be sure to snip off the pointed end of the skewer with a pair of kitchen shears.)

3. Can be placed in a flat storage container and chilled overnight.

Per Serving   Calories: 248 | Fat: 19g | Protein: 14g | Sodium: 348mg | Fiber: 1g | Carbohydrates: 6g | Sugar: 4g

PB and J Kebabs

Who doesn't love peanut butter and jelly?
This is a great snack for kids and adults.

INGREDIENTS | SERVES 2

2 ripe medium bananas, cut into 1" slices
¼ cup Strawberry Chia Seed Jam (see recipe in Chapter 13)
¼ cup peanut butter

Thread banana pieces onto skewers and smear jam and peanut butter onto opposite ends so they touch. Do not put jam or peanut butter on banana pieces that are on outer edge of skewers.

Per Serving   Calories: 405 | Fat: 17g | Protein: 10g | Sodium: 162mg | Fiber: 5g | Carbohydrates: 61g | Sugar: 37g

Maple Almond Strawberry Banana Rice Cake

Dress up bland rice cakes with a few delicious ingredients.

INGREDIENTS | SERVES 1

1 rice cake
1 tablespoon almond butter
½ ripe medium banana, thinly sliced
5 strawberries, thinly sliced
½ tablespoon maple syrup

Top rice cake with almond butter, banana, strawberries, and maple syrup.

Per Serving Calories: 227 | Fat: 9g | Protein: 6g | Sodium: 105mg | Fiber: 4g | Carbohydrates: 35g | Sugar: 18g

CHAPTER 11

Cookies and Bars

Nut-Free Cranberry
Granola Bars
214

Chocolate Coconut Cookies
215

Peanut Butter Cookies
215

Chocolate Coconut Balls
216

Chocolate Chip Cookies
217

Buckwheat Thumbprint Cookies
218

Peppermint Patties
219

Molasses Cookies
220

Quinoa Cookies
221

Coconut Balls
222

Cranberry Walnut Oat Cookies
223

Chai-Spice Cookies
224

Paleo Fudge
225

Nutty Fudge
226

No-Bake Crispy Almond
Pecan Bars
227

Nut-Free Cranberry Granola Bars

These bars are great for most schools that have nut bans and of course for anyone with a nut allergy. Make batches ahead of time to bring to school, work, or while out and about.

INGREDIENTS | MAKES 2 DOZEN

2 cups gluten-free old-fashioned oats
½ cup rice crisp cereal
½ cup plus 2 teaspoons oat flour
2 tablespoons light brown sugar
½ teaspoon Himalayan sea salt
¼ cup ground and milled flaxseed
3 tablespoons coconut oil
½ cup plus 1 tablespoon maple syrup
½ cup no-sugar-added dried cranberries
⅛ cup dark chocolate chips (optional)

1. Preheat oven to 350°F. Line a 9" × 13" baking dish with parchment paper.

2. Add oats, cereal, flour, sugar, salt, and flaxseed to a stand mixer, and mix to combine.

3. In a smaller bowl combine oil, maple syrup, cranberries, and chocolate chips, if using. Add to mixer and mix until combined.

4. Use a spatula to spread mixture out evenly on prepared pan.

5. Place another piece of parchment paper over top of mixture and use a heavy, flat object (such as a book) to press down evenly and firmly. Remove parchment paper and bake 16–18 minutes (don't throw top layer of parchment paper away).

6. Once done, use parchment paper and heavy object to squish down bars again.

7. Place pan on top of a cookie sheet and refrigerate 15–20 minutes. This will allow you to easily cut bars and give bars a slightly more chewy texture. (Leaving pan to cool outside of refrigerator is not recommended.)

Per Serving Calories: 104 | Fat: 3g | Protein: 2g | Sodium: 58mg | Fiber: 2g | Carbohydrates: 18g | Sugar: 8g

Chocolate Coconut Cookies

Missing the taste of homemade chocolate chip cookies?
Try these gluten-free beauties with coconut for extra fiber.

INGREDIENTS | MAKES 2 DOZEN

½ cup unsalted butter at room temperature

¾ cup light brown sugar

1 large egg

2 teaspoons alcohol-free vanilla extract

1 cup plus 2 tablespoons gluten-free all-purpose flour

¼ cup shredded unsweetened coconut

1 cup semisweet chocolate chips

1. Preheat oven to 350°F.

2. Cream together butter and sugar in an electric stand mixer on low speed. Once combined, add egg and vanilla and continue mixing on low speed until combined.

3. Slowly add flour, ¼ cup at a time. Add coconut and chocolate chips. Mix to combine.

4. Roll dough between palms to make 24 balls, about 1" in diameter. Place on a nonstick cookie sheet and bake 13–15 minutes. Edges and bottoms should be lightly browned.

Per Serving   Calories: 121 | Fat: 6g | Protein: 1g | Sodium: 6mg | Fiber: 1g | Carbohydrates: 16g | Sugar: 11g

Peanut Butter Cookies

These cookies are very easy and quick to make. Bake them for your kids, grandkids, nieces, or nephews or have them as a snack to enjoy at work or while on the run.

INGREDIENTS | MAKES 18

1 cup natural peanut butter

1 cup turbinado sugar

1 teaspoon alcohol-free vanilla extract

1 tablespoon maple syrup

1 large egg

¼ teaspoon coarse Himalayan sea salt

1. Preheat oven to 350°F.

2. In a medium bowl, mix together peanut butter, sugar, vanilla, maple syrup, and egg.

3. Spoon out about 1 tablespoon dough for each cookie and place about 1" apart on an ungreased cookie sheet. Use prongs of a fork to gently press down and flatten cookies. Turn fork and press down again to make a crosshatch pattern. Lightly sprinkle salt on top of cookies.

4. Bake 5 minutes, then turn cookie sheet 180° and continue baking. Check on cookies 5 minutes later—they should be golden brown around the edges.

Per Serving   Calories: 138 | Fat: 8g | Protein: 4g | Sodium: 106mg | Fiber: 1g | Carbohydrates: 16g | Sugar: 14g

Chocolate Coconut Balls

These Chocolate Coconut Balls are very easy to make and won't take much of your time. Enjoy them with your sweetie!

INGREDIENTS | MAKES 15

2½ tablespoons melted coconut oil
2 cups shredded unsweetened coconut
2 tablespoons rice flour
⅓ cup egg whites from 2 large eggs
¼ cup pure cane sugar
1 teaspoon alcohol-free vanilla extract
⅛ teaspoon sea salt
1 ounce semisweet chocolate, broken into pieces
½ tablespoon maple syrup

1. Preheat oven to 350°F.

2. Place coconut oil in small bowl in microwave 30–45 seconds.

3. Using a stand mixer, mix coconut oil, coconut shreds, and flour on high speed.

4. In a separate bowl, whisk together egg whites, sugar, vanilla, and salt.

5. In a small saucepan, melt chocolate over medium heat. Chocolate will melt quickly. Stir constantly until completely melted, then add immediately to coconut and flour mixture and mix until chocolate is spread throughout evenly.

6. Add egg mixture to flour mixture and mix on high speed 30–45 seconds. Add maple syrup.

7. Shape mixture into 1" balls and place on a nonstick cookie sheet. Bake 15–20 minutes. Remove from oven and let stand 30–60 minutes.

Per Serving Calories: 89 | Fat: 6g | Protein: 1g | Sodium: 31mg | Fiber: 1g | Carbohydrates: 8g | Sugar: 6g

Chocolate Chip Cookies

Chocolate lovers will swoon over these chocolaty delights!

INGREDIENTS | MAKES 12

2 cups gluten-free all-purpose flour

1 cup light brown sugar, lightly packed

1 teaspoon baking soda

1 teaspoon gluten-free baking powder

½ teaspoon Himalayan salt

½ cup safflower oil

1 tablespoon maple syrup

¼ cup unsweetened almond milk

1¼ tablespoons alcohol-free vanilla extract

1 cup dark chocolate chips

1. Preheat oven to 350°F.

2. In a large bowl combine flour, sugar, baking soda, baking powder, and salt.

3. In bowl of a stand mixer combine oil, maple syrup, almond milk, and vanilla on medium speed.

4. Add dry ingredients and mix on low speed until smooth. Gradually add chocolate chips.

5. Drop rounded tablespoons of dough onto a nonstick cookie sheet. This mixture will be slightly wet.

6. Bake cookies 12–14 minutes. Longer baking yields crispier cookies.

Per Serving Calories: 304 | Fat: 14g | Protein: 3g | Sodium: 254mg | Fiber: 1g | Carbohydrates: 45g | Sugar: 27g

Buckwheat Thumbprint Cookies

These dainty cookies have a hint of cardamom and you'll love the jam baked into the centers.

INGREDIENTS | MAKES 10

¼ cup plus 2 tablespoons softened coconut oil

¾ packed cup light brown sugar

½ tablespoon alcohol-free vanilla extract

1 large egg (or egg replacer)

½ cup buckwheat flour

½ cup sorghum flour

¼ cup tapioca starch

¾ teaspoons xanthan gum

¾ teaspoons baking soda

¼ cup unsweetened cocoa powder

1 teaspoon ground cardamom

½ teaspoon sea salt

2 tablespoons canned coconut milk

3½ tablespoons low-FODMAP jam of your choice

Why Buy Gluten-Free Buckwheat Flour

Buckwheat flour is gluten-free; however, people with celiac disease should look for brands with 100 percent gluten-free certification to avoid the risk of cross-contamination. If gluten is not of concern to you, you can buy buckwheat flour without the certification label.

1. In the bowl of a stand mixer, mix together coconut oil, sugar, and vanilla on medium speed until combined. Add eggs and beat to combine.

2. In a medium mixing bowl, whisk together dry ingredients: flours, tapioca starch, xanthan gum, baking soda, cocoa powder, cardamom, and salt.

3. Gradually add dry ingredients to stand mixer bowl and mix on low speed until doughy, gradually adding coconut milk, 1 tablespoon at a time. Cover bowl with plastic wrap and chill 1 hour.

4. Preheat oven to 350°F. Position a rack in center of oven. Line a cookie sheet with parchment paper.

5. Using a tablespoon or an ice cream scoop, scoop out 10 balls and place about 2" apart on prepared cookie sheet. Press a thumbprint into center of each ball, about ½" deep. Fill each indentation with about 1 teaspoon jam.

6. Bake 12–15 minutes or until golden around edges. Remove cookies and transfer to a cooling rack. Allow to cool.

Per Serving Calories: 241 | Fat: 10g | Protein: 3g | Sodium: 230mg | Fiber: 2g | Carbohydrates: 38g | Sugar: 20g

Peppermint Patties

Put one of these in your child's (or partner's) lunch bag for a sweet, fun treat.

INGREDIENTS | MAKES 24

2 cups shredded unsweetened coconut

¼ cup canned coconut milk

¼ cup coconut oil

½ cup maple syrup

½ teaspoon alcohol-free peppermint extract

2 cups dark chocolate chips

1. In a food processor, process shredded coconut about 30 seconds into a fine texture. Add coconut milk, coconut oil, maple syrup, and peppermint extract to make a paste.

2. Shape paste into 1½" rounds and place on a cookie sheet covered with parchment paper. Place rounds in freezer for 10 minutes. Don't throw away parchment paper.

3. To melt chocolate, place 1" water in a skillet over a burner. Place chocolate chips in a glass heatproof bowl and place bowl directly in water. Bring water to a simmer, then turn off heat and let chocolate sit until melted.

4. Remove patties from freezer. Place patties on tines of a fork and dip into melted chocolate until completely covered. Place patties back on parchment-lined cookie sheet.

5. Allow chocolate shell to cool and harden before serving. Store leftovers in an air-tight container in refrigerator for up to 2 weeks or in freezer for 1–2 months.

Per Serving Calories: 133 | Fat: 9g | Protein: 1g | Sodium: 4mg | Fiber: 1g | Carbohydrates: 15g | Sugar: 12g

Molasses Cookies

Bake these when the weather starts to cool down and enjoy with those you love.

INGREDIENTS | MAKES 18

¾ cup plus 2 tablespoons sorghum flour
½ teaspoon baking soda
1 teaspoon ground cinnamon
1 teaspoon ground ginger
1½ tablespoons softened butter
½ packed cup brown sugar
1 large egg
2 tablespoons molasses
½ cup turbinado sugar

1. Preheat oven to 375°F. Spray a large cookie sheet with cooking spray.

2. In the bowl of a stand mixer, add flour, baking soda, cinnamon, and ginger and mix on low speed. Set aside.

3. In a large bowl, whisk together butter and brown sugar until fluffy. Add egg and beat to incorporate; add molasses and mix until well combined. Add to bowl with dry ingredients. Mix on medium speed.

4. Scoop out dough, roll into a ball, and then flatten into a disk between your hands. Dip each cookie into turbinado sugar, pressing gently if needed to get sugar to stick.

5. Place cookies on prepared baking sheet 1–2" apart and bake 6–8 minutes. Cookies should not be overbaked and should have a gooey texture. Cool on a rack.

Per Serving   Calories: 88 | Fat: 1g | Protein: 1g | Sodium: 43mg | Fiber: 0g | Carbohydrates: 19g | Sugar: 13g

Quinoa Cookies

As you're finding out on the low-FODMAP diet, quinoa can be used for so many things, including delicious cookies!

INGREDIENTS | MAKES 12

½ cup quinoa
1 cup water
1 cup sorghum flour
½ cup turbinado sugar
½ cup shredded unsweetened coconut
1 teaspoon ground cinnamon
1 teaspoon ground nutmeg
1 teaspoon gluten-free baking powder
½ teaspoon sea salt
¼ cup melted coconut oil, at room temperature
2 large eggs
2 teaspoons alcohol-free vanilla extract
1 ripe medium banana, mashed
⅓ cup dried no-sugar-added cranberries
⅓ cup macadamia nut halves

Recipe Substitutions

Instead of adding cranberries you can add ⅓ cup dark chocolate chips; instead of macadamia nuts you could use slivered almonds, walnuts, or crushed Brazil nuts; instead of eggs use 2 flaxseed eggs.

1. Thoroughly rinse quinoa in a sieve. Bring water and quinoa to a boil in a saucepan. Cover saucepan, reduce heat to medium-low, and cook at a simmer until moisture is absorbed completely, 12–15 minutes.

2. Preheat oven to 350°F. Line a cookie sheet with parchment paper.

3. In the bowl of a standing mixer, add flour, sugar, coconut, cinnamon, nutmeg, baking powder, and salt. Mix until well combined.

4. In a medium bowl mix oil, eggs, vanilla, and banana. Add to dry ingredients and mix until well combined. Fold in cranberries and nuts.

5. Use a cookie scoop or tablespoon to drop dough onto cookie sheet in even amounts (about 12 total) and place about 1" apart. Bake 12–14 minutes.

6. Remove from oven and place cookies on cooling rack to cool.

Per Serving Calories: 228 | Fat: 10g | Protein: 4g | Sodium: 156mg | Fiber: 3g | Carbohydrates: 32g | Sugar: 13g

Coconut Balls

Sweet and crunchy, these charming Coconut Balls also look pretty when served. If you're feeling fancy, give them a fine drizzle of melted dark chocolate or lightly sprinkle with cinnamon or confectioners' sugar.

INGREDIENTS | MAKES 15

2 cups shredded unsweetened coconut

2½ tablespoons melted coconut oil

2 tablespoons rice flour

⅓ cup egg whites, about 2 large eggs

¼ cup pure cane sugar

1 teaspoon alcohol-free vanilla extract

⅛ teaspoon sea salt

½ tablespoon maple syrup

1. Preheat oven to 350°F.

2. In the bowl of a stand mixer, add coconut shreds, coconut oil, and rice flour and mix on low speed.

3. In a small mixing bowl, whisk together egg whites, sugar, vanilla, and salt. Add to flour mixture and mix on medium speed 30–45 seconds. Add maple syrup and mix until fully combined.

4. Gently shape mixture into 1" balls and place on a non-stick cookie sheet.

5. Bake 15–20 minutes. Remove from oven and let stand 30–60 minutes. Consuming right away may cause coconut balls to crumble.

Per Serving Calories: 81 | Fat: 6g | Protein: 1g | Sodium: 31mg | Fiber: 1g | Carbohydrates: 7g | Sugar: 4g

Cranberry Walnut Oat Cookies

*Amid all the chocolate during the holidays, these cookies
are a lovely alternative, especially paired with tea.*

INGREDIENTS | MAKES 13

1¼ cup gluten-free old-fashioned rolled oats

1 cup rice flour

½ teaspoon baking soda

¾ teaspoon gluten-free baking powder

¼ teaspoon ground cinnamon

¾ teaspoon kosher salt

½ cup unsalted butter, room temperature

½ cup firmly packed light brown sugar

½ cup turbinado sugar

1 large whole egg

1 large egg yolk

1 teaspoon alcohol-free vanilla extract

1 cup coarsely chopped walnuts

1 cup coarsely chopped no-sugar-added dried cranberries

Where Do I Find Alcohol-Free Vanilla Extract?

You will find alcohol-free vanilla extract used in several low-FODMAP recipes. Many gourmet specialty food purveyors carry alcohol-free vanilla extract and you can also buy it on Amazon.com.

1. Preheat oven to 350°F. Position racks in upper and lower thirds of oven. Line two baking sheets with parchment paper.

2. Combine oats, flour, baking soda, baking powder, cinnamon, and salt in a large bowl.

3. Using a stand mixer, beat butter and sugars together on medium speed until fluffy, about 5 minutes. Add egg, egg yolk, and vanilla and reduce speed to low. Beat until smooth, about 2 minutes.

4. Add flour mixture, walnuts, and cranberries and mix until completely combined.

5. Scoop about ⅓ cup dough for each cookie. Form balls between your palms and arrange on prepared baking sheets about 2" apart. Bake 8–10 minutes, until edges are golden. Let cool 2–3 minutes on baking sheets, and then transfer to wire racks to cool.

Per Serving   Calories: 286 | Fat: 14g | Protein: 3g | Sodium: 241mg | Fiber: 2g | Carbohydrates: 38g | Sugar: 23g

Chai-Spice Cookies

These are the perfect chewy cookies for the holidays.
With a little bit of sweet and spice and all that's nice.

INGREDIENTS | MAKES 15

¾ cup plus 2 tablespoons lightly packed light brown sugar

1¼ teaspoons ground cinnamon

½ teaspoon ground cardamom

½ teaspoon ground ginger

¼ teaspoon ground allspice

⅛ teaspoon freshly ground black pepper

⅛ teaspoon ground cloves

½ cup unsalted butter at room temperature

1¼ cups gluten-free all-purpose flour

¼ teaspoon gluten-free baking powder

½ teaspoon baking soda

¼ teaspoon Himalayan salt

1 egg at room temperature

½ teaspoon alcohol-free vanilla extract

Gluten-Free Flours

When a recipe calls for gluten-free all-purpose flour, it does not consist of one flour, but a few flours in a blend. If you are not comfortable with the world of gluten-free flour, buying all-purpose gluten-free flour will take the guesswork out of baking. See Chapter 16 for gluten-free flour recipes.

1. Preheat oven to 350°F. Line a cookie sheet with parchment paper and set aside.

2. In the bowl of a stand mixer combine sugar, cinnamon, cardamom, ginger, allspice, pepper, and cloves. Remove ⅛ cup of sugar-spice mixture and set aside on a wide plate or rimmed baking sheet. Fit mixer with a paddle attachment and add butter. Beat until fluffy, about 2 minutes.

3. In a large bowl, sift together flour, baking powder, baking soda, and salt and set aside.

4. Add egg and vanilla extract to stand mixer and beat until fully incorporated. Slowly add flour mixture and mix until combined.

5. Take dough between palms and roll dough into 1" balls. Roll each ball in reserved sugar mixture. Transfer balls to prepared baking sheet and place about 1" apart.

6. Bake 8–10 minutes. Cookies should be golden and slightly puffed with a cracked surface. After removing cookies from oven, let stand on cookie sheet 2–3 minutes before transferring to wire racks to cool.

Per Serving Calories: 88 | Fat: 0g | Protein: 1g | Sodium: 93mg | Fiber: 0g | Carbohydrates: 21g | Sugar: 12g

Paleo Fudge

This fudge is low-FODMAP and Paleo, if that's your thing!

INGREDIENTS | MAKES 10

½ cup coconut oil

½ cup smooth peanut butter

½ cup unsweetened cocoa powder

¼ cup maple syrup

½ teaspoon alcohol-free vanilla extract

1. Allow coconut oil to come to room temperature or heat it quickly in microwave to melt. Then blend coconut oil with remaining ingredients in a food processor or blender until smooth.

2. Place 10 muffin liners on a baking sheet or wide plate. Fill each muffin liner ½" full with fudge mixture.

3. Chill 30 minutes or freeze 10 minutes. When firm, remove and cut into 10 pieces. Store fudge in between pieces of wax paper at room temperature in an airtight container 1–2 weeks; store in refrigerator 2–3 weeks; store in freezer 3 months if properly wrapped (store in bags within an airtight container to prevent ice crystals and freezer burn).

Per Serving   Calories: 203 | Fat: 18g | Protein: 4g | Sodium: 61mg | Fiber: 2g | Carbohydrates: 10g | Sugar: 6g

Nutty Fudge

Serve this fudge over the holidays, at birthday parties, or any other joyous occasion!

INGREDIENTS | MAKES 8

1 (13.5-ounce) can coconut milk
¼ cup maple syrup
1¾ cups dark chocolate chips
⅛ teaspoon Himalayan salt
½ tablespoon alcohol-free vanilla extract
½ cup chopped walnuts

1. Line an 8" × 8" baking pan with parchment paper. Set aside.

2. In a medium saucepan over medium-high heat, add coconut milk and bring to a boil. Reduce heat to low and simmer 5–7 minutes, stirring occasionally.

3. Whisk in maple syrup and simmer 25–30 minutes.

4. Remove from heat. Stir in chocolate chips, salt, and vanilla, and continue stirring until chocolate is melted. Stir in nuts to combine. Pour mixture into prepared pan.

5. Refrigerate at least 2 hours or until set. Cut into 1" squares. Store fudge in between pieces of wax paper at room temperature in an airtight container 1–2 weeks; store in refrigerator 2–3 weeks; store in freezer 3 months if properly wrapped (store in bags within an airtight container to prevent ice crystals and freezer burn).

Per Serving   Calories: 461 | Fat: 35g | Protein: 5g | Sodium: 64mg | Fiber: 4g | Carbohydrates: 44g | Sugar: 35g

No-Bake Crispy Almond Pecan Bars

Heavenly. That's all you need to know.

INGREDIENTS | MAKES 8

1⅔ cups marshmallows

⅔ cup almond butter

⅓ cup brown rice syrup

¾ cup dark chocolate chips, divided

¼ teaspoon sea salt

1 tablespoon alcohol-free vanilla extract

¼ cup chopped pecans

3½ cups brown rice cereal

1. Lightly grease an 8" × 8" baking pan with butter or cooking spray.

2. In a large saucepan set over low heat, add marshmallows and stir continuously 1–2 minutes. Add almond butter and stir until smooth and warmed.

3. Add brown rice syrup, ½ cup chocolate chips, and salt. Continuously stir, and once everything is completely melted, stir in vanilla, pecans, and cereal. Stir well to combine and remove from heat.

4. Pour into prepared baking pan and press down with a large spoon to make sure mixture is even throughout pan. Sprinkle on ¼ cup chocolate chips. Refrigerate 25–30 minutes before serving. Cut into 1" squares and enjoy!

Per Serving Calories: 488 | Fat: 25g | Protein: 11g | Sodium: 266mg | Fiber: 5g | Carbohydrates: 63g | Sugar: 23g

CHAPTER 12

Desserts

Mixed Berry Cobbler
230

Strawberry Shortcake
231

Coconut Whipped Cream
232

Buttercream Lactose-Free Icing
233

Dark Chocolate Glaze
233

Pumpkin Doughnuts
234

Pumpkin Spice Cupcakes
235

Maple Cinnamon Coconut Chia
Seed Pudding
236

Pumpkin Bread
236

Vanilla Frosting
237

Blueberry Granola Crisp
237

Vegan Lemon Poppy Seed
Muffins
238

Lemon Poppy Seed Muffins with
Lemon Glaze
239

Sweet Vegan Mixed Berry Tart
240

Carrot Cake with Cream Cheese
Frosting
241

Banana Coconut Nice Cream
242

Banana Cookie Dough
Nice Cream
242

Banana Almond Nice Cream
243

Peanut Butter Chocolate
Mug Cake
243

Pumpkin Pie Mug Cake
244

Pumpkin Spice Pecan Cornbread
244

Mixed Berry Cobbler

Moist and slightly sweet, make this dessert next time you want to show off.

INGREDIENTS | SERVES 8

2 teaspoons ground cinnamon, divided
1 cup gluten-free all-purpose flour mix
½ teaspoon xanthan gum
3 tablespoons granulated sugar
1½ teaspoons gluten-free baking powder
¼ teaspoon salt
1 large egg
1 cup lactose-free milk
3 cups mixed blueberries, raspberries, and sliced strawberries
Zest of ½ large lemon
1 cup gluten-free quick-cooking oats
¼ cup firmly packed brown sugar
8 tablespoons butter, softened

1. Preheat oven to 400°F. Grease an 8" × 8" baking dish.

2. Using a stand mixer on low speed, mix together 1 teaspoon cinnamon, flour, xanthan gum, sugar, baking powder, and salt. Add egg and milk, mixing on medium speed until well combined.

3. Pour into prepared baking dish. Top with fruit and lemon zest.

4. Combine oats, brown sugar, butter, and remaining cinnamon in the stand mixer. Crumble on top of fruit.

5. Bake 35 minutes.

Per Serving   Calories: 300 | Fat: 14g | Protein: 5g | Sodium: 196mg | Fiber: 3g | Carbohydrates: 41g | Sugar: 18g

Strawberry Shortcake

If you're looking for a lighter dessert perhaps to have with tea, this dessert will delight your fancy. Pair with Coconut Whipped Cream (see recipe in this chapter).

INGREDIENTS | SERVES 8

½ pound strawberries, washed, de-stemmed and quartered

1 tablespoon turbinado sugar

1 cup gluten-free all-purpose flour

½ teaspoon xanthan gum

½ teaspoon sea salt

1¼ teaspoons gluten-free baking powder

3 tablespoons butter, cold and cubed

½ cup lactose-free milk

1. Mix strawberries and sugar in a medium bowl. Cover and allow to sit for 2 hours.

2. Preheat oven to 425°F. Grease a 12-cup muffin tin with cooking spray.

3. Mix and sift flour, xanthan gum, salt, and baking powder in a medium bowl. Add to a food processor along with butter and pulse until butter is reduced to small pieces. Add in milk until well combined; mixture will be wet.

4. Use a spoon to drop an even amount of dough mixture into 8 muffin tins. Place in oven and bake for 10–14 minutes. At 10–12 minutes, check shortcakes by piercing with a fork to check for doneness—fork should come out clean.

5. Remove shortcakes from muffin tin and allow to cool for 15 minutes. Once cooled, split shortcakes in half and top with strawberries and coconut whipped cream if desired. Place top half of shortcake on top of whipped cream and cover with more strawberries and whipped cream.

Per Serving   Calories: 128 | Fat: 6g | Protein: 2g | Sodium: 301mg | Fiber: 1g | Carbohydrates: 16g | Sugar: 0g

Coconut Whipped Cream

This recipe makes a lovely topping for French toast, hot dark cocoa, pies, and cakes, as well as chocolate, vanilla, or fruit desserts.

INGREDIENTS | MAKES 2 CUPS

1 (14-ounce) can coconut milk

1 tablespoon maple syrup

1 teaspoon alcohol-free vanilla extract

¼ cup confectioners' sugar

Tips for Coconut Milk and Coconut Cream

Use the leftover clear liquid from the coconut milk can for low-FODMAP smoothies or drink as is (up to ½ cup)!

1. Chill can of coconut milk in refrigerator overnight. While can chills, coconut cream will separate from liquid. Once chilled, remove coconut milk from refrigerator and skim off thick white cream from top using a spoon.

2. Place cream in medium mixing bowl. Beat 1 minute or until creamy.

3. Add maple syrup, vanilla, and confectioners' sugar and mix 1 minute or until creamy.

4. To allow cream to set, refrigerate 30 minutes or longer. You can store cream in an airtight container in refrigerator up to 2 weeks.

Per Serving (1 cup)   Calories: 476 | Fat: 42g | Protein: 4g | Sodium: 27mg | Fiber: 0g | Carbohydrates: 27g | Sugar: 21g

Buttercream Lactose-Free Icing

This lactose-free icing is so yummy!
Use it on a variety of cupcakes, cakes, pumpkin bread, or pumpkin cookies.

INGREDIENTS | MAKES 1¼ CUPS

½ cup dairy-free margarine

2 cups confectioners' sugar

½ teaspoon alcohol-free vanilla extract

1 tablespoon unsweetened almond milk

½ tablespoon lactose-free plain yogurt

1. Using a stand mixer or an electric hand mixer with a large mixing bowl, cream margarine at low speed and gradually add confectioners' sugar until combined.

2. Setting speed to high, add remaining ingredients and beat until smooth and creamy. Be sure to chill 30–60 minutes in refrigerator before using.

Per Serving (2 tablespoons) Calories: 176 | Fat: 9g | Protein: 0g | Sodium: 108mg | Fiber: 0g | Carbohydrates: 24g | Sugar: 24g

Dark Chocolate Glaze

Use this glaze for yummy Pumpkin Doughnuts (see recipe in this chapter) or any other dessert treats you want to make more indulgent.

INGREDIENTS | MAKES 1¾ CUPS

2 tablespoons unsweetened cocoa powder

¾ cup confectioners' sugar

1½ tablespoons lactose-free milk

1 teaspoon alcohol-free vanilla extract

1. In a medium bowl, whisk together cocoa powder and confectioners' sugar.

2. Gradually add milk and vanilla. Whisk until smooth. Add more milk if necessary to ensure glaze is the right consistency for dipping. Refrigerate for up to 7 days.

Per Serving (2 tablespoons) Calories: 29 | Fat: 0g | Protein: 0g | Sodium: 1mg | Fiber: 0g | Carbohydrates: 7g | Sugar: 6g

Pumpkin Doughnuts

If you don't have a doughnut pan, you can use this recipe to make muffins.
Divide the batter evenly in a 24-cup mini-muffin pan and increase the bake time to 18 minutes.
Then follow the recipe for dipping in chocolate.

INGREDIENTS | MAKES 12

½ cup canned chickpeas, rinsed and drained

1 cup canned pumpkin

⅓ cup natural peanut butter

1 teaspoon alcohol-free vanilla extract

1 tablespoon blackstrap molasses

½ cup pure maple syrup

2 large eggs

½ cup oat flour

½ cup almond flour

1 tablespoon pumpkin pie spice

1 teaspoon gluten-free baking powder

¼ teaspoon sea salt

½ cup Dark Chocolate Glaze (see recipe in this chapter)

Choose Natural Peanut Butter

Check the label when purchasing peanut butter. Natural peanut butter should have just one ingredient: peanuts. Other peanut butters may contain added fat, sugar, and hydrogenated oils, all of which may be detrimental to your health. You may see that the oil has separated from the solid in the bottle. Give it a good stir and then refrigerate it after opening.

1. Preheat oven to 350°F. Spray a nonstick 12-cup mini-doughnut pan with coconut oil spray.

2. Add chickpeas to a food processor and blend until smooth. Add pumpkin, peanut butter, vanilla, molasses, maple syrup, and eggs and blend until smooth.

3. In a separate medium bowl, mix together flours, pumpkin pie spice, baking powder, and salt. Add to food processor and pulse just until combined.

4. Divide batter evenly in doughnut pan. Bake 8–10 minutes or until a toothpick inserted in a doughnut comes out clean. Carefully remove doughnuts and transfer to a cooling rack.

5. Line a baking sheet with parchment paper. Warm the chocolate glaze over low heat in a small saucepan. Using a fork or tongs, dip each doughnut into the chocolate to coat all sides. Place on baking sheet.

6. Once all doughnuts are coated, carefully lay sheet in freezer 15 minutes or until chocolate coating is firm and dry to the touch. Transfer to an airtight container and store in refrigerator up to 3 days.

Per Serving Calories: 197 | Fat: 7g | Protein: 6g | Sodium: 148mg | Fiber: 3g | Carbohydrates: 29g | Sugar: 17g

Pumpkin Spice Cupcakes

When pumpkin is available in abundance, take advantage and make this heart-warming recipe. Frost these with Buttercream Lactose-Free Icing (see recipe in this chapter) if desired; let them cool 30 minutes before frosting.

INGREDIENTS | MAKES 24

½ cup butter, room temperature
½ cup turbinado sugar
¼ firmly packed cup light brown sugar
½ cup canned pumpkin
1 large egg
½ teaspoon alcohol-free vanilla extract
1¼ cups gluten-free all-purpose flour
½ teaspoon baking soda
½ teaspoon gluten-free baking powder
1 teaspoon ground cinnamon
¼ teaspoon Himalayan sea salt

1. Preheat oven to 350°F.

2. Using a stand mixer, cream together butter and sugars on medium speed until fluffy. Add pumpkin, egg, and vanilla extract and mix until blended.

3. In a medium bowl stir together flour, baking soda, baking powder, cinnamon, and salt. Combine with butter-sugar mixture on low speed.

4. Using a nonstick, ungreased muffin pan, fill cups ⅔ full with batter.

5. Bake 12 minutes or until a toothpick inserted into the center of a cupcake comes out clean. Remove cupcakes from pan and transfer to racks to cool.

Per Serving Calories: 89 | Fat: 4g | Protein: 1g | Sodium: 67mg | Fiber: 0g | Carbohydrates: 12g | Sugar: 7g

Maple Cinnamon Coconut Chia Seed Pudding

This is a delicious dessert and can also be enjoyed for breakfast.

INGREDIENTS | SERVES 4

¼ cup chia seeds

1 cup unsweetened almond milk

2 tablespoons maple syrup

½ teaspoon alcohol-free vanilla extract

½ teaspoon ground cinnamon

⅛ cup shredded unsweetened coconut

2 medium bananas, sliced

20 medium strawberries, chopped

¼ cup chopped walnuts

1. In a large bowl mix chia seeds, milk, maple syrup, vanilla, cinnamon, and coconut. Allow to sit 10 minutes and then stir every 10–15 minutes three more times. Cover with plastic wrap and refrigerate overnight.

2. Layer bananas, pudding, and then strawberries in 4 ice cream glasses, canning jars, or bowls. Top with walnuts.

Per Serving   Calories: 189 | Fat: 7g | Protein: 4g | Sodium: 39mg | Fiber: 4g | Carbohydrates: 30g | Sugar: 19g

Pumpkin Bread

Perfect for the holidays or a cold weekend, warm pumpkin bread from the oven is so heavenly!

INGREDIENTS | SERVES 8

½ cup butter

1 cup pure cane sugar

2 large eggs

1 teaspoon alcohol-free vanilla extract

1 (15-ounce) can pumpkin purée

2 cups gluten-free all-purpose flour

1 tablespoon orange zest

½ tablespoon ground cinnamon

1½ teaspoons pumpkin pie spice

1 teaspoon baking soda

½ teaspoon salt

1. Preheat oven to 325°F. Lightly grease a 9" × 5" loaf pan.

2. In a stand mixer, cream butter and sugar until light and fluffy. Add eggs, mixing well after each. Add vanilla and pumpkin and mix until well blended.

3. In a separate bowl, mix together flour, orange zest, cinnamon, pumpkin pie spice, baking soda, and salt. Gradually add flour mixture to the pumpkin mixture and mix until combined. Do not overmix.

4. Pour into prepared bread pan and bake 60–70 minutes or until a toothpick inserted into the center comes out clean.

Per Serving   Calories: 351 | Fat: 13g | Protein: 6g | Sodium: 327mg | Fiber: 3g | Carbohydrates: 54g | Sugar: 27g

Vanilla Frosting

This frosting is divine on cupcakes, cakes, and spread onto cookies.

INGREDIENTS | MAKES 1 CUP

2 cups confectioners' sugar

2 tablespoons butter, softened

2 tablespoons lactose-free milk

½ teaspoon alcohol-free vanilla extract

In a medium bowl, combine sugar, butter, milk, and vanilla. Beat on medium speed until smooth and fluffy. Place in an air-tight container in refrigerator for 3–5 days.

Per Recipe Calories: 1,008 | Fat: 24g | Protein: 1g | Sodium: 18mg | Fiber: 0g | Carbohydrates: 203g | Sugar: 203g

Blueberry Granola Crisp

Moist, lightly sweet, and berry delicious! Bring this crisp to a barbecue, winter holiday party, or make to enjoy after brunch. Try with Coconut Whipped Cream (see recipe in this chapter) or with lactose-free, wheat-free ice cream!

INGREDIENTS | SERVES 8

3 cups fresh blueberries

1 tablespoon cornstarch

2½ cups gluten-free rolled oats

⅔ cup melted coconut oil

1 cup brown rice flour

⅓ cup turbinado sugar

¼ cup chopped macadamia nuts

¼ cup chopped walnuts

1 teaspoon ground cinnamon

½ teaspoon ground ginger

¼ teaspoon ground nutmeg

1. Preheat oven to 350°F.

2. In a 9" × 13" baking dish, combine blueberries and cornstarch. Mix well. Set aside.

3. In a large mixing bowl, mix together remaining ingredients until well combined. Spread mixture evenly over blueberries.

4. Bake 50–60 minutes or until top starts to brown. Serve warm.

Per Serving Calories: 445 | Fat: 26g | Protein: 6g | Sodium: 6mg | Fiber: 7g | Carbohydrates: 50g | Sugar: 15g

Vegan Lemon Poppy Seed Muffins

These healthy and vibrant lemony and deliciously vegan muffins will go fast! Enjoy with a smile.

INGREDIENTS | MAKES 10

2 cups gluten-free all-purpose flour

1 tablespoon gluten-free baking powder

½ teaspoon baking soda

¼ teaspoon Himalayan salt

⅓ cup turbinado sugar

2 tablespoons poppy seeds

2 flax eggs (see Chapter 16)

1 cup unsweetened almond milk

1 tablespoon freshly squeezed lemon juice

¼ cup safflower or sunflower oil

2 tablespoons lemon zest

Muffin Tip!

If you do not fill up all muffin cups, fill remaining empty cups halfway with water to allow for even baking.

1. Preheat oven to 400°F. Position rack in center of oven and coat a 12-cup muffin pan with cooking spray. Set aside.

2. Combine flour, baking powder, baking soda, salt, sugar, and poppy seeds in a large bowl. Mix together with a whisk until blended.

3. Whisk together eggs, milk, lemon juice, oil, and zest in a small bowl until well blended. Stir egg mixture into flour mixture until just combined. Batter should look lumpy.

4. Spoon batter into prepared muffin tins, filling each cup ⅔ full.

5. Bake about 20 minutes or until golden brown and a toothpick inserted into the center of a muffin comes out clean. Remove pan from oven and allow to cool.

6. Transfer muffins to a wire rack and let cool completely.

Per Serving   Calories: 205 | Fat: 8g | Protein: 5g | Sodium: 298mg | Fiber: 1g | Carbohydrates: 29g | Sugar: 8g

Lemon Poppy Seed Muffins with Lemon Glaze

Another great version of Lemon Poppy Seed Muffins except these are dressed in a lemony-sweet glaze.

INGREDIENTS | MAKES 10

For the muffins:

2 cups gluten-free all-purpose flour

1 teaspoon xanthan gum

1 teaspoon gluten-free baking powder

½ teaspoon baking soda

½ teaspoon salt

¾ cup turbinado sugar

Zest and juice of 1 large lemon, divided

2 tablespoons poppy seeds

½ cup unsalted butter, at room temperature

1 cup lactose-free sour cream

2 extra-large eggs, beaten

For the lemon glaze:

1 cup confectioners' sugar, sifted

2–3 tablespoons fresh lemon juice

A Word on Gums

Xanthan gum and other gums such as guar gum might cause intestinal discomfort. As of the publication of this book, gums have not been formally analyzed for their FODMAP content, so if they are of concern to you, test your own tolerance by trying a small amount of any baked good containing gums. Omit xanthan gum in this recipe if your gluten-free flour blend already contains it.

1. Preheat oven to 350°F. Grease a 12-cup muffin tin with cooking spray or butter and set aside.

2. In a medium bowl, mix together flour, xanthan gum, baking powder, baking soda, salt, sugar, lemon zest, and poppy seeds.

3. Add butter, sour cream, lemon juice, and eggs, beating well to combine.

4. Fill muffin cups about ¾ full. Place muffin tin in center of preheated oven. Bake 22–24 minutes or until a toothpick or tine of fork inserted into center of a muffin comes out clean.

5. To make lemon glaze: In a small bowl add confectioners' sugar and 1½ tablespoons of lemon juice. Stir to combine and gradually add in remaining lemon juice. Use a spoon to drizzle glaze over muffins. Serve.

Per Serving   Calories: 350 | Fat: 16g | Protein: 5g | Sodium: 268mg | Fiber: 1g | Carbohydrates: 56g | Sugar: 16g

Sweet Vegan Mixed Berry Tart

Get a little dainty and rustic with this lovely berry tart!
It pairs well with white or green decaf tea and makes a great dessert any time of the year.

INGREDIENTS | SERVES 6

½ cup white rice flour, plus extra for rolling dough

3 tablespoons coconut flour

¼ cup potato starch

¼ cup tapioca starch

1 teaspoon xanthan gum

¼ cup turbinado sugar

½ teaspoon sea salt

½ cup cold vegetable shortening

2 tablespoons cold vegan buttery spread, divided

¼ cup plus 2 tablespoons ice water

1 pint strawberries, quartered

½ cup blueberries

½ cup raspberries

1½ tablespoons blueberry jam

½ tablespoon chia seeds

Zest from 1 medium lemon

1 tablespoon lemon juice

1–2 tablespoons coconut oil

1. To make dough, sift together rice flour, coconut flour, potato starch, tapioca starch, and xanthan gum. Add sugar and salt and mix to combine. Fold in cold shortening and vegan spread and cut through flour with a pastry cutter or two knives, or pulse in a food processor.

2. Once crumbles form, create a well and very slowly pour in ice-cold water. Continue folding and cutting (or pulsing in food processor) and adding more water a few tablespoons at a time until dough forms.

3. Remove dough mixture and wrap in plastic wrap. Refrigerate 30 minutes.

4. Place a large piece of wax paper on a clean work surface or a marble board and sprinkle with flour. Remove dough from plastic wrap and place on top of flour on one side of wax paper; sprinkle dough with more flour. Fold other side of wax paper over dough. Get out rolling pin and roll gently back and forth over dough and then turn dough 90°. Roll again gently and turn another 90°. Sprinkle dough with more flour if dough begins to stick to wax paper. Continue to turn and roll dough until dough is thin and about 12" in diameter. Circle should look rustic, not perfect!

5. Preheat oven to 400°F. Grease a baking sheet with vegan butter or cooking spray.

6. Slip hand gently under bottom side of wax paper to flip dough onto baking sheet.

7. In a medium bowl combine half of strawberries with blueberries, raspberries, jam, chia seeds, lemon zest, and juice. Stir gently to combine.

8. Fill middle of dough with berry mixture. Fold over sides of dough. Pinch any cracks together.

9. Brush coconut oil on top of tart.

10. Bake 35–40 minutes or until golden on top. Let sit 20–30 minutes before serving. Divide onto plates and serve with remaining strawberries.

Per Serving Calories: 407 | Fat: 26g | Protein: 2g | Sodium: 211mg | Fiber: 5g | Carbohydrates: 44g | Sugar: 16g

Carrot Cake with Cream Cheese Frosting

This cake with velvety lactose-free frosting will have you loving cake in a new way.

INGREDIENTS | SERVES 10

1 cup coconut oil
1⅓ cups packed light brown sugar
3 large eggs
2 tablespoons almond meal
3 cups gluten-free all-purpose flour
1 cup chopped walnuts
4 cups peeled and shredded carrots
1 teaspoon baking soda
1½ teaspoons ground allspice
¼ cup butter
⅔ cup lactose-free cream cheese
Zest of 1½ medium lemons, divided
Juice of ½ medium lemon
4 cups confectioners' sugar

Why Gluten-Free Baking Powder?

Wheat starch is sometimes used in baking powder in order to help the baking powder to absorb moisture so it doesn't clump. Look for the gluten-free label on baking powders from these brands: *Rumford, Clabber Girl,* and *Ener-G.*

1. Preheat oven to 350°F.

2. Using a stand mixer, mix together oil, sugar, and eggs. Add almond meal, flour, walnuts, carrots, baking soda, and allspice. Mix on low speed until fully combined.

3. Pour batter into a 10" cake pan and bake on middle rack 70 minutes. Remove from oven and cool on a wire rack 20 minutes.

4. Clean bowl of electric mixer. Add butter, cream cheese, zest of 1 lemon, and lemon juice. Gradually add confectioners' sugar. Spread on top of cooled carrot cake. Sprinkle remaining lemon zest on top of cake.

Per Serving   Calories: 974 | Fat: 42g | Protein: 9g | Sodium: 238mg | Fiber: 4g | Carbohydrates: 146g | Sugar: 112g

Banana Coconut Nice Cream

Enjoy ice cream without heavy cream, milk, or tablespoons of sugar.

INGREDIENTS | SERVES 1

1 ripe medium banana, frozen with skin on

¼ teaspoon ground cinnamon

½ teaspoon shredded unsweetened coconut

1 tablespoon unsweetened almond milk

Remove peel from banana. Place banana and remaining ingredients in a blender or food processor and blend until smooth. Enjoy immediately!

Per Serving Calories: 117 | Fat: 1g | Protein: 2g | Sodium: 9mg | Fiber: 4g | Carbohydrates: 28g | Sugar: 15g

Banana Cookie Dough Nice Cream

Banana Nice Cream can be made so many different ways—just choose low-FODMAP ingredients and stick to suitable servings.

INGREDIENTS | SERVES 1

1 ripe medium banana, frozen with skin on

¼ teaspoon ground cinnamon

½ teaspoon shredded unsweetened coconut

1 tablespoon chocolate chip cookie dough (see Chocolate Chip Cookies recipe, Chapter 11), frozen

1. Remove peel from banana. Place banana, cinnamon, and coconut in blender and blend until smooth.

2. Cut frozen dough into chunks and stir into nice cream. Enjoy immediately!

Per Serving Calories: 109 | Fat: 1g | Protein: 1g | Sodium: 1mg | Fiber: 3g | Carbohydrates: 28g | Sugar: 14g

Banana Almond Nice Cream

Take that jar of almond butter out of your pantry and use it for this nice cream recipe!

INGREDIENTS | SERVES 1

1 ripe medium banana, frozen with skin on

½ cup unsweetened almond milk

1 tablespoon almond butter

Remove peel from banana. Place banana and remaining ingredients in a blender or food processor and blend until smooth. Enjoy immediately!

Per Serving   Calories: 265 | Fat: 11g | Protein: 9g | Sodium: 137mg | Fiber: 5g | Carbohydrates: 38g | Sugar: 21g

What Other Milk Alternatives May I Use?

For any nice cream recipes featured in this book you can use hemp milk or soy milk made from soy protein, up to 1 cup per serving.

Peanut Butter Chocolate Mug Cake

When you have a craving for peanut butter and chocolate, try this recipe and feed your craving in less than 5 minutes.

INGREDIENTS | SERVES 1

2 tablespoons gluten-free all-purpose flour

2 tablespoons unsweetened almond milk

1 tablespoon maple syrup

2 tablespoons natural, smooth peanut butter

¼ teaspoon gluten-free baking powder

¼ teaspoon ground nutmeg

¼ teaspoon ground cinnamon

½ teaspoon alcohol-free vanilla extract

1 tablespoon dark chocolate chips

1. Add all ingredients except chocolate chips to a microwave-safe mug and stir well until combined.

2. Place in microwave 1–2 minutes. Microwave ovens vary so check every 30 seconds. Once cake rises, your mug cake is ready. Top with chocolate chips.

Per Serving   Calories: 377 | Fat: 20g | Protein: 11g | Sodium: 289mg | Fiber: 4g | Carbohydrates: 42g | Sugar: 22g

Pumpkin Pie Mug Cake

Mug cakes are a fun way to enjoy cake on the fly! The possibilities in flavors are endless.

INGREDIENTS | SERVES 1

⅓ cup pumpkin purée

1 large egg

1 tablespoon lactose-free milk

½ teaspoon alcohol-free vanilla extract

2 tablespoons light brown sugar

1 teaspoon pumpkin pie spice

⅛ teaspoon salt

2 small gluten-free graham crackers, crushed

¼ cup Coconut Whipped Cream (see recipe in this chapter)

1 tablespoon crushed walnuts

1. In a small bowl, whisk together pumpkin, egg, milk, vanilla, sugar, pumpkin pie spice, and salt. Whisk until smooth.

2. In a microwavable mug, add crushed grahams and press down on bottom of mug. Pour in pumpkin pie mix.

3. Microwave 1½–2 minutes. Microwave ovens vary so check every 30 seconds to ensure mixture is not bubbling over.

4. Carefully remove mug from microwave. Let stand 1–2 minutes to cool.

5. Serve topped with whipped cream and walnuts.

Per Serving   Calories: 537 | Fat: 22g | Protein: 10g | Sodium: 420mg | Fiber: 3g | Carbohydrates: 76g | Sugar: 69g

Pumpkin Spice Pecan Cornbread

This cornbread is great for the holidays or any cold and wintry night.
Serve this bread hot from the oven with a dab of butter.

INGREDIENTS | SERVES 10

1 cup yellow cornmeal

½ cup brown rice flour

½ cup cornstarch

1 tablespoon gluten-free baking powder

½ teaspoon salt

⅛ cup packed light brown sugar

½ teaspoon ground cinnamon

½ teaspoon ground nutmeg

1 cup coarsely chopped pecans

2 large eggs

⅓ cup safflower oil

1 cup unsweetened canned coconut milk

1 cup pumpkin purée

1. Preheat oven to 400°F.

2. Grease an 8" × 8" glass baking dish. Place baking dish in oven as it preheats.

3. In a mixing bowl, whisk together dry ingredients to blend. Add eggs, oil, milk, and pumpkin purée; stir until batter achieves a smooth consistency.

4. Carefully remove baking dish from oven and pour batter into dish.

5. Bake 20–25 minutes or until corn bread is golden brown on top and deep golden brown around the edges. Cut into squares and serve.

Per Serving   Calories: 308 | Fat: 21g | Protein: 5g | Sodium: 138mg | Fiber: 3g | Carbohydrates: 27g | Sugar: 4g

CHAPTER 13

Condiments, Sauces, and Dressings

Raspberry Lemon Chia
Seed Jam
246

Blueberry Chia
Seed Jam
246

Strawberry Chia
Seed Jam
247

Basic Mayonnaise
247

Sweet Barbecue Sauce
248

Artisanal Ketchup
248

Aioli
249

Basil Sauce
249

Tomato Purée
250

Burger Sauce
250

Tomato Paste
251

Roasted Tomato Sauce
251

Basic Marinara Sauce
252

Pesto Sauce
253

Dill Dipping Sauce
253

Tartar Sauce
254

Chermoula
254

Red Curry Paste
255

Clever Curry
Mayonnaise
255

Sweet Chili
Garlic Sauce
256

Tzatziki Dressing
257

Pumpkin Maple Glaze
257

Maple Dressing
258

Maple Mustard
Dressing
258

Tahini Dressing
259

Pumpkin Seed
Dressing
259

Garlic Turmeric
Dressing
260

Caesar Salad Dressing
260

Ginger Sesame Salad
Dressing
261

Pomegranate Salsa
261

Fiesta Salsa
262

Thai Peanut Dressing
263

Simple Brown Syrup
263

Raspberry Lemon Chia Seed Jam

This jam is delicious on a warm scone, on gluten-free toast with butter, or mixed into a tub of lactose-free yogurt.

INGREDIENTS | MAKES 1 CUP

½ pint (or 6 ounces) fresh raspberries
1 tablespoon lemon juice
1 tablespoon lemon zest
2½ tablespoons pure maple syrup
1 tablespoon chia seeds

1. Add fruit, lemon juice, lemon zest, and maple syrup to a small saucepan and cook over medium-high heat. Cover. Stir occasionally until fruit begins to thicken, about 10 minutes.

2. Uncover and bring mixture to a boil until it develops a sauce-like consistency, about 5 minutes.

3. Stir in chia seeds and cook 2 more minutes. Stir again and then remove from heat.

4. Transfer jam to an airtight jar or other container and allow to cool, or refrigerate 2–3 hours before use. The jam will continue to thicken. Can be stored in refrigerator 2 weeks or frozen up to 2 months.

Per Serving (2 tablespoons)   Calories: 32 | Fat: 1g | Protein: 1g | Sodium: 1mg | Fiber: 1g | Carbohydrates: 7g | Sugar: 5g

Blueberry Chia Seed Jam

This jam is delicious on a warm scone, a gluten-free muffin, or gluten-free toast with butter.

INGREDIENTS | MAKES 1 CUP

½ pint (or 6 ounces) fresh blueberries
1 tablespoon lemon juice
2½ tablespoons pure maple syrup
1 tablespoon chia seeds

1. Add fruit, lemon juice, and maple syrup to a small saucepan and cook over medium-high heat. Cover. Stir occasionally until fruit begins to thicken, about 10 minutes.

2. Uncover and bring mixture to a boil until it develops a sauce-like consistency, about 5 minutes.

3. Stir in chia seeds and cook 2 more minutes. Stir again and then remove from heat.

4. Transfer jam to an airtight jar or other container and allow to cool, or refrigerate 2–3 hours before use. The jam will continue to thicken. Can be stored in refrigerator 2 weeks or frozen up to 2 months.

Per Serving (2 tablespoons)   Calories: 34 | Fat: 1g | Protein: 0g | Sodium: 1mg | Fiber: 1g | Carbohydrates: 7g | Sugar: 6g

Strawberry Chia Seed Jam

This jam is delicious on PB and J Kebabs (see recipe in Chapter 10),
a warm scone, a gluten-free muffin, or gluten-free toast with butter.

INGREDIENTS | MAKES 1 CUP

½ pint (or 6 ounces) fresh strawberries

1 tablespoon lemon juice

2½ tablespoons pure maple syrup

1 tablespoon chia seeds

1. Add fruit, lemon juice, and maple syrup to a small saucepan and cook over medium-high heat. Cover. Stir occasionally until fruit begins to thicken, about 10 minutes.

2. Uncover and bring mixture to a boil until it develops a sauce-like consistency, about 5 minutes.

3. Stir in chia seeds and cook 2 more minutes. Stir again and then remove from heat.

4. Transfer jam to an airtight jar or other container and allow to cool, or refrigerate 2–3 hours before use. The jam will continue to thicken. Can be stored in refrigerator 2 weeks or frozen up to 2 months.

Per Serving (2 tablespoons) Calories: 26 | Fat: 0g | Protein: 0g | Sodium: 2mg | Fiber: 1g | Carbohydrates: 6g | Sugar: 5g

Basic Mayonnaise

It can sometimes be hard to find mayonnaise that is low-FODMAP,
but it's easy to make your own at home.

INGREDIENTS | MAKES 2 CUPS

2 large eggs

2 tablespoons Dijon mustard

1⅓ cups safflower or sunflower oil

2 tablespoons freshly squeezed lemon juice

¼ teaspoon salt

¼ teaspoon freshly ground black pepper

1. Use a food processor fitted with a blade attachment to combine eggs and mustard. Process until evenly combined.

2. Keep food processor running and add oil in a slow stream until completely combined.

3. Add lemon juice, salt, and pepper and pulse until smooth. If storing, place in a jar or container with a tight-fitting lid in refrigerator up to 3 days.

Per Serving (1 tablespoon) Calories: 86 | Fat: 9g | Protein: 0g | Sodium: 34mg | Fiber: 0g | Carbohydrates: 0g | Sugar: 0g

Sweet Barbecue Sauce

In this recipe you can use specialty ingredients such as smoked sea salt or smoked paprika to suit a preference for a smokier barbecue sauce flavor.

INGREDIENTS | MAKES 1 CUP

1 cup Tomato Purée (see recipe in this chapter)

1 tablespoon Dijon mustard

1 tablespoon blackstrap molasses

1½ tablespoons pure maple syrup

½ teaspoon ground cinnamon

½ teaspoon ground cumin

½ teaspoon dried oregano

½ teaspoon white wine vinegar

½ teaspoon arrowroot powder

½ teaspoon paprika

⅛ teaspoon ground red pepper

⅛ teaspoon ground nutmeg

⅛ teaspoon sea salt

Bring all ingredients just to a boil in a small saucepan over medium-high heat. Lower heat and simmer, uncovered, 5–10 minutes or until sauce thickens.

Per Serving (2 tablespoons) Calories: 25 | Fat: 0g | Protein: 1g | Sodium: 100mg | Fiber: 1g | Carbohydrates: 6g | Sugar: 5g

Artisanal Ketchup

The best thing about making your own ketchup is that you can flavor it to suit your dishes and taste preferences. This recipe features a sweet and savory spice blend, but you can substitute thyme and bay leaf for the spices in this recipe to achieve a woodsier effect.

INGREDIENTS | MAKES ¾ CUP

¾ cup Tomato Paste (see recipe in this chapter)

1 tablespoon white wine vinegar

1 tablespoon Simple Brown Syrup (see recipe in this chapter)

¼ teaspoon dried oregano

⅛ teaspoon ground cumin

⅛ teaspoon ground cinnamon

Water (as needed)

Blend all ingredients in a food processor, adding water ¼ cup at a time until desired consistency is achieved.

Per Serving (2 tablespoons) Calories: 53 | Fat: 2g | Protein: 1g | Sodium: 55mg | Fiber: 1g | Carbohydrates: 8g | Sugar: 6g

Aioli

This aioli tastes delicious spread on sandwiches, burgers, or used as a dip for appetizers.

INGREDIENTS | MAKES 1¼ CUPS

1 teaspoon Dijon mustard
1 large egg
¼ cup garlic-infused olive oil
¾ cup olive oil
2 teaspoons freshly squeezed lemon juice
¼ teaspoon kosher salt
⅛ teaspoon freshly ground black pepper

1. Place mustard and egg in the bowl of a food processor fitted with a blade attachment.

2. With the motor running, slowly add garlic-infused oil followed by olive oil until completely combined, about 2 minutes.

3. Stop processor; add lemon juice, salt, and pepper and pulse until thoroughly mixed. If necessary, stop and scrape down the sides of the bowl using a rubber spatula to get any extra aioli, then continue to pulse until well combined.

4. Let aioli sit 30 minutes before using. If storing, place in a container with a tight-fitting lid in refrigerator up to 3 days.

Per Serving (1 tablespoon)   Calories: 99 | Fat: 11g | Protein: 0g | Sodium: 36mg | Fiber: 0g | Carbohydrates: 0g | Sugar: 0g

Basil Sauce

Use this Basil Sauce on top of fish, chicken, or on Salmon Cakes (see recipe in Chapter 8).

INGREDIENTS | MAKES 1 CUP

¼ cup tahini
¼ cup fresh flat-leaf parsley leaves
¼ cup coarsely chopped fresh chives
1 packed cup fresh basil
Juice of 2 medium lemons
¼ cup olive oil
¼ teaspoon sea salt
¼ teaspoon freshly ground black pepper

Add all ingredients to a food processor. Blend until smooth. Store in an air-tight container in refrigerator for 5–7 days or in freezer for 3–4 months.

Per Serving (1 tablespoon)   Calories: 56 | Fat: 5g | Protein: 1g | Sodium: 42mg | Fiber: 1g | Carbohydrates: 2g | Sugar: 0g

Tomato Purée

Due to the concern about excessive fructose in canned tomato purée, it is a good idea to make your own. This is a basic recipe, but feel free to experiment with FODMAP-friendly seasonings such as basil, oregano, or parsley.

INGREDIENTS | MAKES 1½ CUPS

1 tablespoon garlic-infused olive oil

5 ripe medium tomatoes, cored, seeded, and diced

1 teaspoon sea salt

¼ teaspoon freshly ground black pepper

Canned Tomatoes and the Low-FODMAP Diet

Although tomatoes are allowed on the low-FODMAP diet, this does not mean that all tomato products are okay. Canned tomato paste and purée may have excessive levels of fructose. It is best to use fresh tomatoes or canned tomatoes with thin, watery juice.

1. Heat oil on medium-low in a large saucepan. Add tomatoes and stir. Season with salt and pepper. Sauté, stirring occasionally, 15–20 minutes or until tomatoes are soft and broken down. Remove from heat and let cool.

2. Transfer cooled tomatoes to a food processor and blend completely. Set a large strainer over a large bowl and strain mixture. Press down with a large spoon to completely separate solids in strainer from purée in bowl.

3. Transfer to an airtight container and store in refrigerator for 5–7 days or in freezer for 3–4 months.

Per Serving (¼ cup) Calories: 39 | Fat: 3g | Protein: 1g | Sodium: 398mg | Fiber: 1g | Carbohydrates: 4g | Sugar: 3g

Burger Sauce

Change up your burger and try this sauce instead!

INGREDIENTS | MAKES 1 CUP

2 tablespoons relish

½ cup Basic Mayonnaise (see recipe in this chapter)

¼ cup Artisanal Ketchup (see recipe in this chapter)

1 teaspoon paprika

1 tablespoon Dijon mustard

1 teaspoon freshly ground black pepper

1⁄16 teaspoon wheat-free asafetida powder

Stir together all ingredients in a medium bowl. Store in an air-tight container in refrigerator for up to 2 weeks.

Per Serving (1 tablespoon) Calories: 57 | Fat: 6g | Protein: 0g | Sodium: 113mg | Fiber: 0g | Carbohydrates: 2g | Sugar: 1g

Tomato Paste

Tomato paste is a pantry staple—used to thicken and flavor many tomato-based recipes. Store in an airtight container in the refrigerator up to 3 days or in the freezer for several months.

INGREDIENTS | MAKES ⅓ CUP

1½ cups Tomato Purée (see recipe in this chapter)

1. Preheat oven to 300°F. Pour purée into an ovenproof skillet.

2. Bake uncovered about 2 hours, stirring every 20 minutes until it reaches a paste-like consistency.

3. Let cool completely.

Per Serving (1 tablespoon) Calories: 46 | Fat: 3g | Protein: 1g | Sodium: 478mg | Fiber: 2g | Carbohydrates: 5g | Sugar: 3g

Roasted Tomato Sauce

This sauce makes a lovely summer supper served over gluten-free pasta. The more varieties of fresh, colorful tomatoes you use, the prettier this sauce gets.

INGREDIENTS | MAKES 2 CUPS

2 tablespoons garlic-infused olive oil
1 teaspoon salt
1½ pounds fresh tomatoes, cored, seeded, and diced
1 bay leaf
⅛ teaspoon crushed red pepper flakes

1. Preheat oven to 400°F. Line a roasting pan with parchment paper.

2. Place all ingredients in a medium bowl and toss to thoroughly combine. Transfer to roasting pan and spread tomatoes in a thin layer.

3. Roast 20 minutes, tossing halfway through. Remove and discard bay leaf. Transfer to a bowl and stir. Use immediately or transfer to an airtight container and store in the refrigerator for 3–4 days or in freezer for 5–6 months.

Per Serving (½ cup) Calories: 91 | Fat: 7g | Protein: 2g | Sodium: 598mg | Fiber: 2g | Carbohydrates: 7g | Sugar: 5g

Basic Marinara Sauce

If you've been following the low-FODMAP diet you know most marinara and pasta sauces are made with high FODMAPs such as onions and garlic. This sauce is a lifesaver!

INGREDIENTS | MAKES 4¼ CUPS

16 Roma tomatoes, chopped, or 1 (35-ounce) can San Marzano tomatoes

1 tablespoon garlic-infused olive oil

1 tablespoon plus 2 teaspoons extra-virgin olive oil

¼ teaspoon of red pepper flakes

1 teaspoon salt

20 leaves fresh basil, chopped

1. Add tomatoes to a large mixing bowl. Using your hands or a potato masher, crush the tomatoes and break up into small pieces.

2. Heat a 2-quart pot on medium-high. Pour both oils into pot and stir with red pepper flakes. Wait 1 minute and then add crushed tomatoes; stir well.

3. Increase heat to high and sprinkle in salt. Add basil and stir to combine.

4. Bring sauce to a boil and cover. Reduce heat to medium-high and cook 10–12 minutes, keeping sauce at a rolling simmer.

5. Uncover and cook another 5 minutes. Remove from heat. Use immediately or transfer to an airtight container and store in refrigerator for 3–4 days or in freezer for 5–6 months.

Per Serving (½ cup)   Calories: 59 | Fat: 5g | Protein: 1g | Sodium: 283mg | Fiber: 1g | Carbohydrates: 5g | Sugar: 3g

Pesto Sauce

Minus the high FODMAPs, this pesto is still delicious.
Use it in pasta, salads, and sandwiches or mix it with brown rice and top with an egg, sunny-side up.

INGREDIENTS | MAKES 1⅛ CUPS

¾ packed cup fresh basil leaves
⅛ cup garlic-infused olive oil
¼ cup pine nuts
⅛ cup extra-virgin olive oil
½ cup freshly grated Parmesan cheese
⅛ teaspoon sea salt
⅛ teaspoon freshly ground black pepper

1. Combine basil, garlic oil, and pine nuts in a food processor and pulse until coarsely chopped.

2. Add extra-virgin olive oil, cheese, salt, and pepper and process until fully incorporated and smooth. Use immediately or transfer to an airtight container and store in refrigerator for 4–5 days or in freezer for 1–2 months.

Per Serving (2 tablespoons) Calories: 142 | Fat: 13g | Protein: 5g | Sodium: 237mg | Fiber: 1g | Carbohydrates: 2g | Sugar: 0g

Dill Dipping Sauce

This sauce is great on fish as well as gluten-free fried appetizers.
Serve with homemade chicken fingers or gluten-free sweet potato fries.

INGREDIENTS | MAKES ¾ CUP

3 tablespoons chopped fresh dill
1 tablespoon lemon juice
7 ounces lactose-free sour cream
¼ teaspoon salt

In a food processor combine all ingredients and process until smooth. Use immediately or transfer to an airtight container and store in refrigerator for 3–4 days.

Per Serving (2 tablespoons) Calories: 64 | Fat: 7g | Protein: 1g | Sodium: 125mg | Fiber: 0g | Carbohydrates: 1g | Sugar: 1g

Tartar Sauce

This low-FODMAP sauce pairs well with some fish and seafood recipes in Chapter 8.

INGREDIENTS | MAKES ½ CUP

3 tablespoons Basic Mayonnaise (see recipe in this chapter)

3 tablespoons lactose-free plain yogurt

1/16 teaspoon wheat-free asafetida powder

1 tablespoon relish

1 teaspoon granulated sugar

Add all ingredients to a small bowl. Stir well with a spoon. If storing, place in a container with a tight-fitting lid in refrigerator up to 3 days.

Per Serving (1 tablespoon) Calories: 44 | Fat: 4g | Protein: 0g | Sodium: 53mg | Fiber: 0g | Carbohydrates: 1g | Sugar: 1g

Chermoula

You can find Chermoula used in a variety of cuisines including Algerian, Libyan, Moroccan, and Tunisian. It is usually used to flavor fish or seafood, but it can be used on other meats or vegetables.

INGREDIENTS | MAKES 1 CUP

1 teaspoon coriander seeds

2 cups fresh cilantro leaves

1½ cups fresh flat-leaf parsley leaves

½ teaspoon salt

1 teaspoon paprika

½ teaspoon ground cumin

⅛ teaspoon saffron

⅛ teaspoon cayenne pepper

¼ cup freshly squeezed lemon juice

⅓ cup garlic-infused olive oil

1. Prepare coriander seeds: Put seeds in a small dry skillet and set over medium heat 3–4 minutes or until fragrant. Grind seeds in a mortar and pestle until fine. Set aside.

2. Place cilantro and parsley in a food processor fitted with a steel blade. Pulse until finely chopped. Add ground coriander, salt, paprika, cumin, saffron, cayenne, and lemon juice. Pulse to combine.

3. Continue running food processor and slowly pour in oil through feed tube. Pulse to combine.

4. Use immediately or store in an airtight container in refrigerator up to 2 days.

Per Serving (2 tablespoons) Calories: 88 | Fat: 9g | Protein: 1g | Sodium: 158mg | Fiber: 1g | Carbohydrates: 2g | Sugar: 1g

Red Curry Paste

This garlic-free recipe makes it easy for you to enjoy your own homemade curry dishes and other Asian meals at home.

INGREDIENTS | MAKES ¼ CUP

4 dried red chilies

¼ teaspoon ground cumin

3 green onions, green part only, chopped

1 tablespoon garlic-infused olive oil

1 tablespoon chopped fresh gingerroot

1 teaspoon lemon juice

Juice of 1 medium lime

Zest of ½ medium kaffir lime

2 teaspoons ground coriander

½ teaspoon white pepper

4 teaspoons gluten-free fish sauce

½ teaspoon shrimp paste

½ teaspoon salt

Place all ingredients in a food processor and grind to a smooth consistency. Store in an air-tight container in the refrigerator for 2–3 months.

Per Serving (1 tablespoon) Calories: 65 | Fat: 4g | Protein: 2g | Sodium: 765mg | Fiber: 2g | Carbohydrates: 9g | Sugar: 4g

Clever Curry Mayonnaise

This recipe is very simple if you have low-FODMAP mayonnaise handy. It's great on beef, chicken, or turkey burgers or as a dipping sauce.

INGREDIENTS | MAKES 1 CUP

1 cup Basic Mayonnaise (see recipe in this chapter)

2 teaspoons curry powder (without onions or garlic)

½ tablespoon fresh lime juice

½ tablespoon fresh lemon juice

⅛ teaspoon cayenne pepper

⅛ teaspoon paprika

Place all ingredients in a food processor and pulse to a smooth consistency. If storing, place in a container with a tight-fitting lid in refrigerator up to 3 days.

Per Serving (1 tablespoon) Calories: 100 | Fat: 11g | Protein: 0g | Sodium: 79mg | Fiber: 0g | Carbohydrates: 1g | Sugar: 0g

Sweet Chili Garlic Sauce

Use this sauce for Coconut Shrimp with Pineapple Sauce (see recipe in Chapter 3), on top of salmon, in stir fry, as a sauce for a Thai-inspired pizza, or use as a dipping sauce with panko-crusted chicken.

INGREDIENTS | MAKES 2½ CUPS

1 pound fresh chili peppers, ends trimmed

1/16 teaspoon wheat-free asafetida powder

2 tablespoons safflower oil or other cooking oil

¼ cup rice wine vinegar

¼ cup brown sugar

¼ cup gluten-free fish sauce

1. In a food processor add in chili peppers and asafetida powder. Process until minced.

2. In a medium sauté pan heat oil until shimmering on medium-high heat. Add in chili pepper mixture and cook 1 minute. Add in vinegar, sugar, and fish sauce and stir to combine. Turn heat to low and cook 25 minutes.

3. Before removing from heat taste sauce to see if you'd like it sweeter (add 1 tablespoon or more of brown sugar), saltier (add 1 tablespoon or more of fish sauce) or tangier (add 1 tablespoon or more of vinegar). Pour in an air-tight container or canning jar and store in pantry for 1 month or in refrigerator for up to 6 months.

Per Serving (½ cup) Calories: 133 | Fat: 6g | Protein: 2g | Sodium: 1,129mg | Fiber: 1g | Carbohydrates: 19g | Sugar: 16g

Tzatziki Dressing

This smooth dressing can be drizzled over grilled meats, fish, or salads. It captures the flavors and nutrients of traditional tzatziki sauce. Even garlic plays a role via infused oil.

INGREDIENTS | MAKES 1 CUP

½ medium cucumber, seeded and diced

½ cup lactose-free plain yogurt

1 teaspoon garlic-infused olive oil

1 tablespoon freshly squeezed lemon juice

1 tablespoon chopped fresh dill

Place all ingredients in a blender and process until smooth. Store in an air-tight container in the refrigerator for up to 2 days.

Per Serving (¼ cup)   Calories: 35 | Fat: 2g | Protein: 1g | Sodium: 16mg | Fiber: 0g | Carbohydrates: 3g | Sugar: 2g

Pumpkin Maple Glaze

It doesn't have to be fall for you to dazzle your family or guests as you dress up your carved roast chicken with this fast, delicious autumnal glaze.

INGREDIENTS | MAKES ½ CUP

2 tablespoons butter

¼ cup hulled pumpkin seeds

⅛ teaspoon sea salt

3 tablespoons pure maple syrup, divided

1 tablespoon Dijon mustard

1. Melt butter in a small saucepan over medium heat and set aside.

2. Preheat broiler. Spread pumpkin seeds on a lined baking sheet. Drizzle 1 tablespoon melted butter over pumpkin seeds. Sprinkle on salt. Toss seeds to coat. Broil 1–2 minutes or until seeds start to brown lightly. Remove from oven. Move seeds to serving dish and mix in 1 tablespoon maple syrup.

3. Return saucepan that contains the remaining tablespoon butter to cooktop. Over medium heat, add remaining maple syrup and mustard. Bring just to a boil, then lower heat and simmer, uncovered, 1–2 minutes more to thicken.

4. The glaze and roasted seeds can be used to top any roasted poultry.

Per Serving (1 tablespoon)   Calories: 71 | Fat: 5g | Protein: 1g | Sodium: 60mg | Fiber: 0g | Carbohydrates: 6g | Sugar: 5g

Maple Dressing

When making your own dressings at home, maple syrup, rice wine vinegar, and extra-virgin olive oil can actually be a great base for different varieties. Experiment!

INGREDIENTS | MAKES ⅜ CUP

2 tablespoons pure maple syrup

2 tablespoons rice wine vinegar

2 tablespoons extra-virgin olive oil

Combine all ingredients in a bowl or glass condiment jar and stir until completely combined. Store in an air-tight container at room temperature for 1–2 weeks.

Per Serving (2 tablespoons)   Calories: 51 | Fat: 5g | Protein: 0g | Sodium: 1mg | Fiber: 0g | Carbohydrates: 3g | Sugar: 3g

Maple Mustard Dressing

This dressing tastes divine on salad, chicken, or as a dip.

INGREDIENTS | MAKES 1⅛ CUPS

½ cup Dijon mustard

½ cup maple syrup

1¼ tablespoons rice wine vinegar

¼ teaspoon salt

Combine all ingredients in a small bowl or glass condiment jar and stir until completely combined. Store in an air-tight container at room temperature for 1–2 weeks.

Per Serving (2 tablespoons)   Calories: 56 | Fat: 1g | Protein: 1g | Sodium: 225mg | Fiber: 0g | Carbohydrates: 13g | Sugar: 11g

Tahini Dressing

This nutty dressing pairs well with Lemon Kale Salad (see recipe in Chapter 4).

INGREDIENTS | MAKES ABOUT ¾ CUP

¼ cup tahini

¼ cup water

2 tablespoons fresh lemon juice

1 tablespoon maple syrup

¼ teaspoon pink Himalayan salt

¼ teaspoon freshly ground black pepper

Combine all ingredients in a blender or food processor. Store in an air-tight container at room temperature for 1–2 weeks.

Per Serving (2 tablespoons)   Calories: 70 | Fat: 5g | Protein: 2g | Sodium: 111mg | Fiber: 1g | Carbohydrates: 5g | Sugar: 2g

Pumpkin Seed Dressing

Pour this dressing over salad, grains, or fish.

INGREDIENTS | MAKES ½ CUP

¼ cup hulled green pumpkin seeds

1/16 teaspoon wheat-free asafetida powder

1/8 cup extra-virgin olive oil

1/8 cup water

1 tablespoon fresh lemon juice

¼ teaspoon salt

1 tablespoon finely chopped fresh cilantro

1. Toast pumpkin seeds in a small skillet over medium heat, stirring frequently until just about browned, about 5 minutes.

2. Transfer to a plate to cool 2–3 minutes.

3. Purée seeds in a blender with remaining ingredients. Blend until smooth. Store in an air-tight container in refrigerator for 1–2 weeks.

Per Serving (2 tablespoons)   Calories: 109 | Fat: 11g | Protein: 3g | Sodium: 157mg | Fiber: 1g | Carbohydrates: 1g | Sugar: 0g

Garlic Turmeric Dressing

This earthy dressing has a taste of garlic from the asafetida powder and a bit of healthy turmeric, which has been used in Ayurvedic and traditional Chinese medicine for its many health benefits.

INGREDIENTS | MAKES ABOUT ¾ CUP

¼ cup tahini

3 tablespoons fresh lemon juice

2 tablespoons fresh orange juice

1 tablespoon extra virgin olive oil

1 tablespoon garlic-infused olive oil

½ teaspoon ground turmeric

¼ teaspoon paprika

Pinch kosher salt

½ teaspoon freshly ground black pepper

In a small blender or food processer blend all ingredients until completely combined. Store in an air-tight container in refrigerator for 3–4 weeks.

Per Serving (2 tablespoons) Calories: 105 | Fat: 10g | Protein: 2g | Sodium: 406mg | Fiber: 1g | Carbohydrates: 4g | Sugar: 1g

Caesar Salad Dressing

All hail Caesar! It's Caesar Salad Dressing, the low-FODMAP way.

INGREDIENTS | MAKES 1½ CUPS

6 anchovy fillets packed in oil, drained and chopped

¹⁄₁₆ teaspoon wheat-free asafetida powder

2 large egg yolks

2 tablespoons fresh lemon juice

¾ teaspoon Dijon mustard

2 tablespoons garlic-infused olive oil

½ cup extra virgin olive oil

3 tablespoons finely grated Parmesan cheese

¼ teaspoon kosher salt

1 teaspoon freshly ground black pepper

1. In a small bowl, mash anchovies and asafetida into a paste, then place in a medium bowl.

2. Whisk in egg yolks, lemon juice, and mustard. Slowly whisk in garlic-infused oil and then olive oil.

3. Whisk in Parmesan, salt, and pepper. Store in an air-tight container in refrigerator for 3–4 days.

Per Serving (2 tablespoons) Calories: 74 | Fat: 7g | Protein: 3g | Sodium: 306mg | Fiber: 0g | Carbohydrates: 1g | Sugar: 0g

Ginger Sesame Salad Dressing

Dress tofu with this dressing or use it for any Asian-inspired salad or to top vegetables in collard green wraps.

INGREDIENTS | MAKES 1 CUP

½ cup extra-virgin olive oil

¼ cup rice wine vinegar

2 tablespoons gluten-free soy sauce (tamari)

2 tablespoons demerara sugar

1 teaspoon sesame oil

1" piece fresh gingerroot, minced

Blend all ingredients in a blender or food processor until smooth. Dressing can be stored 1 week in refrigerator. Bring to room temperature before serving.

Per Serving (2 tablespoons) Calories: 141 | Fat: 14g | Protein: 0g | Sodium: 226mg | Fiber: 0g | Carbohydrates: 4g | Sugar: 3g

Pomegranate Salsa

Use this beautiful-looking and tasty salsa on fish, poultry, or scooped up with gluten-free tortilla chips.

INGREDIENTS | MAKES 4 CUPS

1⅓ cups diced cucumber

2½ cups pomegranate seeds

¼–⅓ cup finely chopped cilantro

Juice of ½ medium lime

1 tablespoon maple syrup

2 tablespoons slivered almonds

⅛ teaspoon sea salt

1. Add cucumber and pomegranate to a medium serving bowl.

2. Combine cilantro, lime juice, maple syrup, almonds, and salt in a small bowl; stir to combine.

3. Add to bowl with cucumber and pomegranate and toss gently to combine.

Per Serving (1 cup) Calories: 32 | Fat: 1g | Protein: 1g | Sodium: 20mg | Fiber: 1g | Carbohydrates: 7g | Sugar: 5g

Fiesta Salsa

Use this salsa as a dip for tortilla chips or nachos, mix it with mayonnaise for a bold kick, stir into scrambled eggs, or use it with Mexican Egg Brunch (see recipe in Chapter 2).

INGREDIENTS | SERVES 6

1 (10-ounce) can diced tomatoes, drained

1 (14.5-ounce) can diced tomatoes with green chilies

1 tablespoon garlic-infused extra-virgin olive oil

¼ cup chopped green onions, green part only

¼ cup chopped fresh cilantro

¼ cup chopped fresh flat-leaf parsley

⅛ teaspoon wheat-free asafetida powder

¼ teaspoon ground cumin

¼ teaspoon coriander

¼ teaspoon dried oregano

¼ teaspoon smoked paprika

¼ teaspoon sea salt

½ teaspoon freshly ground black pepper

Juice of 1 medium lime

Add all ingredients to a medium serving bowl. Stir well to combine. Store in an airtight container in refrigerator 5–7 days.

Per Serving Calories: 46 | Fat: 3g | Protein: 1g | Sodium: 265mg | Fiber: 2g | Carbohydrates: 6g | Sugar: 3g

Important Tip!

When shopping for canned tomatoes, especially made with chilies, make sure the ingredients do not include high FODMAPs such as onions, garlic, onion powder, or garlic powder.

Thai Peanut Dressing

Use this dressing in Collard Green Wraps with Thai Peanut Dressing (see recipe in Chapter 9) or add to salads, other wraps, and sandwiches.

INGREDIENTS | MAKES ABOUT 1 CUP

¼ cup natural creamy peanut butter

2 tablespoons rice wine vinegar

Juice from 1 medium lime

1 tablespoon gluten-free soy sauce (tamari)

2 tablespoons maple syrup

2½ tablespoons light brown sugar

1/16 teaspoon wheat-free asafetida powder

1½ tablespoons grated fresh gingerroot

1 teaspoon Himalayan salt

¼ teaspoon chili powder

Place all ingredients in a food processor and pulse until combined. Store in an air-tight container in refrigerator for up to 3 days.

Per Serving (2 tablespoons) Calories: 82 | Fat: 4g | Protein: 2g | Sodium: 447mg | Fiber: 1g | Carbohydrates: 11g | Sugar: 1g

Simple Brown Syrup

You can experiment with the thickness and flavor of this sweet liquid beverage base by varying the sugar-to-water ratio. Using demerara or muscovado sugar will intensify the flavor.

INGREDIENTS | MAKES 1½ CUPS

1 cup turbinado sugar

1 cup filtered water

Heat sugar and water in a saucepan over low heat, stirring often, just until crystals dissolve. Remove from heat and bring to room temperature or cool before using.

Per Serving (1 teaspoon) Calories: 28 | Fat: 0g | Protein: 0g | Sodium: 1mg | Fiber: 0g | Carbohydrates: 5g | Sugar: 4g

CHAPTER 14

Snacks

Gluten-Free Cinnamon and
Sugar Soft Pretzels
266

Kale Chips
267

Coconut Cinnamon Popcorn
267

Chocolate Chip Energy Bites
268

Roasted Pumpkin Seeds
269

Roasted Pumpkin Seeds with
Cinnamon and Sugar
269

Dark Chocolate–Covered
Pretzels
270

Banana Nut Boat
270

Gluten-Free Cinnamon and Sugar Soft Pretzels

Get the whole family together and make these chewy, buttery, and slightly sweet pretzels.

INGREDIENTS | SERVES 8

2½ cups gluten-free all-purpose flour, plus extra for dusting

1 teaspoon salt

1 teaspoon turbinado sugar

2¼ teaspoons instant yeast

1 cup boiling water

2 tablespoons baking soda

2 tablespoons light brown sugar

1 tablespoon ground cinnamon

3 tablespoons unsalted butter, melted

1. Add flour, salt, turbinado sugar, and yeast to the bowl of a stand mixer and beat until well combined. Knead dough with flat beater attachment 5 minutes (or if you don't have a beater attachment, knead dough by hand). Knead until dough is soft and smooth. Sprinkle flour on dough and place in a bag or wrap in plastic wrap; allow to rest for 1 hour until dough is doubled in size.

2. While dough is resting, combine boiling water and baking soda in a medium bowl, stirring until soda is almost completely dissolved. Set aside.

3. Once dough is close to finally rising, preheat oven to 475°F. Coat a baking sheet with cooking spray.

4. Lightly grease a clean work surface with coconut oil, olive oil, or butter. Divide dough into 8 equal pieces. Allow pieces to rest 5 minutes.

5. Pour baking soda mixture into a 9" square pan.

6. On your work surface, roll a piece of dough into a long, thin rope (about 28" long) and twist rope into a pretzel by crossing ends, twisting once, and bringing twisted ends up to rest on top of pretzel. Repeat with remaining dough to make 8 large pretzels.

7. Take half of pretzels and place them in pan with baking soda mixture. Use a spoon to splash water over tops; allow to rest in water 2 minutes (no longer) before placing on baking sheet. Repeat with remaining 4 pretzels.

8. Transfer pretzels to prepared baking sheet and allow to rest 5 minutes.

9. In a small bowl, mix together brown sugar, cinnamon, and butter. Heat in microwave until butter is melted; 20 seconds or more depending on microwave. Stir to combine.

10. Brush pretzels thoroughly with melted butter mixture. Be sure to coat pretzels entirely, otherwise white spots from dough will show. Spreading enough butter allows for a beautiful and tasty pretzel!

11. Bake pretzels 8–9 minutes or until golden brown. Serve immediately.

Per Serving Calories: 200 | Fat: 5g | Protein: 5g | Sodium: 1,302mg | Fiber: 2g | Carbohydrates: 35g | Sugar: 4g

Kale Chips

There's no need to buy expensive kale chips from the store when you can make your own earthy and delicious version. Kale chips may have an anti-inflammatory effect on IBS symptoms or other causes for inflammation, so munch away!

INGREDIENTS | SERVES 4

1 large bunch curly kale, torn into bite-sized pieces (stems removed)
2 tablespoons olive oil
¼ teaspoon ground turmeric
½ teaspoon curry powder
½ teaspoon chili powder
½ teaspoon ground cumin
⅛ teaspoon coarse salt

1. Preheat oven to 350°F. Line 2 baking sheets with parchment paper.

2. Put kale in a large bowl and drizzle with oil. Add turmeric, curry powder, chili powder, and cumin. Massage kale until evenly coated. Add more oil if all pieces are still not evenly coated.

3. Spread kale pieces in a single layer on baking sheets and sprinkle with salt.

4. Bake 16 minutes, rotating pans after first 8 minutes. Bake until crispy but not burning. Serve immediately.

Per Serving Calories: 66 | Fat: 7g | Protein: 0g | Sodium: 81mg | Fiber: 0g | Carbohydrates: 1g | Sugar: 0g

Coconut Cinnamon Popcorn

When made the right way, popcorn can be very healthy and it also has 3.6 grams of fiber per ounce. It can also help relieve constipation! Try this recipe on your next movie night.

INGREDIENTS | SERVES 2

2 tablespoons coconut oil
½ tablespoon ground cinnamon
4 cups freshly popped natural popcorn (or 3 tablespoons popcorn kernels)

Choosing the Right Popcorn

When choosing microwavable popcorn, choose a brand that does not include anything other than popcorn kernels. Stay away from brands that use added salt, diacetyl (a synthetic butter flavoring) or other artificial flavorings, partially hydrogenated soybean oil, TBHQ (tertiary butylhydroquinone, a fat preservative), and propyl gallate (an artificial food additive).

1. Add coconut oil and cinnamon to a microwave-safe measuring cup. Microwave 30 seconds or until coconut oil has melted. Stir to combine.

2. If making microwavable popcorn, carefully pour coconut and cinnamon mixture into bag, then shake well. If making popcorn in a pot on the stove, once popcorn has popped, remove pot from stove and add oil mixture to popcorn as you shake pot back and forth.

Per Serving Calories: 186 | Fat: 14g | Protein: 2g | Sodium: 1mg | Fiber: 3g | Carbohydrates: 14g | Sugar: 0g

Chocolate Chip Energy Bites

When you need a little bit of energy on an active day, try these energy bites.

INGREDIENTS | MAKES 24

½ cup gluten-free oat bran
½ cup almond butter
⅓ cup maple syrup
1½ cups gluten-free quick-cooking oats
¼ cup pumpkin seeds
¼ cup dark chocolate chips
¼ cup no-sugar-added dried cranberries
¼ cup ground walnuts

1. Preheat oven to 375°F.

2. Add oat bran to a baking sheet and toast 5–7 minutes or until lightly brown.

3. Using a handheld or stand mixer, mix together almond butter and maple syrup on low speed until well combined.

4. Gradually add oats until combined, and then add pumpkin seeds, chocolate chips, cranberries, and walnuts. Mix until well combined.

5. Line a baking sheet with parchment paper.

6. Break up mixture into 24 even pieces. Gently roll each into a ball.

7. Roll balls in toasted oat bran. Refrigerate 2 hours to set or consume immediately. Can be stored in a freezer bag in freezer up to 2 weeks.

Per Serving   Calories: 95 | Fat: 5g | Protein: 3g | Sodium: 26mg | Fiber: 1g | Carbohydrates: 11g | Sugar: 5g

Roasted Pumpkin Seeds

When making pumpkin, don't throw away the seeds. Use them for roasting—so delish!

INGREDIENTS | SERVES 1 CUP

1 cup pumpkin seeds, rinsed and dried
1 tablespoon olive oil
½ teaspoon salt

1. Preheat oven to 300°F. Line a rimmed baking sheet with parchment paper.

2. In a medium bowl, toss together all ingredients. Spread mixture in a single layer on baking sheet.

3. Bake 50–60 minutes, stirring every 15 minutes until seeds are crisp. Let cool completely before serving. Store at room temperature.

Per Serving   Calories: 101 | Fat: 6g | Protein: 3g | Sodium: 701mg | Fiber: 3g | Carbohydrates: 8g | Sugar: 0g

Roasted Pumpkin Seeds with Cinnamon and Sugar

Roasting seeds at home is very easy to do. Pumpkin seeds, whether roasted or raw, can be beneficial to health as they contain magnesium, zinc, protein, and healthy fiber.

INGREDIENTS | SERVES 6

2 cups pumpkin seeds, rinsed and dried
¼ cup butter, melted
1 tablespoon light brown sugar
½ teaspoon ground cinnamon
⅛ teaspoon salt
2 tablespoons turbinado sugar

1. Preheat oven to 350°F. Line a rimmed baking sheet with parchment paper.

2. Combine pumpkin seeds, butter, brown sugar, cinnamon, and salt in a small bowl; stir to coat seeds. Spread seeds in a single layer on baking sheet.

3. Bake 50–60 minutes, stirring every 15 minutes until seeds are crisp. After about 40 minutes of baking, stir in remaining sugar. Let cool completely before serving. Store at room temperature.

Per Serving   Calories: 351 | Fat: 30g | Protein: 14g | Sodium: 55mg | Fiber: 3g | Carbohydrates: 12g | Sugar: 7g

Dark Chocolate–Covered Pretzels

Who doesn't love chocolate-covered pretzels? Have these on hand when you need a sweet and salty fix.

INGREDIENTS | MAKES 12

3 ounces dark chocolate chips

1 tablespoon vegetable shortening

12 gluten-free mini pretzels

1. Melt chocolate and shortening over a double boiler. Stir until smooth and combined.

2. Remove from heat. Dip each pretzel in chocolate, allowing excess to drip off.

3. Place on a cookie sheet lined with wax paper and chill in refrigerator until firm.

Per Serving Calories: 66 | Fat: 3g | Protein: 1g | Sodium: 82mg | Fiber: 1g | Carbohydrates: 9g | Sugar: 4g

Banana Nut Boat

This is a great snack for adults or kids, and so many different low-FODMAP toppings can work with a delicious ripe banana boat as your canvas!

INGREDIENTS | SERVES 1

1 ripe medium banana, cut in half lengthwise

1 tablespoon almond butter

1 tablespoon shredded unsweetened coconut

1. Place banana cut side up on a plate or shallow dish.

2. Spread on almond butter.

3. Sprinkle with coconut.

Per Serving Calories: 217 | Fat: 10g | Protein: 5g | Sodium: 76mg | Fiber: 4g | Carbohydrates: 31g | Sugar: 16g

What Other Nut Butters Can I Use?

You can use other low-FODMAP nut butters such as peanut butter or allergen-friendly sunflower butter.

CHAPTER 15

Drinks

Warm Ginger Tea
272

Ginger Maple Tea
272

Cucumber Melon Water
273

Aloe Vera Rewind
273

Carrot Pineapple Ginger Juice
274

Strawberry Coconut Almond
Smoothie
274

Gut-Friendly Smoothie
275

Jeremy's Revival Smoothie
275

Blueberry Ginger Water
276

Paixão Smoothie
276

Blue Moon Smoothie
277

Peanut Butter Lover Smoothie
277

Shamrock Shake
278

Banana-Nut Smoothie
278

Strawberry Morning Smoothie
279

Pineapple Turmeric Smoothie
279

Warm Ginger Tea

When your gut is having a bad day, sit down with this cup of tea. Sip slowly and relax.

INGREDIENTS | SERVES 1

1 cup boiling water
2" piece fresh gingerroot, grated
Juice of ½ medium lemon
1 teaspoon pure maple syrup
¼ teaspoon freshly ground black pepper
¼ teaspoon Himalayan salt

Pour water into teacup and add all ingredients. Let sit 2–3 minutes.

Per Serving Calories: 27 | Fat: 0g | Protein: 0g | Sodium: 597mg | Fiber: 1g | Carbohydrates: 8g | Sugar: 5g

Ginger Maple Tea

Sooth your tummy with the best comforts of ginger, lemon, cinnamon, and maple syrup.

INGREDIENTS | SERVES 1

1 cup water
1 teaspoon freshly grated gingerroot
2 slices lemon
1 teaspoon ground cinnamon
1 tablespoon maple syrup

1. Boil water and pour ¾ into mug. Add ginger, lemon, cinnamon, and maple syrup and allow to steep 10 minutes.

2. Add remaining ¼ cup boiling water. Relax and sip slowly.

Per Serving Calories: 68 | Fat: 0g | Protein: 0g | Sodium: 10mg | Fiber: 2g | Carbohydrates: 18g | Sugar: 12g

Cucumber Melon Water

When you're tired of water, this drink will leave you cool as a cucumber!

INGREDIENTS | SERVES 1

2½ cups cold water with ice
½ cup sliced cucumber
½ cup cubed honeydew melon
Juice of ½ medium lime
4 mint leaves

Mix together all ingredients in a small pitcher and refrigerate 3–4 hours.

Per Serving Calories: 88 | Fat: 1g | Protein: 4g | Sodium: 82mg | Fiber: 6g | Carbohydrates: 20g | Sugar: 8g

Aloe Vera Rewind

Got acid reflux, constipation, or ulcerative colitis? This drink may help, as it contains aloe and turmeric, which have both been known to help fight inflammation.

INGREDIENTS | SERVES 1

2 tablespoons aloe vera gel
½ cup chopped cucumber
Juice of 1 medium lime
8 ounces cold water
¼ teaspoon ground turmeric

Place all ingredients in a blender. Blend well and add to glass. Cover glass with plastic wrap and chill in refrigerator 1 hour before consuming.

Per Serving Calories: 30 | Fat: 0g | Protein: 1g | Sodium: 9mg | Fiber: 2g | Carbohydrates: 9g | Sugar: 2g

Carrot Pineapple Ginger Juice

*When you need some help getting your digestive tract moving,
this juice is refreshing and delightful for the tummy.*

INGREDIENTS | SERVES 2

2 cups pineapple chunks
1 large carrot, peeled and chopped
3 tablespoons freshly grated gingerroot
½ teaspoon cayenne pepper

Add all ingredients to a juicer or food processor. Blend well and strain through a sieve. Serve in glasses.

Per Serving Calories: 126 | Fat: 1g | Protein: 2g | Sodium: 29mg | Fiber: 4g | Carbohydrates: 31g | Sugar: 18g

Strawberry Coconut Almond Smoothie

This smoothie is great for breakfast, lunch, or after a workout.

INGREDIENTS | SERVES 1

½ cup ice cubes
½ cup chopped strawberries
½ cup unsweetened almond milk
¼ cup shredded unsweetened coconut
1 tablespoon smooth almond butter
1 scoop protein powder

Place all ingredients in a blender and blend until smooth.

Per Serving Calories: 359 | Fat: 17g | Protein: 34g | Sodium: 181mg | Fiber: 5g | Carbohydrates: 20g | Sugar: 12g

Gut-Friendly Smoothie

Per a published study, turmeric extract may help reduce IBS symptoms. The curcumin content in turmeric may help with inflammation. This smoothie was created especially for those suffering from IBS. Enjoy and relax!

INGREDIENTS | SERVES 1

1 cup canned coconut milk
1 tablespoon coconut oil
1 tablespoon chia seeds
½ ripe medium banana
½ teaspoon ground turmeric
½ teaspoon ground cinnamon

Blend all ingredients thoroughly in a blender and enjoy immediately.

Per Serving   Calories: 676 | Fat: 67g | Protein: 7g | Sodium: 31mg | Fiber: 3g | Carbohydrates: 24g | Sugar: 7g

Jeremy's Revival Smoothie

When you need something filling to make in a flash or want a post-workout meal, this smoothie is it.

INGREDIENTS | SERVES 1

2 cups spinach
10 frozen blueberries
½ ripe medium banana, frozen
1 tablespoon chia seeds
½ tablespoon hemp seeds
1 scoop protein powder
½ cup water
1 teaspoon unsweetened cocoa powder

Place all ingredients in a blender and blend until combined.

Per Serving   Calories: 245 | Fat: 7g | Protein: 30g | Sodium: 141mg | Fiber: 5g | Carbohydrates: 21g | Sugar: 9g

Blueberry Ginger Water

*This refreshing drink will complement a day in the shade and it's
great when you want something other than water.*

INGREDIENTS | MAKES 1 CUP

1 cup coarsely chopped gingerroot,
unpeeled

1 cup turbinado sugar

3 cups water

1 tablespoon lime juice (per serving)

¼ cup blueberries (per serving)

1. Place ginger in a food processor and process until rough in texture.

2. Place ginger, sugar, and water in a medium saucepan. Bring to a boil, then reduce heat to low and simmer; cook 1 hour or until liquid has reduced to 1 cup of glossy liquid.

3. Place a sieve over a medium bowl. Strain syrup through sieve, pushing gently on ginger. Allow syrup to cool slightly before storing in a glass jar. Before using refrigerate for several hours. Keep refrigerated 2–3 weeks.

4. Once you're ready to use the syrup, measure 1 tablespoon into an 8-ounce glass with water and ice. Add lime juice and blueberries.

Per Recipe   Calories: 858 | Fat: 3g | Protein: 6g |
Sodium: 96mg | Fiber: 11g | Carbohydrates: 212g | Sugar: 200g

Paixão Smoothie

*This smoothie is dedicated to the passionfruit and the warm, colorful beaches of Brazil.
It's a perfect smoothie after a surf, swim, or paddleboard session.*

INGREDIENTS | SERVES 2

½ medium passionfruit

½ ripe medium banana

1 (6-ounce) tub lactose-free vanilla
yogurt

1½ cups unsweetened coconut milk

1 tablespoon coconut cream

1 tablespoon maple syrup

1½ cups crushed ice

Scoop out fruit and seeds from passionfruit and place in blender with remaining ingredients. Blend until smooth. Add more milk or ice if necessary. Enjoy!

Per Serving   Calories: 526 | Fat: 39g | Protein: 9g |
Sodium: 85mg | Fiber: 2g | Carbohydrates: 44g | Sugar: 31g

Blue Moon Smoothie

For those who love blueberries and chia seeds, this smoothie is a true fit.

INGREDIENTS | SERVES 1

½ cup unsweetened coconut milk

10 frozen blueberries

½ ripe medium banana

1 tablespoon chia seeds

1 cup crushed ice

Place milk in blender followed by other ingredients and blend until smooth. Add more milk or ice if desired. Enjoy!

Per Serving Calories: 289 | Fat: 24g | Protein: 3g | Sodium: 16mg | Fiber: 2g | Carbohydrates: 20g | Sugar: 10g

Peanut Butter Lover Smoothie

Yummy peanut butter, banana, and avocado make for a creamy and awesome smoothie! If peanut butter is not your thing you can use other low-FODMAP nut butters.

INGREDIENTS | SERVES 1

¾ cup unsweetened coconut milk

½ frozen ripe medium banana

⅛ medium avocado

2 tablespoons peanut butter

½ cup lactose-free plain yogurt

½ cup crushed ice

Place milk in blender followed by other ingredients and blend until smooth. Add more milk or ice if desired. Enjoy!

Per Serving Calories: 693 | Fat: 58g | Protein: 19g | Sodium: 258mg | Fiber: 5g | Carbohydrates: 35g | Sugar: 19g

Shamrock Shake

Try this smoothie and top o' the morning to you and your day!

INGREDIENTS | SERVES 1

½ cup lactose-free milk

½ frozen ripe medium banana

⅛ medium avocado

1–2 leaves romaine lettuce or a handful of baby spinach

¼ teaspoon alcohol-free vanilla extract

⅛ teaspoon alcohol-free peppermint extract

Place milk in blender first followed by a ½ cup ice and remaining ingredients and blend until smooth. Add more milk or add ice if desired. Enjoy!

Per Serving   Calories: 158 | Fat: 5g | Protein: 6g | Sodium: 60mg | Fiber: 4g | Carbohydrates: 24g | Sugar: 15g

Banana-Nut Smoothie

This smoothie is great for breakfast and is made with walnuts, which are a good source of magnesium, vitamin B_6, and calcium. Garnish with a ripe, red strawberry for a colorful presentation.

INGREDIENTS | SERVES 1

½ cup soy milk

½ ripe frozen medium banana

5 frozen strawberries

10 walnut halves

1 cup crushed ice

Place milk in blender first followed by other ingredients; blend until smooth. Enjoy!

Per Serving   Calories: 269 | Fat: 16g | Protein: 8g | Sodium: 64mg | Fiber: 5g | Carbohydrates: 29g | Sugar: 15g

Strawberry Morning Smoothie

Another great filling and delicious smoothie that is excellent for breakfast.

INGREDIENTS | SERVES 1

½ cup unsweetened coconut milk
½ ripe frozen medium banana
5 frozen strawberries
¼ cup gluten-free quick-cooking oats
½ teaspoon alcohol-free vanilla extract

Place milk in blender first followed by other ingredients and blend until smooth. Enjoy!

Per Serving   Calories: 377 | Fat: 26g | Protein: 6g | Sodium: 17mg | Fiber: 5g | Carbohydrates: 35g | Sugar: 11g

Pineapple Turmeric Smoothie

This anti-inflammatory smoothie may help suppress symptoms from an IBS attack. Enjoy slowly.

INGREDIENTS | SERVES 1

1 cup coconut water
1 cup chopped pineapple
½ teaspoon ground turmeric
½ teaspoon ground cinnamon
¼ teaspoon freshly ground black pepper
1 tablespoon chia seeds
1 tablespoon shredded unsweetened coconut
¼ teaspoon freshly grated gingerroot
½ medium lime, peeled, seeds removed

Place coconut water in a blender, plus a ½ cup ice, then add other ingredients and blend until smooth. Add more ice if desired.

Per Serving   Calories: 225 | Fat: 6g | Protein: 3g | Sodium: 35mg | Fiber: 7g | Carbohydrates: 53g | Sugar: 39g

CHAPTER 16

From Scratch

Gluten-Free All-Purpose
1-to-1 Flour
282

Flour Mix 1 for Gluten-
Free Bread
282

Flour Mix 2 for Gluten-
Free Bread
283

Flax Egg, Egg Replacer
283

Pie Crust
284

Gluten-Free Pizza Dough
285

Vanilla Maple Almond Butter
286

Toasted Coconut Flake Butter
286

Vegan Parmesan Cheez
287

How to Soak Almonds
287

Gluten-Free All-Purpose 1-to-1 Flour

Use this flour for sandwich breads, pancake mix, crepes, waffles, pie crust, and more.

INGREDIENTS | MAKES 20 CUPS

3 cups sweet white rice flour

3 cups brown rice flour

3 cups white rice flour

2½ cups tapioca flour/starch

2½ tablespoons xanthan gum

In a large bowl, whisk ingredients together until well combined. Store in an airtight container.

Per Serving (1 cup) Calories: 269 | Fat: 1g | Protein: 3g | Sodium: 14mg | Fiber: 2g | Carbohydrates: 60g | Sugar: 1g

Flour Mix 1 for Gluten-Free Bread

If your supermarket doesn't carry gluten-free bread in the freezer section or you just feel like baking, use this mix as a base to then add your starch of choice, yeast, salt, and other ingredients.

INGREDIENTS | MAKES 5 CUPS

1 cup millet flour

1 cup sorghum flour

1 cup potato flour

2 cups rice flour

Combine all flours in a large container with a lid. Stir to combine or cover and shake. Store in refrigerator for freshness. Allow to come to room temperature before using.

Per Serving (1 cup) Calories: 626 | Fat: 4g | Protein: 15g | Sodium: 22mg | Fiber: 9g | Carbohydrates: 135g | Sugar: 1g

Gluten-Free Bread Tips

Using high-protein flours such as millet and sorghum adds structure and flavor to bread, which is key to making great gluten-free bread.

Flour Mix 2 for Gluten-Free Bread

Brown rice flour adds stability to this mix and imparts a neutral flavor while the sorghum flour provides the protein structure for the bread.

INGREDIENTS | MAKES 3 CUPS

1¼ cups brown rice flour
¾ cup potato starch
½ cup tapioca flour
½ cup sorghum flour

Put all flours into a large container with a lid. Stir to combine or cover and shake. Store in refrigerator for freshness. Allow to come to room temperature before using.

Per Serving (1 cup) Calories: 407 | Fat: 2g | Protein: 8g | Sodium: 30mg | Fiber: 5g | Carbohydrates: 93g | Sugar: 2g

Flax Egg, Egg Replacer

Add this egg replacement mixture to recipes calling for 1 large egg. Purchase ground flaxseed meal or grind your own at home in a blender.

INGREDIENTS | MAKES 1 "EGG"

1 tablespoon flaxseed meal
3 tablespoons water

Combine flaxseed meal and water in a small bowl and allow to sit 5 minutes.

Per Serving Calories: 35 | Fat: 3g | Protein: 2g | Sodium: 1mg | Fiber: 2g | Carbohydrates: 2g | Sugar: 0g

Pie Crust

*Use this delicious gluten-free recipe to make pies
or for Chicken Potpie (see recipe in Chapter 10).*

INGREDIENTS | MAKES 2 (9") PIE CRUSTS

2½ cups gluten-free all purpose flour

⅓ cup white sugar

½ teaspoon salt

½ teaspoon xanthan gum (unless your flour blend already contains it)

¾ cup butter or dairy-free margarine

¼ cup vegetable shortening

1 large egg white

5 tablespoons ice-cold water

1. Add flour, sugar, salt, and xanthan gum to food processor and pulse to fully incorporate.

2. Add butter, shortening, egg white, and 4 tablespoons of ice-cold water to food processor. Pulse to fully incorporate. Dough should be smooth; if dough isn't smooth, add 1 more tablespoon of water. Pulse again to fully incorporate. Dough will be smoother and stickier than dough that is not gluten-free.

3. Divide dough into two portions. On a clean surface, place two pieces of plastic wrap. Shape dough into two discs and individually wrap both in pieces of plastic wrap. Refrigerate for 1 hour to allow dough to rest.

4. Remove 1 disc from refrigerator. Place a large piece of wax paper (two times larger than the shape of your pie tin or baking dish) on working surface (or marble board) and sprinkle flour on top of wax paper. Remove plastic wrap from disc of dough. Place dough on one half of floured wax paper and pull other half of wax paper over to cover dough. Get out rolling pin and roll gently back and forth over dough and then turn dough 90°. Roll again gently and turn another 90°. Sprinkle dough with more flour if dough begins to stick to wax paper. Continue to turn and roll dough until dough is thin and slightly larger than your pie tin or baking dish.

5. Slip hand gently under bottom side of wax paper to flip dough into pie tin, and press dough into pan. If dough cracks, gently mold and press back together. Press dough into sides of pie tin or if placing in a baking dish, press into sides of dish. Cut off any remaining dough over edges (if making a pie) with a knife. You can use remaining dough to decorate top of pie. Pierce bottom of dough with fork. Place in refrigerator for 10 minutes to cool and set.

6. Fill tin or dish with pie filling.

7. Repeat steps above to roll out second disc of dough.

8. Add top layer of pie crust dough to pie tin or dish. Slit top layer with knife to vent.

Per Serving (1 crust) Calories: 1,549 | Fat: 96g | Protein: 19g | Sodium: 639mg | Fiber: 5g | Carbohydrates: 154g | Sugar: 34g

Gluten-Free Pizza Dough Recipe

Try making your own dough at home and get creative—
there are many low-FODMAP possibilities for toppings.

INGREDIENTS | MAKES 1 CRUST

1 cup warm water
1 teaspoon light brown sugar
1 tablespoon active dry yeast
2½ cups gluten-free all-purpose flour
¼ teaspoon gluten-free baking powder
¾ teaspoon salt
2½ tablespoons olive oil

1. Mix water, sugar, and yeast in a shallow bowl.

2. Mix flour, baking powder, and salt in a stand mixer on low speed.

3. Add yeast mixture. Increase mixing speed to medium and slowly add 1½ tablespoons oil.

4. Grease dough with 1 tablespoon of olive oil and add to a bowl. Cover bowl with a towel, and allow to rise in a warm area until doubled in size, about 1½ hours. If making dough to use at a later time, shape into ½-pound balls, wrap tightly and store in refrigerator up to 2 weeks. If freezing, place wrapped plastic balls of dough into a plastic bag in freezer up to 3 weeks.

5. When ready to make pizza, prebake crust at 350°F for 25–30 minutes. Remove from oven and add toppings. Bake 15–20 minutes or until toppings are warmed through.

Per Serving (1 crust) Calories: 1,492 | Fat: 37g | Protein: 37g | Sodium: 1,911mg | Fiber: 12g | Carbohydrates: 248g | Sugar: 5g

Vanilla Maple Almond Butter

This almond butter tastes so good on top of bananas, in smoothies, on crackers, or with jam!

INGREDIENTS | MAKES 2 CUPS

2 cups raw almonds

2 tablespoons maple syrup

3 teaspoons coconut oil at room temperature, divided

½ teaspoon ground cinnamon

1 teaspoon alcohol-free vanilla extract

⅛ teaspoon sea salt

1. Preheat oven to 350°F.

2. Place almonds on a rimmed baking sheet and toss with maple syrup and 2 teaspoons coconut oil. Roast for about 30 minutes, stirring halfway through. Allow to cool 10–15 minutes.

3. Place roasted almonds in food processor and process until smooth, about 5 minutes. Stop when needed to scrape down nut butter from sides.

4. Add cinnamon, vanilla, salt, and remaining coconut oil. Process until well combined. Store in an air-tight container for 6–8 weeks in refrigerator or freeze for up to 4 months.

Per Serving (1 cup)   Calories: 667 | Fat: 54g | Protein: 20g | Sodium: 150mg | Fiber: 12g | Carbohydrates: 35g | Sugar: 16g

Toasted Coconut Flake Butter

If you love coconut, now you can add it to your smoothie or spread it on your gluten-free bread, bagel, or fruit!

INGREDIENTS | MAKES 2 CUPS

1 pound shredded unsweetened coconut

1 teaspoon ground cinnamon

1. Preheat oven to 350°F.

2. Spread coconut evenly on a rimmed baking sheet. Bake 8 minutes or until light golden brown; stir occasionally. Or, place coconut shreds in a medium skillet and heat on medium-heat heat, stirring frequently until a beautiful golden brown color.

3. Add toasted coconut flakes and cinnamon to a food processor and blend on high speed 4–6 minutes or until the consistency of nut butter. Store at room temperature for up to 1 year. Before use, stir well with a spoon.

Per Serving (1 cup)   Calories: 795 | Fat: 75g | Protein: 8g | Sodium: 45mg | Fiber: 21g | Carbohydrates: 35g | Sugar: 14g

Vegan Parmesan Cheez

Many vegan cheeses are made with cashews, which as you may know are high in FODMAPs. In this recipe, Brazil nuts provide a nice consistency and earthiness that make this cheese a winner to sprinkle on your favorite vegan dishes.

INGREDIENTS | MAKES 1 CUP

¾ cup Brazil nuts

¼ teaspoon sea salt

1 tablespoon nutritional yeast

1 tablespoon chopped fresh flat-leaf parsley

1 tablespoon fresh lemon juice

1. Preheat oven to 275°F. Line a baking sheet with parchment paper.

2. Process nuts in a food processor until just crumbly. Place in a medium bowl and add salt, nutritional yeast, parsley, and lemon juice. Stir well until combined.

3. Bake 35–40 minutes, tossing at least 3 times during baking. When finished, the cheez should become golden around edges.

4. Remove cheez from oven and allow to cool. May be refrigerated in an airtight container for up to 2 months.

Per Serving   Calories: 687 | Fat: 66g | Protein: 19g | Sodium: 1,245mg | Fiber: 8g | Carbohydrates: 15g | Sugar: 3g

How to Soak Almonds

Soaking almonds releases the enzyme lipase, which is beneficial for digestion of fats. The brown skin, which contains tannins, inhibits nutrient absorption but it falls off during soaking, making almonds easier to digest.

INGREDIENTS | MAKES 1 CUP

1 cup raw unsalted almonds

2 cups water

2 teaspoons sea salt

Soaking Nuts

Use the same method described here for soaking any nut, always a 2:1 ratio of water to nuts. Know that soaking and drying times differ for other nuts. You can find several soaking and drying charts on the Internet to help you estimate times.

1. Place almonds in a medium bowl. Cover with water. Add salt.

2. Cover with a cheesecloth or thin breathable cloth and allow to sit on countertop for about 8–12 hours. Throw out any nuts that float to the top as they may be rancid.

3. Drain nuts and rinse thoroughly until water is clear. Spread out in single layer on a baking sheet to dehydrate. Using a dehydrator or oven, dry at a low temperature no greater than 150°F for 12–24 hours.

Per Serving   Calories: 546 | Fat: 47g | Protein: 20g | Sodium: 4,730mg | Fiber: 12g | Carbohydrates: 21g | Sugar: 4g

Sample Menu Plans and Snack Suggestions

There are plenty of foods on the low-FODMAP diet that you can make ahead of time to then use throughout the week for soups, salads, sandwiches, snacks, entrées, and more. Though planning does take some time at first, it will save time later when you are too exhausted to cook. Planning will keep you from staring blindly into your refrigerator wondering what to make. You will be less apt to make poor choices in food or eat high-FODMAP meals.

Remember this tip—when you are making a dish that includes buckwheat, rice, rice pasta or other gluten-free pastas, quinoa, stock, or pasta sauce, make extra to use in other recipes included in this book.

Meat-Eater 5-Day Plan

	Day One	Day Two	Day Three	Day Four	Day Five
Breakfast	Peanut Butter Lover Smoothie (Chapter 15)	Omelet with mozzarella cheese and spinach, GF bread with ⅛ avocado	Overnight Carrot Cake Oats and Walnuts (Chapter 2)	Turkey sausage with brown rice and Parmesan cheese	Ham and Cheese Crepes (Chapter 2) with blueberries
Snack	6 ounces lactose-free vanilla yogurt with 10 blueberries	1 medium navel orange, 10 almonds	Dark Chocolate–Covered Pretzels (Chapter 14)	1 slice American cheese, rice crackers, baby carrots	1 slice turkey with 1 slice Cheddar cheese, 1 cup grapes
Lunch	Turkey sandwich on GF bread with 1 slice Havarti cheese, spinach, mustard, and mayonnaise	Beef with Buckwheat Soup (Chapter 4)	Barbecue Chicken Wrap (Chapter 6)	Turkey Pesto Wrap (Chapter 6)	Ham and Cheddar sandwich on GF bread
Snack	1 slice Havarti cheese with rice crackers	2 small imperial mandarins, GF crackers	½ cup GF cereal (dry), 2 small kiwifruit	1 cup grapes (any variety)	1 cup Coconut Cinnamon Popcorn (Chapter 14)
Dinner	Pork Chops with Carrots and Toasted Buckwheat (Chapter 7)	Roast Beef Tenderloin with Parmesan Crust (Chapter 7)	Victor's Chicken Parmesan (Chapter 7)	Turkey Bolognese with Pasta (Chapter 7)	Orange Chicken and Broccoli Stir-Fry (Chapter 7)

Vegetarian 5-Day Plan

	Day One	Day Two	Day Three	Day Four	Day Five
Breakfast	Lactose-free vanilla yogurt topped with Cinnamon Spice Granola (Chapter 2) and raspberries	Green Dragon Smoothie Bowl (Chapter 2)	Coconut Cacao Hazelnut Smoothie Bowl (Chapter 2)	Eggs Baked in Heirloom Tomatoes (Chapter 2)	1 cup quinoa flakes with ½ cup almond milk and strawberries
Snack	Feta Cheese Dip (Chapter 3), green bell pepper, and rice crackers	Millet bread, 1 ounce mozzarella cheese, ½ tablespoon pesto	1 ounce tortilla chips, Pomegranate Salsa (Chapter 13)	⅔ cup Savory Baked Tofu (Chapter 9), ¼ cup brown rice	1 rice cake, 1 tablespoon almond butter

Lunch	Collard Green Wraps with Thai Peanut Dressing (Chapter 9)	Avocado, Goat Cheese, and Spinach Panini (Chapter 6)	Curry Chickpea and Vegetable Spread Sandwich (Chapter 6)	Baba Ghanoush Sandwich (Chapter 6)	Cucumber Goat Cheese Sandwich (Chapter 6)
Snack	Banana Nut Boat (Chapter 14)	Kale Chips (Chapter 14)	Roasted Pumpkin Seeds with Cinnamon and Sugar (Chapter 14)	Gluten-Free Cinnamon and Sugar Soft Pretzels (Chapter 14)	1 slice 100% spelt sourdough bread, pesto
Dinner	Lemon and Mozzarella Polenta Pizza (Chapter 9)	Vegan Carrot, Leek, and Saffron Soup (Chapter 4)	Fish Curry (Chapter 4)	Orange Tempeh and Rice Salad (Chapter 9)	Lentil Pie (Chapter 9)

Vegan 5-Day Plan

	Day One	Day Two	Day Three	Day Four	Day Five
Breakfast	Autumn Breakfast Chia Bowl (Chapter 2) with almond milk	Raspberry Lemon Oatmeal Bars (Chapter 2)	Cranberry Almond Granola (Chapter 2), hemp milk, and blueberries	Green Dragon Smoothie Bowl (Chapter 2)	Overnight Banana Chocolate Oats (Chapter 2)
Snack	2 tablespoons Roasted Pumpkin Seeds (Chapter 14)	1 piece GF bread, ⅛ avocado, dash of salt	10 Brazil nuts	1 ounce tortilla chips, Pomegranate Salsa (Chapter 13)	Kale Chips (Chapter 14)
Lunch	Vegetable Nori Roll (Chapter 9)	Quinoa Tabbouleh (omit feta cheese) (Chapter 5)	Baked Tofu and Vegetables (Chapter 9)	Vegan Potato Salad, Cypriot-Style (Chapter 9)	Summer Vegetable Pasta (Chapter 9)
Snack	Carrots, green peppers, 1 tablespoon tahini	1 tablespoon Roasted Pumpkin Seeds (Chapter 14), 5 Brazil nuts, 2 small kiwifruit	1 tablespoon no-sugar-added dried cranberries, 10 walnut halves	1 Maple Almond Strawberry Banana Rice Cake (Chapter 10)	Banana Nut Boat (Chapter 14)
Dinner	Tempeh Coconut Curry Bowls (Chapter 9)	Latin Quinoa-Stuffed Peppers (Chapter 9)	Orange Tempeh and Rice Salad (Chapter 9)	Mac 'n' Cheeze (Chapter 9)	Vegan Pad Thai (Chapter 9)

Basic Snack Servings and Snack Combo Ideas

Seeds, Nuts, and Grains Snacks

2 tablespoons pumpkin seeds

10 walnut halves

10 Brazil nuts

1 cup quinoa flakes

¼ cup rice flakes

1 slice gluten-free bread, millet bread, or 100% spelt sourdough bread

½ medium banana with 1 tablespoon almond butter

⅓ cup cubed tofu

1 rice cake with 1 tablespoon almond butter

1 ounce tortilla chips with Pomegranate Salsa (Chapter 13)

Vegetable Snacks

1 medium carrot

¼ medium stalk celery

½ cup sliced cucumber

½ cup sliced zucchini

1 medium carrot chopped with ½ cup sliced green peppers and 1 tablespoon tahini

Fruit Snacks

½ medium breadfruit

10 dried banana chips

½ cup cubed cantaloupe

½ cup fresh coconut pieces

1 tablespoon no-sugar-added dried cranberries

1 medium dragon fruit

2 segments durian

1 cup grapes (any variety)

2 small kiwifruit

5 longans

2 small imperial mandarins

1 medium prickly pear

1 medium navel orange

1 passionfruit

1 cup chopped pineapple

10 raspberries

1 medium starfruit (carambola)

10 strawberries

Cheese and Yogurt Snack Combos

2 Camembert wedges with ½ cup grapes

1 slice Cheddar cheese with 5 rice crackers

1 slice Cheddar cheese with ½ cup mini gluten-free pretzels

2 ounces mozzarella cheese on gluten-free crackers (refer to serving size on package) with ½ tablespoon pesto

1 slice melted Havarti cheese on gluten-free bread

Feta Cheese Dip (Chapter 3) with ½ cup sliced green bell peppers and gluten-free crackers (refer to serving size on package)

6 ounces lactose-free yogurt with ¼ cup pomegranate seeds

6 ounces lactose-free yogurt with 20 blueberries

Low- and High-FODMAP Foods List

Included in this section you will find a low-FODMAP foods list containing all the delicious foods you can incorporate into your low-FODMAP diet every day. Serving sizes have been listed next to each food. Remember to balance your plate with fruit (1 serving per meal), vegetables, protein, grains, as well as nuts and/or seeds. You can also download a printable Low-FODMAP Grocery List (*www.FODMAPLife.com*).

Following the low-FODMAP foods list you will find the high-FODMAP foods list.

If you have undergone hydrogen breath testing and your doctor has confirmed that you do not have an issue with malabsorption of lactose, fructose, and/or polyols, you will not have to avoid those FODMAPs in any phase of the diet. Without that testing, you should avoid all high-FODMAP foods during the Elimination Phase.

During the Challenge Phase you will choose from the high-FODMAPs list to re-challenge your tolerance levels one FODMAP at a time. This is one of the best phases of the diet because it can finally enable you to truly know which FODMAPs have been causing the most discomfort, however many years it has been for you. From that knowledge, you will reintroduce FODMAPs that your gut can tolerate, creating a modified low-FODMAP diet you can follow long-term. Knowing the type of FODMAPs, which combination of FODMAPs and the overall load (total amount or threshold) of FODMAPs you can have can empower you and your gut to be happier and healthier.

Low-FODMAP Foods List

Please note: In the first parentheses you will see the low-FODMAP serving size for each food. If you see any food listed as moderate, in the second parentheses the type of FODMAP it contains is listed in moderate amounts. It is also noted whether intake should be limited or avoided. If a food has only one amount in parentheses (like Boysenberry) it means there are no low-FODMAP servings for the food. As always, FODMAPs affect everyone differently, so it's important to keep a food and symptom diary to record any symptoms experienced from food or stress. The FODMAP Life food and symptom diary also helps you to keep track of bowel movements and other possible triggers, aside from food.

Fruit

Avocado

(one ⅛ slice of whole avocado)

Banana, ripe (1 medium)

Banana, dried (10 chips)

Blueberries (20 berries)

Boysenberry (5 berries, moderate) *contains moderate amounts of excess fructose. Limit intake if you malabsorb fructose.*

Breadfruit (½ fruit)

Cantaloupe (½ cup)

Cherries (3, moderate) *contains moderate amounts of excess fructose. Limit intake if you malabsorb fructose.*

Cranberry (1 tablespoon dried no sugar added) (2 tablespoons, moderate)

Clementine (1 medium)

Coconut (½ cup) (1 cup moderate)*contains moderate amounts of polyol-sorbitol. Limit intake.*

Dragon fruit (1 medium)

Durian (2 segments)

Grapes (1 cup)

Grapefruit (½ medium, moderate)*contains moderate amounts of oligos-fructans. Limit intake.*

Kiwi (2 small, peeled)

Lemon (1 small)

Lime (1 small)

Longon (5)

Orange, Mandarin (2 small, peeled)

Orange, Navel (1 medium)

Melon, Honeydew (½ cup)

Passionfruit (1 whole pulp)

Papaya (a.k.a. Paw paw—1 cup, chopped)

Pear, prickly (1 medium)

Pineapple (1 cup, chopped)

Plantain (1 medium, peeled)

Pomegranate (¼ cup seeds)

Rambutan (2)

Raspberry (10 berries)

Rhubarb (1 cup, chopped)

Star fruit (a.k.a. Carambola, 1 medium)

Strawberry (10 medium, chopped)

Tamarind (4 fruits)

Vegetables

Artichoke hearts (canned ⅛ cup hearts)

Asparagus (1 spear, moderate) *contains moderate amounts of excess fructose. Limit intake if you malabsorb fructose.*

Bean sprouts (½ cup)

Beans, green (12 beans)

Beetroot (2 slices) (3 slices, moderate) *contains moderate amounts of oligos-fructans and GOS. Limit intake.*

Bell pepper green/red (½ cup)

Bok choy (1 cup)

Broccoli (½ cup) (⅔ cup, moderate) *contains moderate amounts of polyol-sorbitol. Limit intake.*

Brussels sprouts (2 sprouts)

Butternut squash (¼ cup diced) (½ cup diced, moderate) *contains moderate amounts of polyols-mannitol and oligos-GOS. Limit intake.*

Cabbage, red/common (1 cup)

Callaloo (tinned in brine, 4 pieces)

Carrot (1 medium)

Cassava (½ cup diced)(¾ cup diced, moderate) *contains moderate amounts of oligos-GOS. Limit intake.*

Celeriac (½ medium stalk)

Celery (¼ medium stalk) (½ medium, moderate) *contains moderate amounts of* polyols-mannitol. Avoid moderate amount if you malabsorb mannitol.

Chicory leaves (½ cup)

Chili green/red (11cm long)

Chives (1 tablespoon)

Cho cho (½ cup)

Choko (½ cup diced)

Choy sum (1 cup chopped)

Collard greens (1 cup chopped)

Corn, sweet (½ cob) (¾ cob moderate) *contains moderate amounts of oligos-GOS and polyol-sorbitol. Limit intake.

Cucumber, common (½ cup)

Eggplant (½ cup)

Endive (4 leaves)

Fennel (½ cup bulb)

Gai Lan (1 cup chopped)

Galangal (1 × 3.5 cm piece)

Ginger root (1 teaspoon)

Kale (1 cup chopped)

Karela (¼ sliced, moderate) *contains moderate amounts of oligos-GOS. Limit intake.

Leek (½ leek)

Leek (½ cup chopped leaves)

Lettuce, all (1 cup)

Olives green/black (15 small)

Parsnip (½ cup)

Seaweed, nori (2 sheets)

Sweet potato (½ cup) (¾ cup, moderate) *contains moderate amounts of polyol-mannitol. Avoid if you malabsorb mannitol.

Potato (1 medium)

Pumpkin, butternut (¼ cup) (½ cup diced, moderate) *contains moderate amounts of polyols-mannitol and oligos-GOS. Limit intake.

Pumpkin, canned (¼ cup) (½ cup moderate) *contains moderate amounts of oligos-fructans and GOS. Limit intake.

Pumpkin, jap (½ cup diced)

Radish (2)

Silverbeet (1 cup chopped)

Spaghetti squash (cooked, 1 cup)

Spinach, baby (1 cup)

Squash (2 squash)

Swiss chard (1 cup chopped)

Taro (½ cup diced)

Tomato, canned (½ cup)

Tomato, cherry (4)

Tomato, common (1 small)

Tomato, roma (1 small)

Tomato, sun-dried (4 pieces)

Turnip (1 cup diced)

Water chestnuts (½ cup sliced)

Witloof (4 leaves)

Yam (1 cup diced)

Zucchini (½ cup chopped)

Nuts, Seeds

Almonds (up to 10)

Chestnuts (20 boiled)

Hazelnuts (up to 10) (20 nuts moderate) *contains moderate amounts of oligos-GOS and fructans. Limit intake.

Linseed, sunflower, almond mix (1 tablespoon)

Macadamia (20)

Mixed nuts (18 assorted nuts)

Brazil nuts (10)

Peanuts (32)

Pecans (10 halves)

Pine nuts (1 tablespoon)

Chia seeds (black/white 2 tablespoons)

Egusi seeds (2 tablespoons) (3 tablespoons moderate) *contains moderate amounts of oligos-fructans and GOS. Limit intake.*
Poppy seeds (black/white 2 tablespoons)
Pumpkin seeds (2 tablespoons)
Sesame seeds (1 tablespoon)
Sunflower (2 teaspoons, hulled)
Walnuts (10 halves)
Nut or seed butters (2 tablespoons)

Pulses, Legumes, Vegetarian Substitutes

Butter beans, canned (¼ cup) (3 tablespoons moderate) *contains moderate amounts of oligos-GOS. Limit intake.*
Chana dal, boiled (½ cup)
Chickpeas, canned (¼ cup) (½ cup moderate) *contains moderate amounts of oligos-GOS. Limit intake.*
Lentils, canned (½ cup)
Lentils, green and red, boiled (¼ cup) (½ cup moderate) *contains moderate amounts of oligos-GOS and fructans. Limit intake.*
Lima beans, boiled (¼ cup) (⅓ cup moderate) *contains moderate amounts of oligos-GOS and fructans. Limit intake.*
Mung beans, boiled (¼ cup)
Urad dal, boiled (½ cup)
Mince, quorn (75g, 2½ oz.)
Tempeh, plain (1 slice 100g)
Tofu, plain (⅔ cup, cubed)

Lactose-free Alternatives, Cheese, and Dairy

Almond milk (1 cup)
Coconut milk, canned (½ cup)
Coconut (UHT—ultra high temperature) (½ cup) (150 ml, moderate)
Oat milk (⅛ cup)
Hemp milk (1 cup)
Soy milk (soy protein 1 cup)
Soya milk unsweetened (hulled soya beans) (¼ cup) (½ cup moderate) *contains moderate amounts of oligos-GOS. Limit intake.*

Cheese

Brie (2 wedges)
Camembert (2 wedges)
Cheddar (2 slices)
Colby (2 slices)
Cottage (4 tablespoons)
Cream cheese (2–4 tablespoons moderate) *contains moderate amounts of lactose. Limit intake if you malabsorb lactose.*
Feta (½ cup crumbled)
Goat (½ cup crumbled)
Haloumi (2 slices)
Havarti (2 slices) (4 slices moderate) *contains moderate amounts of lactose. Limit intake if you malabsorb lactose.*
Mozzarella (½ cup grated)
Pecorino (½ cup grated)
Ricotta (2 tablespoons) (4 moderate) *contains moderate amounts of lactose. Limit intake if you malabsorb lactose.*
Swiss (2 slices)

Dairy

Cream, pure (regular ¼ cup, moderate) *contains moderate amounts of lactose. Limit intake if you malabsorb lactose.*

Ice cream (1 scoop moderate) *contains moderate amounts of lactose. Limit intake if you malabsorb lactose.*

Sour cream (¼ cup moderate) *contains moderate amounts of lactose. Limit intake if you malabsorb lactose.*

Whipped cream (½ cup)

Yogurt, lactose-free (6 ounces about 1 small tub)

Yogurt, lactose-free, strawberry (6 ounces, about 1 small tub)

Yogurt, lactose-free, vanilla flavored (3 ounces, about ½ tub) *contains moderate amounts of lactose. Limit intake if you malabsorb lactose.*

Confectionary

Chocolate, dark (5 squares/30g)

Chocolate, milk (1 fun size bar) (5 squares moderate) *contains moderate amounts of lactose. Limit intake if you malabsorb lactose.*

Chocolate, white (1 fun size bar) (5 squares moderate) *contains moderate amounts of lactose. Limit intake if you malabsorb lactose.*

Sugars and Sweeteners

Jaggery (Sri Lanka ½ tablespoon)

Stevia powder (2 sachets)

Sugar, brown (1 tablespoon)

Sugar, palm (1 tablespoon)

Sugar, raw (1 tablespoon)

Sugar, white (1 tablespoon)

Maple syrup (2 tablespoons)

Rice malt syrup (1 tablespoon)

Treacle, coconut (½ tablespoon) (1 tablespoon moderate) *contains moderate amounts of oligos-fructans. Limit intake.*

Fats and Oils

Butter (1 tablespoon)

Dairy blend 70% butter, 30% oil (1 tablespoon)

Margarine (1 tablespoon)

Mayonnaise low and regular fat (2 tablespoons)

Avocado oil (1 tablespoon)

Canola oil (1 tablespoon)

Coconut oil (1 tablespoon)

Olive oil (1 tablespoon)

Extra-virgin olive oil (1 tablespoon)

Peanut oil (1 tablespoon)

Rice bran oil (1 tablespoon)

Sesame oil (1 tablespoon)

Sunflower oil

Vegetable oil (1 tablespoon)

Meats and Fish

Beef (1 small fillet)

Chicken (1 small fillet)

Eggs (2)

Fish (100g cooked)

Kangaroo (1 small fillet)

Lamb (1 small fillet)

Pork (1 small fillet)

Prawns, peeled (10)

Salmon, plain, canned in brine (105g drained)

Sardines, plain, canned in oil (110g drained)

Tuna, plain, canned in brine (185g drained)

Tuna, plain, canned in oil (185g drained)

Cereals

Amaranth, puffed (¼ cup)

Flakes of corn (gluten-free, 1 cup)

Granola made with honey (¼ cup)

Quinoa flakes (1 cup)

Rice flakes (¼ cup)

Rice, puffed/popped (½ cup)

Oats, quick-cooking, dry (¼ cup)

Pastas and Grains

Bourghal, cooked (¼ cup)

Bran, oat, unprocessed (2 tablespoons)

Bran, rice, unprocessed (2 tablespoons)

Bran, wheat, processed (½ tablespoon) (¾ tablespoon) *contains moderate amounts of oligos-fructans. Limit intake.*

Bran, wheat, unprocessed (½ tablespoon)

Buckwheat groats, cooked (U.S., ¾)

Buckwheat kernels, cooked (⅛ cup) (¼ cup moderate) *contains moderate amounts of oligos-fructans. Limit intake.*

Couscous, rice, corn, cooked (¼ cup) (⅓ cup moderate) *contains moderate amounts of oligos-fructans. Limit intake.*

Millet, hulled, cooked (1 cup)

Noodles, rice stick, cooked (1 cup)

Pasta, gluten-free, cooked (1 cup)

Pasta, quinoa, cooked (1 cup)

Pasta, spelt, cooked (½ cup) (⅔ cup moderate) *contains moderate amounts of oligos-fructans. Limit intake.*

Pasta, wheat, cooked (½ cup) (⅔ cup moderate) *contains moderate amounts of oligos-fructans. Limit intake.*

Polenta, cornmeal, cooked (1 cup)

Quinoa, black, red, white, cooked (1 cup)

Rice, basmati, cooked (1 cup)

Rice, brown, white, cooked (1 cup)

Snacks, Biscuits, and Cookies

Bar, granola, oat and honey (1 bar moderate) *contains moderate amounts of oligos-fructans. Limit intake.*

Biscuit/cookie, chocolate chip (1) (1½ biscuits moderate) *contains moderate amounts of oligos-fructans. Limit intake.*

Biscuit, cream filled, chocolate coating (1) (2 moderate) *contains moderate amounts of oligos-fructans. Limit intake.*

Biscuit, savory plain or wholemeal (2)

Biscuit, shortbread (1) (2 moderate) *contains moderate amounts of oligos-fructans. Limit intake.*

Biscuit, sweet, plain (2)

Chips, corn, plain (small packet)

Chips, potato, plain (small packet), if on gluten-free diet look for gluten-free

Chips, potato straws, salted (small packet)

Corn thins, flavored, sour cream and chives (1)

Crackers, saltines (U.S., 5)

Pretzels (½ cup rings)

Rice cakes, flavored, sour cream and chives (1)

Rice cakes, plain (2)

Breads and Tortillas

Gluten-free (2 slices)

Gluten-free, white (2 slices)

Gluten-free, wholemeal (2 slices)

Gluten-free high fiber (U.S., 1 slice) (2 slices moderate) *contains moderate amounts of excess fructose. Limit intake.*

Gluten-free, multigrain (U.S., 1 slice) (1½ slices moderate) *contains moderate amounts of excess fructose. Limit intake.*

Gluten-free, multi-grain, sprouted (1 slice) (2 slices moderate) *contains moderate amounts of excess fructose. Limit intake.*

Multi-grain, sprouted (U.S., 1 slice)

Millet (2 slices)

Rice chia, gluten-free (1 slice) (2 slices moderate) *contains moderate amounts of oligos-fructans. Limit intake.*

Sourdough, oat (1 slice) (2 slices moderate) *contains moderate amounts of oligos-fructans and GOS. Limit intake.*

Sourdough, 100% spelt (2 slices)

Spelt, 100% spelt flour (1 slice moderate) *contains moderate amounts of excess fructose. Limit intake.*

Wheat, white (1 slice) (1½ slices moderate) *contains moderate amounts of oligos-fructans. Limit intake.*

Wheat, white, sourdough (2 slices)

Wheat, wholegrain (1 slice moderate) *contains moderate amounts of excess fructose. Limit if you malabsorb fructose.*

Wheat, wholemeal (1 slice) (1½ slices) *contains moderate amounts of oligos-fructans. Limit intake.*

Wheat, wholemeal, sourdough (2 slices)

Tortillas, corn (2)

Cakes

Wheat-free, gluten-free (read labels for any FODMAPs)

Flours and Starches

Almond, meal (¼ cup)

Flour, buckwheat (⅔ cup)

Flour, buckwheat, wholemeal (⅔ cup)

Flour, corn (⅔ cup)

Flour, maize (⅔ cup)

Flour, millet (⅔ cup)

Flour, quinoa (⅔ cup)

Flour, rice (⅔ cup)

Flour, rice, roasted (⅔ cup)

Flour, sorghum (⅔ cup)

Flour, spelt, organic, sieved (⅔ cup)

Flour, teff (⅔ cup)

Flour, yam, pounded (⅔ cup)

Starch, maize (⅔ cup)

Starch, potato (⅔ cup)

Starch, tapioca (⅔ cup)

Beverages
Fruit or Vegetable Beverages

Coconut water, fresh (100 ml) (163ml moderate) *contains moderate amounts of polyol-sorbitol and oligos-fructans. Limit intake.*

Coconut water, packaged (100 ml) (150ml moderate) *contains moderate amounts of polyol-sorbitol. Limit intake.*

Cranberry (1 glass/250 ml)

Orange, 99% blend, reconstituted, fresh (½ glass/125 ml) (¾ glass moderate) *contains moderate amounts of excess fructose. Limit intake if you malabsorb fructose.*

Vegetable blend, tomato juice base (1 glass/200 ml)

Coffee

Caffeine when consumed in excess can also aggravate the gut and trigger symptoms.

Remember caffeine is also present in chocolate.

Espresso, decaf with low-FODMAP milk (1 shot/30 ml)

Espresso, decaf, black (2 shots/60 ml)

Espresso, regular with low-FODMAP milk (1 shot/30 ml)

Instant, decaf with low-FODMAP milk (2 teaspoons and 100 ml milk)

Instant, decaf, black (2 teaspoons)

Instant, regular with low-FODMAP milk (2 teaspoons and 100 ml milk)

Instant, regular, black (2 teaspoons)

Tea

Caffeine when consumed in excess can also aggravate the gut and trigger symptoms. Remember caffeine is also present in chocolate.

Black, strong with cow's milk (250 ml)

Black, strong with low-FODMAP milk (250 ml)

Black, strong with soy milk—soy beans (180 ml moderate) *contains moderate amounts of oligos-fructans and GOS. Limit intake.*

Black, strong with water (180 ml) (250ml moderate) *contains moderate amounts of oligos-fructans. Limit intake.*

Black, weak with water (250 ml)

Black, weak with cow's milk (250 ml)

Black, weak with low-FODMAP milk (250 ml)

Black, weak with soy milk (soy beans) (250 ml)

Chai, weak with water (250 ml)

Chai, strong made with water (180 ml moderate) *contains moderate amounts of oligos-fructans. Limit intake.*

Chai, strong made with low-FODMAP milk (180 ml moderate) *contains moderate amounts of oligos-fructans and GOS. Limit intake.*

Chai, weak with cow's milk (250 ml)

Chai, weak with low-FODMAP milk (250 ml)

Chai, weak with soy milk (soy beans) (180 ml) (250 ml moderate) *contains moderate amounts of oligos-GOS. Intake should be avoided.*

Chamomile, weak made with water (180 ml moderate) *contains moderate amounts of oligos-fructans. Limit intake.*

Dandelion, weak with water (250 ml)

Dandelion, strong with water (180 ml) *contains moderate amounts of oligos-fructans. Limit intake.*

Green, strong with water (250 ml)

Herbal, weak with water (180 ml) (250 ml moderate) *contains moderate amounts of oligos-fructans. Limit intake.*

Peppermint, strong with water (250 ml)

White, strong made with water (250 ml)

Alcohol

Alcohol is an irritant to the gut. It is allowed on the low-FODMAP diet, however, consider having just one glass, and limit consumption for the entirety of the diet.

Wine—Red, Sparkling, Sweet, White, Dry – (½ glass/75 ml to 1 glass/150 ml)

Beer—(½ can/188 ml) or (1 can/375 ml)

Gin—(½ serving/15 ml) or (1 serving/30 ml)

Vodka—(½ serving/15 ml) or (1 serving/30 ml)

Whiskey—(½ serving/15 ml) or (1 serving/30 ml)

Chocolate Beverages

Cacao powder (2 heaped teaspoons)

Carob powder (1 heaped teaspoon) (1½ heaped tablespoons moderate) *contains moderate amounts of oligos-fructans. Limit intake.*

Cocoa powder (2 heaped teaspoons)

Drinking chocolate 23% cocoa powder (2 heaped teaspoons)

Drinking chocolate 60% cocoa powder (2 heaped teaspoons)

Drinking chocolate 70% cocoa powder (2 heaped teaspoons)

Malted, chocolate flavored beverage (1.5 heaped teaspoons) (3 heaped teaspoons moderate) *contains moderate amounts of lactose. Limit intake if you malabsorb lactose.*

Other Beverages

Protein supplement, plant based (U.S., 1 sachet)

Condiments

Sauces and Spreads

Asafoetida/Asafetida Powder/Hing (*wheat-free ¼ teaspoon)

Barbecue sauce (2 tablespoons)

Cream sauce, pasta (¼ cup moderate) *contains moderate amounts of lactose. Limit intake if you malabsorb lactose.*

Fish sauce (1 tablespoon)

Ketchup with HFCS (U.S., 1 sachet) (1½ sachets moderate) *contains moderate amounts of oligos-fructans. Limit intake.*

Ketchup with sucrose (U.S., 1 sachet) (1½ sachets moderate) *contains moderate amounts of oligos-fructans. Limit intake.*

Miso paste (2 sachets)

Oyster sauce (1 tablespoon)

Pesto sauce (½ tablespoon) (1 tablespoon moderate) *contains moderate amounts of oligos-fructans. Limit intake.*

Quince paste (½ tablespoon) (1 tablespoon moderate) *contains moderate amounts of oligos-fructans. Limit intake.*

Shrimp paste (2 teaspoons)

Soy sauce (2 tablespoons)

Sweet and sour sauce (2 tablespoons)

Tamarind paste (Sri Lanka ½ tablespoon)

Tomato sauce (2 sachets)

Balsamic vinegar (1 tablespoon) (2 tablespoons moderate) *contains moderate amounts of excess fructose. Intake should be limited if you malabsorb fructose.*

Rice wine vinegar (2 tablespoons)

Worcestershire sauce (gluten-free) (2 tablespoons)

Dips and Spreads

Caviar dip (1 tablespoon moderate) *contains moderate amounts of lactose. Limit intake if you malabsorb lactose.*

Eggplant dip (2 tablespoons)

Hummus/Hommus dip (1 tablespoon moderate) *contains moderate amounts of oligos-GOS and fructans. Limit intake.*

Tahini paste (1 tablespoon) (1½ tablespoons moderate) *contains moderate amounts of oligos-fructans. Limit intake.*

Jam, marmalade (2 tablespoons)

Jam, mixed berries (1 tablespoon moderate)

Jam, strawberry (2 tablespoons)

Peanut butter (2 tablespoons)

Vegemite (1 teaspoon)

Mustard/Pickles

Capers in vinegar (1 tablespoon)

Capers, salted (1 tablespoon)

Chutney (1 tablespoon)

Mustard (1 tablespoon)

Relish (1 tablespoon) (1½ tablespoons moderate) *contains moderate amounts of oligos-fructans. Limit intake.*

Vegetable relish (1 tablespoon)

Wasabi (1 teaspoon)

Fresh Herbs

Basil (1 cup)

Cilantro (1 cup)

Coriander (1 cup)

Curry leaves (1 cup)

Fenugreek leaves (1 cup)

Gotukala (½ bundle)

Lemongrass (1 × 10 cm stalk)

Pandan leaves (1 × 2.5 cm leaf)

Parsley (1 cup)

Rampa leaves (1 × 2.5 cm leaf)

Rosemary (1 cup)

Tarragon (1 cup)

Thyme (1 cup)

Spices

Allspice (1 teaspoon)

Cardamom (1 teaspoon)

Chilli powder (1 teaspoon)

Cinnamon (1 teaspoon)

Cloves (1 teaspoon)

Coriander seeds (1 teaspoon)

Cumin (1 teaspoon)

Curry powder, garlic-free (1 teaspoon)

Fennel seeds (1 teaspoon)

Fenugreek seeds (2 tablespoons)

Five spice (1 teaspoon)

Goraka (1 average piece)

Mustard seeds (1 teaspoon)

Nutmeg (1 teaspoon)

Paprika (1 teaspoon)

Pepper, black (1 teaspoon)

Saffron (1 packet)

Star anise (2 cloves)

Turmeric (1 teaspoon)

High-FODMAP Foods to Avoid

All foods included in this list are HIGH in FODMAPs and should be avoided during the Elimination Phase, the first phase of the low-FODMAP diet. If you see a serving size next to a food on this list it represents the high-FODMAP serving but also means that food can be low in FOD-MAPs, but in a smaller serving. When that is the case, please refer to the Low-FODMAP Foods List for the appropriate low-FODMAP serving size.

Fruit

Apples (fresh or dried)
Applesauce
Apricots (fresh or dried)
Asian pears
Blackberries
Boysenberries
Cherries
Currants
Dates
Feijoa
Figs (fresh or dried)
Goji berries (dried)
Grapefruit
Lychee
Mangoes (fresh or dried)
Nectarines
Peaches (all)
Pears (dried or Asian, Nashi, packham—firm or ripe)
Persimmon
Pineapple (dried only)
Plums
Prunes
Raisins
Sultanas
Tamarillo
Watermelon

Vegetables

Artichokes (Jerusalem, globe)
Asparagus (1 spear, moderate)
Beetroot
Cabbage, savoy
Cassava
Cauliflower
Cho cho
Choko
Corn, sweet
Garlic
Karela
Leeks
Mushroom, button
Onions, shallots (all including onion powder)
Peas, snow
Peas, sugar snap
Peas, thawed
Scallion, spring onion bulbs (only use green tips)
Snow peas
Sugar snap peas
Taro

Legumes, Beans

Baked beans
Black beans, boiled
Borlotti beans

Broad beans

Four bean mix

Haricot beans

Kidney beans

Chickpeas and Lentils

- Low as long as they are canned, drained and rinsed. Canning helps to leach out FODMAPs. Refer to Low-FODMAP Foods List for serving size.

Lima beans (½ cup)

Mung beans (½ cup)

Red kidney beans (boiled)

Soya beans (boiled)

Split peas (boiled)

Vegetarian Substitutes

Falafel

Lentil burger

Mince (containing onion)

Nuts, Seeds

Almonds (20 nuts)

Pistachios

Cashews

Meat

- Meats containing onion, garlic, onion or garlic powders, dehydrated powders, bread crumbs, dried fruits.
- Marinades/sauces/gravies when prepared with meats may contain high FODMAPs

Dairy, Cheese

Buttermilk

Condensed milk

Cream cheese (2 tablespoons, moderate)

Crème fraîche

Custard

Ice cream

Kefir

Milk

- Evaporated
- Regular
- Full cream
- Cow, full cream, reduced fat, skim
- Goat, full cream
- Skim

Milk Alternatives (high in FODMAPs)

- Oat
- Rice
- Soy (soy beans/sweetened/ unsweetened)

Milk powder (milk solids)

Pudding

Soft cheeses

- More than 2 tablespoons is HIGH

Yogurt

- Indian
- Low-fat
- Regular
- Flavored
- Made from cow/goat/sheep's milk

Confectionary

- Chocolate when consumed in high amounts can irritate the gut due to its fat, sugar, and caffeine content. *Refer to Low-FODMAP Foods List for serving sizes.*

Fruit bar (½ bar)

Snacks, Biscuits, and Cookies

Bar, cereal, wheat-based

Bar, granola, oat and honey (2 bars)

Bar, muesli-based with fruit (½ bar)

Biscuit/cookie, chocolate chip (2)

Biscuit, fruit filled

Cookies, chocolate crème sandwich (U.S., 1 cookie)

Corn thins, flavored, sour cream and chives (4)

Rice cakes, flavored, sour cream and chives (4)

Rye crispbread (1)

Breads, Cakes, Flours
Breads

- Gluten-free, multigrain (U.S., 2 slices)
- Gluten-free, wholegrain, sweetened with pear juice (U.S., 1 slice)
- Multi-grain, sprouted (U.S., 2 slices)
- Naan or roti
- Oatmeal (U.S., 1 slice)
- Pumpernickel (1 slice)
- Raisin toast
- Rye, rye dark, rye sourdough
- Sourdough, kamut, wholemeal
- Spelt, 100% spelt flour (2 slices)
- Wheat, 100% whole wheat (U.S., 1 slice)
- Wheat, high fiber (U.S., 1 slice)
- Wheat, multigrain (2 slices)
- Wheat, white (2 slices)
- Wheat, white (U.S., 2 slices)
- Wheat, white (Norway, 1 slice)
- Wheat, wholegrain (2 slices)
- Wheat, wholegrain (U.S., 2 slices)
- Wheat, wholemeal (2 slices)
- Wheat, wholemeal (Norway, 1 slice)
- Wheat, wholemeal and oatmeal (U.S., 1 slice)

Cakes

Wheat-based or made with other high-FODMAP flours below or including any other high FODMAPs (like dried fruits, honey, agave, etc.):

- Bread crumbs
- Cakes
- Cookies
- Croissants
- Muffins
- Pastries containing wheat/rye

Flours

- Almond, meal (½ cup)
- Khorasan (kamut) whole-wheat flour
- Amaranth
- Barley
- Chickpea flour (may be okay in small amounts)
- Couscous
- Durum
- Einkorn, organic
- Emmer
- Lupin
- Lentil flour (may be okay in small amounts)
- Multigrain flour
- Pea flour (may be okay in small amounts)
- Rye
- Spelt, organic, white or wholemeal
- Soy flour (may be okay in small amounts)
- Triticale
- Wheat bran
- Wheat flour
- Wheat germ

Grains and Pastas

Barley, pearl

Bourghal, cooked (½ cup)

Bran, wheat, processed and unprocessed (1 tablespoon)

Couscous, rice and corn, cooked (½ cup)

Couscous, wheat, cooked (½ cup)

Freekeh, cooked (¼ cup)

Noodles, wheat

Pasta, spelt, cooked (1 cup)

Pasta, wheat, cooked (1 cup)

Gnocchi, wheat

Granola, fruit and nut

Rice crisps (U.S., 1 cup)

Cereals

Flakes of corn (U.S., 1 cup)

Flakes of wheat, corn, rice, oats, dried fruit, nuts (½ cup)

Flakes, barley or spelt or gluten-free rice flakes with psyllium

Muesli, plain, or free of yeast, wheat, gluten, dairy, nut (all HIGH)

Oatmeal (fine, organic, Denmark, 1 cup)

Wheat-based multi-grain breakfast cereal

Wheat bran, pellets

Whole-wheat grain biscuit

Sweeteners

Agave nectar

Corn syrup solids

Fructose

Fruit juice concentrate

High fructose corn syrup (HFCS)

Honey

Pear juice

Sugar alcohols
- Isomalt
- Maltitol
- Mannitol
- Sorbitol
- Xylitol

Condiments, Dressings, Sauces

Many condiments are made with FODMAPs, but you can make your own at home! Refer to recipes in Chapter 13 for ideas. Always read ingredient labels for any condiments you purchase.
- Chutneys
- Gravies
- Chicken, vegetable, beef stock
- Vegetable and beef bouillon cubes
- Dressings
- Sauces
- Brand-made relishes
- Oil-based sauces and condiments

Drinks, Juices

More than ½ cup of any fruit juice is HIGH

Apple

Apple and raspberry cordial

Berry fruit blend (from juice bar)

Pear

Tropical and mango juices

Orange
- 98% reconstituted
- 99% blend
- Orange cordials

Coffee
- Chicory-based coffee substitutes
- Espresso decaf or regular

- Made with cow or soy milk (soy beans)
- Instant decaf or regular
- Made with cow or soy milk (soy beans)

Teas—(250 ml)

- Black—Strong made with soy milk (soy beans)
- Dandelion—Strong made with water
- Fennel tea—Strong or weak made with water
- Chamomile tea—Strong or weak made with water
- Chai tea—Strong made with water, cow's milk, low-FODMAP milk alternatives, soy milk (soy beans)
- Herbal tea—Strong made with water
- Oolong tea—Strong or weak made with water

Coconut water, fresh (250 ml)
Coconut water, packaged (250 ml)
Carob powder (for drinking)
Alcohol

- Rum
- Wine—sweet, dessert, "sticky"

Diet, Sugar-free, Low Carb

Label warnings that say: "Excess consumption may have a laxative effect" and other products containing polyol additives as artificial sweeteners:

Sorbitol
Mannitol
Maltitol
Xylitol
Polydextrose
Isomalt
Mints
Candy
Desserts

APPENDIX C

Sources

Barrett, J.S., et al. "Dietary Poorly Absorbed, Short-Chain Carbohydrates Increase Delivery of Water and Fermentable Substrates to the Proximal Colon." *Alimentary Pharmacology & Therapeutics* 31, no. 8 (2010): 874–82. *www.ncbi.nlm.nih.gov/pubmed/20102355*.

Brogan, K. "From Gut to Brain: The Inflammation Connection." KellyBroganMD.com, 2013. *http://kellybroganmd.com/article/from-gut-to-brain-the-inflammation-connection*.

Brown, K., DeCoffe, D., Molcan, E., and Gibson, D. "Diet-Induced Dysbiosis of the Intestinal Microbiota and the Effects on Immunity and Disease." *Nutrients* 4, no. 8 (2012): 1095–1119. *www.ncbi.nlm.nih.gov/pmc/articles/PMC3448089*.

Canavan, C., J. West, and T. Card. "The Epidemiology of Irritable Bowel Syndrome." *Clinical Epidemiology* 6 (2014): 71–80. *www.ncbi.nlm.nih.gov/pmc/articles/PMC3921083*.

Gibson, P., and S. Shepherd. "Evidence-Based Dietary Management of Functional Gastrointestinal Symptoms: The FODMAP Approach." *Journal of Gastroenterology and Hepatology* 25, no. 2 (2010): 252–58. *www.ncbi.nlm.nih.gov/pubmed/20136989*.

Hadhazy, A. "Think Twice: How the Gut's 'Second Brain' Influences Mood and Well-Being." *Scientific American* (February 12, 2010). *www.scientificamerican.com/article/gut-second-brain*.

Harvard Health Publications, Harvard Medical School. "The gut-brain connection." *www.health.harvard.edu/healthbeat/the-gut-brain-connection*.

Hawrelak, J.A. and Myers, S.P. "The Causes of Intestinal Dysbiosis: A Review." *Altern Med Review* 9, no. 2 (2004): 180–97. *www.ncbi.nlm.nih.gov/pubmed/15253677*.

Hulisz, D. "The Burden of Illness of Irritable Bowel Syndrome: Current Challenges and Hope for the Future." *Journal of Managed Care & Specialty Pharmacy* 10, no. 4 (2004): 299–309. *www.ncbi.nlm.nih.gov/pubmed/15298528*.

Jamma, S., Rubio-Tapia, R., Kelly, C., Murray, J., Sheth, S., Schuppan, D., Dennis, M., and Leffler, D. "Celiac Crisis Is a Rare but Serious Complication of Celiac Disease in Adults." Clinical Gastroenterol Hepatol 8, no. 7 (2010) 587–590. *www.ncbi.nlm.nih.gov/pmc/articles/PMC2900539*.

Kennedy, P.J., et al. "Irritable Bowel Syndrome: A Microbiome-Gut-Brain Axis Disorder?" *World Journal of Gastroenterology* 20, no. 39 (2014): 14105–14125. *www.ncbi.nlm.nih.gov/pmc/articles/PMC4202342*.

Lapind, N., "Ordering Gluten-Free in a Chinese Restaurant." About.com Celiac Disease & Gluten Sensitivity Expert. *http://celiacdisease.about.com/od/socializingwithoutgluten/tp/ChineseRestaurants.htm*.

Layton, J.M., and Larsen, L. "How to Establish a Safe, Gluten-Free Kitchen." Gluten-Free Baking

For Dummies. *www.dummies.com/how-to/ content/how-to-establish-a-safe-glutenfree- kitchen.html.*

Monash University Low-FODMAP Diet app. *www.med.monash.edu.au/cecs/gastro/ fodmap/iphone-app.html.*

Muir, J.G. PhD., and Gibson, P.R. MD. "The Low FODMAP Diet Treatment of Irritable Bowel Syndrome and Other Gastrointestinal Disorders." *Gastroenterol Hepatol* 9, no. 7 (2013): 450–452. *www.ncbi.nlm.nih.gov/pmc/ articles/PMC3736783.*

Nyrop, K.A., et al. "Costs of Health Care for Irritable Bowel Syndrome, Chronic Constipation, Functional Diarrhoea and Functional Abdominal Pain." *Alimentary Pharmacology & Therapeutics* 26, no. 2 (2007): 237–48. *http://onlinelibrary.wiley.com/ doi/10.1111/j.1365-2036.2007.03370.x/full.*

Pimentel, M. *A New IBS Solution: Bacteria— The Missing Link in Treating Irritable Bowel Syndrome* (Sherman Oaks, CA: Health Point Press, 2006).

Scarlata, K. 2010. "The FODMAPs Approach— Minimize Consumption of Fermentable Carbs to Manage Functional Gut Disorder Symptoms." *Today's Dietitian* 12, no. 8 (2010): 30. *www.todaysdietitian.com/ newarchives/072710p30.shtml.*

Shepherd, S., and P. Gibson. *The Complete Low-FODMAP Diet: A Revolutionary Plan for Managing IBS and Other Digestive Disorders* (New York: Penguin, 2013).

Silk, D.B. "Impact of Irritable Bowel Syndrome on Personal Relationships and Working Practices." *European Journal of Gastroenterology & Hepatology* 13, no. 11 (2001): 1327–32. *www.ncbi.nlm.nih.gov/ pubmed/11692059.*

Additional Resources

BonCalme
www.BonCalme.com

Crohn's & Colitis Foundation of America (CCFA)
www.ccfa.org

Digestive Health Alliance (DHA)
www.dha.org

Dr. Barbara Bolen
www.drbarbarabolen.com

FODMAP Life
Blog: *www.fodmaplife.com*
Facebook: *www.facebook.com/fodmaplife*
Instagram: *www.instagram.com/fodmaplife*
Pinterest: *www.pinterest.com/fodmaplife*
Twitter: *www.twitter.com/fodmaplife*

IBS Awareness—American College of Gastroenterology
http://gi.org/acg-institute/ibs-awareness

International Foundation for Functional Gastrointestinal Disorders
www.aboutibs.org

Irritable Bowel Syndrome—KidsHealth
http://kidshealth.org/teen/diseases_conditions/digestive/ibs.html

Irritable Bowel Syndrome—National Library of Medicine
www.nlm.nih.gov/medlineplus/irritablebowelsyndrome.html

Kate Scarlata, RDN
www.katescarlata.com

Monash University, Department of Gastroenterology
www.med.monash.edu/cecs/gastro/fodmap

The Naturopathic Approach to Digestive Disorders—American Association of Naturopathic Physicians
www.naturopathic.org/article_content.asp?article=784

Patsy Catsos, MS, RD, LD
www.ibsfree.net

Shepherd Works
http://shepherdworks.com.au/disease-information/low-fodmap-diet

Standard U.S./Metric Measurement Conversions

VOLUME CONVERSIONS

U.S. Volume Measure	Metric Equivalent
⅛ teaspoon	0.5 milliliter
¼ teaspoon	1 milliliter
½ teaspoon	2 milliliters
1 teaspoon	5 milliliters
½ tablespoon	7 milliliters
1 tablespoon (3 teaspoons)	15 milliliters
2 tablespoons (1 fluid ounce)	30 milliliters
¼ cup (4 tablespoons)	60 milliliters
⅓ cup	90 milliliters
½ cup (4 fluid ounces)	125 milliliters
⅔ cup	160 milliliters
¾ cup (6 fluid ounces)	180 milliliters
1 cup (16 tablespoons)	250 milliliters
1 pint (2 cups)	500 milliliters
1 quart (4 cups)	1 liter (about)

WEIGHT CONVERSIONS

U.S. Weight Measure	Metric Equivalent
½ ounce	15 grams
1 ounce	30 grams
2 ounces	60 grams
3 ounces	85 grams
¼ pound (4 ounces)	115 grams
½ pound (8 ounces)	225 grams
¾ pound (12 ounces)	340 grams
1 pound (16 ounces)	454 grams

OVEN TEMPERATURE CONVERSIONS

Degrees Fahrenheit	Degrees Celsius
200 degrees F	95 degrees C
250 degrees F	120 degrees C
275 degrees F	135 degrees C
300 degrees F	150 degrees C
325 degrees F	160 degrees C
350 degrees F	180 degrees C
375 degrees F	190 degrees C
400 degrees F	205 degrees C
425 degrees F	220 degrees C
450 degrees F	230 degrees C

BAKING PAN SIZES

American	Metric
8 x 1½ inch round baking pan	20 x 4 cm cake tin
9 x 1½ inch round baking pan	23 x 3.5 cm cake tin
11 x 7 x 1½ inch baking pan	28 x 18 x 4 cm baking tin
13 x 9 x 2 inch baking pan	30 x 20 x 5 cm baking tin
2 quart rectangular baking dish	30 x 20 x 3 cm baking tin
15 x 10 x 2 inch baking pan	30 x 25 x 2 cm baking tin (Swiss roll tin)
9 inch pie plate	22 x 4 or 23 x 4 cm pie plate
7 or 8 inch springform pan	18 or 20 cm springform or loose bottom cake tin
9 x 5 x 3 inch loaf pan	23 x 13 x 7 cm or 2 lb narrow loaf or pate tin
1½ quart casserole	1.5 liter casserole
2 quart casserole	2 liter casserole

Index

Note: Page numbers in **bold** indicate recipe
category lists.

Aioli, 249
Alcohols, sugar (polyols), 22
Almonds. *See* Nuts and seeds
Aloe Vera Rewind, 273
Amaranth Breakfast, 60
Ants on a Trunk, 195
Appetizers, **63**–75
    about: low-FODMAP list of dips and
      spreads, 301–2
    Baba Ghanoush, 64
    Baked Camembert and Rosemary, 74
    Chicken Lettuce Cups, 67
    Coconut Shrimp with Pineapple Sauce, 69
    Feta Cheese Dip, 73
    Herbes de Provence Almonds, 73
    Indian-Spiced Mixed Nuts, 71
    Mini Baked Eggplant Pizza Bites, 66
    Mini Polenta Pizzas, 65
    Pão de Queijo (Cheese Bread), 72
    Quinoa, Corn, and Zucchini Fritters, 70
    Smoked Salmon Hand Rolls, 68
    Vegetable Nori Roll, 179
    Vietnamese Summer Rolls, 75
Asafetida powder, 65
Aunt Bete's Chicken Tart, 150
Autumn Breakfast Chia Bowl, 38
Avocado
    about: FODMAP levels, 27
    Avocado, Goat Cheese, and Spinach Panini,
      123
    Latin Quinoa-Stuffed Peppers, 178
    Mexican Risotto, 173
    Smoked Salmon Hand Rolls, 68
    Tempeh Tacos, 190
    Vegetable and Cream Cheese Sandwich,
      199
    Vegetable Nori Roll, 182
Baba Ghanoush, 64
Baba Ghanoush Sandwich, 122
Baked Camembert and Rosemary, 74
Baked Cornflake-Crusted Chicken Tenders
    with Maple Mustard, 196
Baked Moroccan-Style Halibut, 170
Baked Tofu and Vegetables, 183
Baking powder, gluten-free, 241
Bananas
    Ants on a Trunk, 195
    Banana Almond Nice Cream, 243
    Banana Coconut Nice Cream, 242
    Banana Cookie Dough Nice Cream, 242
    Banana Nut Boat, 270
    Maple Almond Strawberry Banana Rice
      Cake, 212
    Overnight Banana Chocolate Oats, 59
    pancakes with. *See* Pancakes and crepes

PB and J Kebabs, 211
Peanut Butter Banana Quesadilla, 202
Raspberry Banana Mint Chia Pudding, 45
smoothies with. *See* Smoothies and
    smoothie bowls
Barbecue Chicken Pizza, 205
Barbecue Chicken Wrap, 126
Barbecue Pork Macaroni and Cheese, 148
Barbecue sauce, sweet, 248
Basil
    Basil Sauce, 249
    Basil Walnut Sauce, 168
    Pesto Sauce, 253
    Warm Basil and Walnut Potato Salad, 98
    Zoodles with Pesto, 114
Beans and other legumes
    about: canned chickpeas and FODMAPs,
      54; high-FODMAP to avoid, 303–4; low-
      FODMAP list of, 296
    Curry Chickpea and Vegetable Spread
      Sandwich, 125
    Eggs with Spinach and Chickpeas, 54
    Lentil Chili, 85
    Lentil Pie, 174
    Root-a-Burgers, 113
    Shakshuka for Two, 50
    Swiss Chard with Lentils, Pine Nuts, and
      Feta Cheese, 186
Beef
    about: buying tenderloin, 130
    Beef with Buckwheat Soup, 92
    Beef with Spinach and Sweet Potatoes, 135
    Citrus Flank Steak, 131
    Fiesta Nachos, 198
    Filet Mignon Salad, 104
    Mac 'n' Cheese Taco Bake, 204
    Meatloaf Muffins, 203
    Roast Beef Tenderloin with Parmesan
      Crust, 130
    Sourdough Meatballs, 149
    Sweet and Savory Brazilian Meat and
      Cheese Tart, 145
    Zucchini Lasagna with Meat Sauce, 146
Berries
    about: softening cranberries, 57
    Banana-Nut Smoothie, 278
    Blueberry Chia Seed Jam, 246
    Blueberry Ginger Water, 276
    Blueberry-Glazed Chicken, 144
    Blueberry Granola Crisp, 237
    Blue Moon Smoothie, 277
    Chicken, Ham, and Blueberry Melt, 199
    Cranberry Almond Granola, 57
    Cranberry Walnut Oat Cookies, 223
    Fruit and Cheese Kebabs, 211
    Glorious Strawberry Salad, 88
    Jeremy's Revival Smoothie, 275
    Maple Almond Strawberry Banana Rice

      Cake, 212
    Mixed Berry Cobbler, 230
    Nut-Free Cranberry Granola Bars, 214
    Prosciutto di Parma Salad, 100
    Quinoa Cookies, 221
    Raspberry Banana Mint Chia Pudding, 45
    Raspberry Lemon Chia Seed Jam, 246
    Raspberry Lemon Oatmeal Bars, 51
    Strawberry Chia Seed Jam, 247
    Strawberry Coconut Almond Smoothie,
      274
    Strawberry Morning Smoothie, 279
    Strawberry Shortcake, 231
    Strawberry Toast, 194
    Sweet Vegan Mixed Berry Tart, 240
    Turmeric Rice with Cranberries, 185
Blueberries. *See* Berries
Bok choy, 118, 183
Bowls. *See also* Smoothies and smoothie
  bowls
    Autumn Breakfast Chia Bowl, 38
    Mixed Grains, Seeds, and Vegetable Bowl,
      179
    Pesto Eggs Rice Bowl, 51
    Tempeh Coconut Curry Bowls, 172
    Vegetable and Rice Noodle Bowl, 184
Breads. *See also* Pizza
    about: buying for low-FODMAP diet, 194;
      gluten-free panko crumbs, 66; gluten-
      free tips, 282; low-FODMAP list of, 299;
      sourdough, 61
    flours for. *See* Flours, gluten-free
    Pão de Queijo (Cheese Bread), 72
    Pumpkin Bread, 236
    Pumpkin Spice Pecan Cornbread, 244
    Quinoa, Egg, Ham, and Cheese Breakfast
      Muffins, 52
    Savory Sourdough Strata, 61
    Strawberry Toast, 194
    Vegan Lemon Poppy Seed Muffins, 238
Breakfast, **37**–61. *See also* Eggs; Pancakes
  and crepes; Smoothies and smoothie bowls
    about: high-FODMAP cereals to avoid, 306;
      low-FODMAP list of cereals, 298; menu
      plans, 289–90; symptom diary for, 23
    Amaranth Breakfast, 60
    Autumn Breakfast Chia Bowl, 38
    Cinnamon Spice Granola, 38
    Collard Green Eggs and Ham Breakfast
      Wrap, 209
    Cranberry Almond Granola, 57
    Cream of Muesli, 48
    Jubilant Muesli Mix, 47
    Overnight Banana Chocolate Oats, 59
    Overnight Carrot Cake Oats and Walnuts,
      59
    Overnight Peanut Butter Pumpkin Spice
      Oats, 58

Raspberry Banana Mint Chia Pudding, 45
Raspberry Lemon Oatmeal Bars, 51
Brie and Orange Marmalade Sandwich, 125
Broccoli
    about: low-FODMAP servings, 208;
        precautionary tip, 28
    Broccoli and Cheddar Quesadilla, 208
    Broccoli Greenballs, 180
    Mediterranean Buckwheat Salad, 109
    Orange Chicken and Broccoli Stir-Fry, 134
    Vegan Pad Thai, 188
    Vegetable and Rice Noodle Bowl, 184
Brown syrup, simple, 263
Buckwheat
    about: gluten-free flour, 218; make-ahead
        items, 30; storing, 30–31
    Beef with Buckwheat Soup, 92
    Buckwheat Thumbprint Cookies, 218
    Mediterranean Buckwheat Salad, 109
    Mixed Grains, Seeds, and Vegetable Bowl,
        179
    Orange, Red, and Green Buckwheat Salad,
        89
    Pork Chops with Carrots and Toasted
        Buckwheat, 136
    Vegan Buckwheat Crepes, 42
Burger Sauce, 250
Buttercream Lactose-Free Icing, 233
Cabbage, 90, 181, 190
Caesar Salad Dressing, 260
Carrots
    Carrot and Ginger Soup, 84
    Carrot Cake with Cream Cheese Frosting,
        241
    Carrot Pineapple Ginger Juice, 274
    Garlicky Parsnip and Carrot Fries, 110
    Moroccan-Inspired Carrot Ginger Soup, 91
    Overnight Carrot Cake Oats and Walnuts,
        59
    Pork Chops with Carrots and Toasted
        Buckwheat, 136
    Roasted Maple Dill Carrots, 116
    Root-a-Burgers, 113
    Vegan Carrot, Leek, and Saffron Soup, 94
    Vegetable and Cream Cheese Sandwich,
        199
Celiac disease, 15–16
Cereals. See Breakfast
Chai-Spice Cookies, 224
Challenge Phase, 23–24, 25, 293
Cheese
    about: high-FODMAP to avoid, 304; lactose-
        free alternatives FODMAP levels, 296;
        low-FODMAP list of, 296–97; snack
        servings and suggestions, 292
    Baked Camembert and Rosemary, 74
    Broccoli and Cheddar Quesadilla, 208
    Cream Cheese Frosting, 241
    eggs with. See Eggs; Pancakes and crepes
    Feta Cheese Dip, 73
    Fruit and Cheese Kebabs, 211

Goat Cheese and Potato Tacos with Red
    Chili Cream Sauce, 182
Pão de Queijo (Cheese Bread), 72
pasta with. See Pasta
pizzas with. See Pizza
salads with. See Salads
sandwiches with. See Sandwiches and
    wraps
Shrimp and Cheese Casserole, 157
Spinach and Feta-Stuffed Chicken Breast,
    137
Swiss Chard with Lentils, Pine Nuts, and
    Feta Cheese, 186
Vegan Parmesan Cheez, 287
Victor's Chicken Parmesan, 139
Chermoula, 254
Chicken
    Aunt Bete's Chicken Tart, 150
    Baked Cornflake-Crusted Chicken Tenders
        with Maple Mustard, 196
    Baked Papaya and Chicken Salad with
        Cilantro-Lime Dressing, 101
    Barbecue Chicken Pizza, 205
    Barbecue Chicken Wrap, 126
    Blueberry-Glazed Chicken, 144
    Chicken, Ham, and Blueberry Melt, 199
    Chicken, Sweet Potato, and Spinach Curry,
        151
    Chicken and Dumplings Soup, 81
    Chicken Burgers, 128
    Chicken Lettuce Cups, 67
    Chicken Piccata, 140
    Chicken Pizza Quesadilla, 207
    Chicken Potpie, 206
    Chicken Tortilla Soup, 96
    Coq au Vin, 143
    Cornflake-Crusted Chicken Wraps, 197
    Crispy Baked Chicken with Gravy, 153
    Easy Onion- and Garlic-Free Chicken
        Stock, 78
    Easy Pan Chicken, 141
    Lemon Thyme Chicken, 137
    Mom's Chicken Salad, 102
    Mustard and Thyme Roasted Chicken, 152
    Orange Chicken and Broccoli Stir-Fry, 134
    Parmesan-Crusted Chicken, 144
    Polenta-Crusted Chicken, 149
    Prosciutto-Stuffed Chicken, 132
    Pumpkin Maple Roast Chicken, 147
    Slow Cooker Chicken Tagine, 93
    Spinach and Feta-Stuffed Chicken Breast,
        137
    Victor's Chicken Parmesan, 139
Chickpeas. See Beans and other legumes
Chocolate and cacao
    about: high-FODMAP to avoid, 304; low-
        FODMAP list of, 297, 301
    Banana Cookie Dough Nice Cream, 242
    Chocolate Chip Cookies, 217
    Chocolate Chip Energy Bites, 268
    Chocolate Coconut Balls, 216

Chocolate Coconut Cookies, 215
Coconut Cacao Hazelnut Smoothie Bowl,
    45
Dark Chocolate–Covered Pretzels, 270
Dark Chocolate Glaze, 233
Grilled S'mores Sandwich, 197
Nutty Fudge, 226
Overnight Banana Chocolate Oats, 59
Paleo Fudge, 225
Peanut Butter Chocolate Mug Cake, 243
Peppermint Patties, 219
Cilantro-Lime Dressing, 101
Cinnamon, 33–34
Cinnamon Spice Granola, 38
Citrus
    about: as digestive aid, 34; lemon water
        benefits, 34
    Brie and Orange Marmalade Sandwich,
        125
    Cilantro-Lime Dressing, 101
    Citrus Fennel and Mint Salad, 89
    Citrus Flank Steak, 131
    Citrusy Swordfish Skewers, 167
    Lemon and Mozzarella Polenta Pizza, 176
    Lemon Kale Salad, 99
    Lemon Poppy Seed Muffins with Lemon
        Glaze, 239
    Lemon Thyme Chicken, 137
    Orange Chicken and Broccoli Stir-Fry, 134
    Orange Tempeh and Rice Salad, 181
    Raspberry Lemon Chia Seed Jam, 246
    Raspberry Lemon Oatmeal Bars, 51
    Vegan Lemon Poppy Seed Muffins, 238
Cobbler, mixed berry, 230
Coconut
    about: aminos as soy alternative, 101;
        ready-made cream, 94; toasting, 46
    Banana Coconut Nice Cream, 242
    Chocolate Coconut Balls, 216
    Chocolate Coconut Cookies, 215
    Coconut Balls, 222
    Coconut Cacao Hazelnut Smoothie Bowl,
        45
    Coconut Cinnamon Popcorn, 267
    Coconut-Crusted Fish with Pineapple
        Relish, 162
    Coconut Curry Lemongrass Soup, 86
    Coconut Rice, 106
    Coconut Shrimp with Pineapple Sauce, 69
    Coconut Whipped Cream, 232
    Maple Cinnamon Coconut Chia Seed
        Pudding, 236
    Panko-Coconut Fish Sticks, 201
    Strawberry Coconut Almond Smoothie,
        274
    Tempeh Coconut Curry Bowls, 172
    Toasted Coconut Almond Millet, 112
    Toasted Coconut Flake Butter, 286
Collard Green Wraps with Thai Peanut
    Dressing, 191
Collard Green Eggs and Ham Breakfast Wrap,

209

Condiments. *See* Sauces, dressings, and condiments

Cookies and bars, **213–27**
    about: alcohol-free vanilla extract for, 223; high-FODMAP to avoid, 304–5; low-FODMAP list of, 298–99
    Buckwheat Thumbprint Cookies, 218
    Chai-Spice Cookies, 224
    Chocolate Chip Cookies, 217
    Chocolate Coconut Balls, 216
    Chocolate Coconut Cookies, 215
    Coconut Balls, 222
    Cranberry Walnut Oat Cookies, 223
    Molasses Cookies, 220
    No-Bake Crispy Almond Pecan Bars, 227
    Nut-Free Cranberry Granola Bars, 214
    Nutty Fudge, 226
    Paleo Fudge, 225
    Peanut Butter Cookies, 215
    Peppermint Patties, 219
    Quinoa Cookies, 221

Coq au Vin, 143

Corn and cornmeal
    about: low-FODMAP diet and, 166; popcorn selection, 267; precautionary tip, 28; roasting corn in oven, 133
    Baked Cornflake-Crusted Chicken Tenders with Maple Mustard, 196
    Coconut Cinnamon Popcorn, 267
    Confetti Corn, 114
    Cornflake-Crusted Chicken Wraps, 197
    Cornmeal-Crusted Tilapia, 165
    Goat Cheese and Potato Tacos with Red Chili Cream Sauce, 182
    Mexican Risotto, 173
    Mini Polenta Pizzas, 65
    Polenta-Crusted Chicken, 149
    Pumpkin Spice Pecan Cornbread, 244
    Quinoa, Corn, and Zucchini Fritters, 70
    Stuffed Peppers with Ground Turkey, 133

Corn syrup, high-fructose, 22

Cranberries. *See* Berries

Cream of Muesli, 48

Creamy Halibut, 164

Crepes. *See* Pancakes and crepes

Crispy Baked Chicken with Gravy, 153

Cucumbers
    Aloe Vera Rewind, 273
    Cucumber Goat Cheese Sandwich, 122
    Cucumber Melon Water, 273
    Open-Faced Shrimp Salad Sandwich with Cucumbers, 124

Cumin Turkey with Fennel, 138

Curry
    about: pastes and FODMAPs, 172
    Chicken, Sweet Potato, and Spinach Curry, 151
    Clever Curry Mayonnaise, 255
    Coconut Curry Lemongrass Soup, 86
    Curry Chickpea and Vegetable Spread

Sandwich, 125
    Fish Curry, 95
    Red Curry Paste, 255
    Tempeh Coconut Curry Bowls, 172

Dairy products
    high-FODMAP to avoid, 304
    lactose-free alternatives FODMAP levels, 296
    lactose levels, 20–21
    low-FODMAP list of, 297

Desserts, **229–44**. *See also* Cookies and bars; Snacks
    about: gums and FODMAP content, 239; high-FODMAP to avoid, 305; symptom diary for, 23
    Banana Almond Nice Cream, 243
    Banana Coconut Nice Cream, 242
    Banana Cookie Dough Nice Cream, 242
    Blueberry Granola Crisp, 237
    Buttercream Lactose-Free Icing, 233
    Carrot Cake with Cream Cheese Frosting, 241
    Coconut Whipped Cream, 232
    Dark Chocolate Glaze, 233
    Lemon Poppy Seed Muffins with Lemon Glaze, 239
    Maple Cinnamon Coconut Chia Seed Pudding, 236
    Mixed Berry Cobbler, 230
    Peanut Butter Chocolate Mug Cake, 243
    Pie Crust, 284
    Pumpkin Bread, 236
    Pumpkin Doughnuts, 234
    Pumpkin Pie Mug Cake, 244
    Pumpkin Spice Cupcakes, 235
    Pumpkin Spice Pecan Cornbread, 244
    Strawberry Shortcake, 231
    Sweet Vegan Mixed Berry Tart, 240
    Vanilla Frosting, 237
    Vegan Lemon Poppy Seed Muffins, 238

Digestion, foods aiding, 33–35

Digestive disorders (FGIDs), 13, 35. *See also specific disorders*

Dill Dipping Sauce, 253

Dill sauce, fresh, 162

Dinner, menu plans, 289–90

Dinner, symptom diary for, 23

Dips and spreads. *See* Appetizers

Disaccharides, 20–21

Doughnuts, pumpkin, 234

Dragon fruit smoothie, 39

Dressings. *See* Sauces, dressings, and condiments

Drinks, **271–79**. *See also* Smoothies and smoothie bowls
    about: high-FODMAP to avoid, 306–7; low-FODMAP list of, 299–301
    Aloe Vera Rewind, 273
    Blueberry Ginger Water, 276
    Carrot Pineapple Ginger Juice, 274
    Cucumber Melon Water, 273

Ginger Maple Tea, 272
    Warm Ginger Tea, 272

Eating out, 31–33

Eggplants
    Baba Ghanoush, 64
    Baba Ghanoush Sandwich, 122
    Mediterranean Noodles, 185
    Mini Baked Eggplant Pizza Bites, 66
    Summer Vegetable Pasta, 177

Egg replacer, flax, 283

Eggs. *See also* Pancakes and crepes
    about: precautionary tip, 28
    Basic Mayonnaise, 247
    Butter Lettuce Salad with Poached Egg and Bacon, 103
    Collard Green Eggs and Ham Breakfast Wrap, 209
    Delicioso Breakfast Tacos, 55
    Eggs Baked in Heirloom Tomatoes, 49
    Eggs with Spinach and Chickpeas, 54
    Mexican Egg Brunch, 53
    Pesto Eggs Rice Bowl, 51
    Quinoa, Egg, Ham, and Cheese Breakfast Muffins, 52
    Roman Egg Drop Soup, 80
    Savory Sourdough Strata, 61
    Shakshuka for Two, 50
    Tomato and Leek Frittata, 56
    Tomato Spinach Frittata Muffins, 40

Elimination Phase, 23, 24–25, 27, 293, 303

Fats and oils, 297

Fennel
    Citrus Fennel and Mint Salad, 89
    Cumin Turkey with Fennel, 138
    Fennel Pomegranate Salad, 88
    Mixed Grains, Seeds, and Vegetable Bowl, 179
    Pork and Fennel Meatballs, 128

Fermentation process, 19

Fermented foods, 34

Fiber supplements, 34–35

Filet Mignon Salad, 104

Fish and shellfish, **155–70**
    about: cornmeal uses, 165; poaching salmon, 159
    Atlantic Cod with Basil Walnut Sauce, 168
    Bacon-Wrapped Maple Scallops, 167
    Baked Moroccan-Style Halibut, 170
    Basic Baked Scallops, 164
    Citrusy Swordfish Skewers, 167
    Coconut-Crusted Fish with Pineapple Relish, 162
    Coconut Shrimp with Pineapple Sauce, 69
    Cornmeal-Crusted Tilapia, 165
    Creamy Halibut, 164
    Fish and Chips, 166
    Fish Curry, 95
    Grilled Swordfish with Pineapple Salsa, 157
    Light Tuna Casserole, 160
    Maple-Glazed Salmon, 169
    Mediterranean Flaky Fish with Vegetables,

161
Open-Faced Shrimp Salad Sandwich with Cucumbers, 124
Panko-Coconut Fish Sticks, 201
Poached Salmon with Tarragon Sauce, 159
Rita's Linguine with Clam Sauce, 163
Salmon Cakes with Fresh Dill Sauce, 162
Salmon with Herbs, 158
Seafood Piccata, 140
Seafood Risotto, 156
Seafood Stock, 79
Seared Sesame Tuna, 158
Shrimp and Cheese Casserole, 157
Shrimp Puttanesca with Linguine, 168
Smoked Salmon Hand Rolls, 68
Sole Meunière, 163
Vietnamese Summer Rolls, 75
Flourless Banana Cinnamon Pancakes, 41
Flourless Vegan Banana Peanut Butter Pancakes, 41
Flours, gluten-free
about, 224; buying gluten-free buckwheat, 218
Flour Mix 1 for Gluten-Free Bread, 282
Flour Mix 2 for Gluten-Free Bread, 283
Gluten-Free All-Purpose 1-to-1 Flour, 282
Gluten-Free Pizza Dough, 285
Pie Crust, 284
Flours, high-FODMAP, 305
Flours, low-FODMAP, 299
FODMAPs
acronym explained, 17
defined, 17–18
disaccharides, 20–21
fermentation process, 19
groups of, 19–22
low- and high- foods list, 292–307
malabsorption possibility, 19
moderate levels explained, 27, 293
monosaccharides, 21–22
oligosaccharides and fructans, 19–20
polyols, 22
Food allergy/intolerance, 15
Food labels, reading, 25–26
Fructans and oligosaccharides, 19–20
Fructo-oligosaccharides (FOS), 20
Fructose malabsorption, 21–22
Fruit. See also specific fruit
about: best time to eat, 21; fructose malabsorption and, 21–22; high-FODMAP to avoid, 303; low-FODMAP list of, 294; snack servings and suggestions, 292; storing, 31
Fruit and Cheese Kebabs, 211
Functional gastrointestinal disorders (FGIDs), 13, 35. See also specific disorders
Galacto-oligosaccharides (GOS), 20
Garlic, cooking with, 20
Garlic, substitute for, 65
Garlicky Parsnip and Carrot Fries, 110
Garlic sauce, sweet chili, 256

Garlic Turmeric Dressing, 260
Gas, preventing, 33
Gibson, Dr. Peter, 12
Ginger
about: as digestive aid, 34
Blueberry Ginger Water, 276
Carrot and Ginger Soup, 84
Carrot Pineapple Ginger Juice, 274
Ginger Maple Tea, 272
Ginger Sesame Salad Dressing, 261
Moroccan-Inspired Carrot Ginger Soup, 91
Sesame and Ginger Bok Choy, 118
Tamari-Ginger Dressing, 97
Warm Ginger Tea, 272
Gluten and wheat, 28–30
Gluten-free baking powder, 241
Gluten-Free Cinnamon and Sugar Soft Pretzels, 266
Gluten-free flours. See Flours
Gluten-Free Pizza Dough, 285
Gluten intolerance, 16. See also Celiac disease
Grains, FODMAP levels, 298, 305–6
Granola. See Oats
Greek Pasta Salad, 87
Greek Salad Wrap, 124
Green beans, lemon pepper, 118
Green Dragon Smoothie Bowl, 39
Grilled S'mores Sandwich, 197
Gums, about, 239
Gut-Friendly Smoothie, 275
Halibut, 164, 170
Ham
Chicken, Ham, and Blueberry Melt, 199
Collard Green Eggs and Ham Breakfast Wrap, 209
Ham and Cheese Crepes, 43
Prosciutto di Parma Salad, 100
Prosciutto-Stuffed Chicken, 132
Quinoa, Egg, Ham, and Cheese Breakfast Muffins, 52
Hasselback Potatoes, 117
Herbed Mashed Potatoes, 106
Herbed Yellow Squash, 108
Herbes de Provence Almonds, 73
Herbs, FODMAP levels, 302
High-fructose corn syrup (HFCS), 22
Indian-Spiced Mixed Nuts, 71
Irritable bowel syndrome (IBS)
diagnosing, 14
digestive aids, 33–35
living with, 9–10
low-FODMAP diet and, 10, 11, 12, 27, 29
mild symptoms, 10
prevalence of, 10, 19
Rome III criteria for, 14
symptoms, 9, 10, 14
wellness tips, 33–36
working with doctor, 16–17
Jams. See Sauces, dressings, and condiments
Jeremy's Revival Smoothie, 275
Kale

about: precautionary tip, 28
Abundantly Happy Kale Salad, 90
Kale Chips, 267
Kale Sesame Salad with Tamari-Ginger Dressing, 97
Lemon Kale Salad, 99
Potato and Kale Gratin, 111
Turkey Pasta with Kale, 154
Kebabs and skewers, 167, 211
Ketchup, artisanal, 248
Kids, snacks and main dishes for, **193**–212
Ants on a Trunk, 195
Baked Cornflake-Crusted Chicken Tenders with Maple Mustard, 196
Barbecue Chicken Pizza, 205
Broccoli and Cheddar Quesadilla, 208
Chicken, Ham, and Blueberry Melt, 199
Chicken Pizza Quesadilla, 207
Chicken Potpie, 206
Collard Green Eggs and Ham Breakfast Wrap, 209
Cornflake-Crusted Chicken Wraps, 197
Fiesta Nachos, 198
Fruit and Cheese Kebabs, 211
Grilled S'mores Sandwich, 197
Mac 'n' Cheese Taco Bake, 204
Maple Almond Strawberry Banana Rice Cake, 212
Meatloaf Muffins, 203
Panko-Coconut Fish Sticks, 201
PB and J Kebabs, 211
Peanut Butter Banana Quesadilla, 202
Pumpkin Parfait, 194
Quinoa Pizza Muffins, 210
Spaghetti and Meatballs, 202
Strawberry Toast, 194
SunButter and Jelly Crepes, 195
Turkey Sloppy Joes, 200
Vegetable and Cream Cheese Sandwich, 199
Kombucha, 34
Labels (food), reading, 25–26
Lactose, dairy and, 20–21
Latin Quinoa-Stuffed Peppers, 178
Leeks, in Tomato and Leek Frittata, 56
Leeks, in Vegan Carrot, Leek, and Saffron Soup, 94
Lemon. See Citrus
Lemongrass, in Coconut Curry Lemongrass Soup, 86
Lemon Pepper Green Beans, 118
Lentils. See Beans and other legumes
Lettuce cups, chicken, 67
Low-FODMAP diet
celiac disease and, 15–16
Challenge Phase, 23–24, 25, 293
defined, 11
development of, 12
eating out, 31–33
Elimination Phase, 23, 24–25, 27, 293, 303
food allergy/intolerance and, 15

foods to avoid, 26, 303–7
gluten intolerance and, 16
IBS and, 10, 11, 12, 14, 27, 29
low-FODMAP foods that might be
    troublesome, 28
make-ahead items, 30–31
reading food labels for, 25–26
reasons for going on, 13, 17
reintroducing foods, 25
serving amounts, 26–28
sources for lists of foods on, 13
wellness tips, 33–36
wheat, gluten and, 28–30
Lunch, menu plans, 289–90
Lunch, symptom diary for, 23
Mac 'n' Cheese, 189
Mac 'n' Cheese Taco Bake, 204
Make-ahead items, 30–31
Maple Almond Strawberry Banana Rice Cake,
    212
Maple Cinnamon Coconut Chia Seed Pudding,
    236
Maple Dressing, 258
Maple glaze, pumpkin, 257
Maple-Glazed Salmon, 169
Maple Mustard Dipping Sauce, 196
Maple Mustard Dressing, 258
Mayonnaise recipes, 247, 255
Measurement conversions, 312
Meatballs, 128, 129, 149, 202
Meatloaf Muffins, 203
Meats and animal proteins. See also specific
    meats
    high-FODMAP to avoid, 304
    low-FODMAP list of, 297–98
    make-ahead items, 30
    precautionary tip, 28
Mediterranean Buckwheat Salad, 109
Mediterranean Flaky Fish with Vegetables, 161
Mediterranean Noodles, 185
Melon, in Cucumber Melon Water, 273
Menu plans and snack suggestions, 288–91
Mexican Egg Brunch, 53
Mexican Risotto, 173
Millet
    about: nutritional benefits, 112
    Fish and Chips with, 166
    Flour Mix 2 for Gluten-Free Bread, 282
    Toasted Coconut Almond Millet, 112
Mini Baked Eggplant Pizza Bites, 66
Mini Polenta Pizzas, 65
Mint
    about: as digestive aid, 34
    Citrus Fennel and Mint Salad, 89
    Peppermint Patties, 219
    Raspberry Banana Mint Chia Pudding, 45
Mixed Grains, Seeds, and Vegetable Bowl, 179
Molasses Cookies, 220
Mom's Chicken Salad, 102
Monosaccharides, 21–22
Moroccan-Inspired Carrot Ginger Soup, 91

Moroccan-style halibut, baked, 170
Muesli recipes, 47, 48
Mustard and maple. See Maple Mustard
    Dipping Sauce; Maple Mustard Dressing
Mustard and Thyme Roasted Chicken, 152
Nachos, 198
No-Bake Crispy Almond Pecan Bars, 227
Nori roll, vegetable, 179
Nut-Free Cranberry Granola Bars, 214
Nuts and seeds. See also Peanuts and peanut
    butter
    about: aiding digestion, 34; almond
        milk and FODMAPs, 189; flaxseeds,
        34; grinding seeds, 48; high-FODMAP
        to avoid, 304; low-FODMAP list of, 296;
        low-FODMAP serving of nuts, 71; snack
        servings and suggestions, 292; soaking
        nuts, 47, 285; SunButter, 195
    Amaranth Breakfast, 60
    Ants on a Trunk, 195
    Autumn Breakfast Chia Bowl, 38
    Banana Almond Nice Cream, 243
    Banana Nut Boat, 270
    Basil Walnut Sauce, 168
    Blueberry Chia Seed Jam, 246
    Blueberry Granola Crisp, 237
    Broccoli Greenballs, 180
    Cranberry Almond Granola, 57
    Cranberry Walnut Oat Cookies, 223
    Cream of Muesli, 48
    Flax Egg, Egg Replacer, 283
    Ginger Sesame Salad Dressing, 261
    Herbes de Provence Almonds, 73
    Indian-Spiced Mixed Nuts, 71
    Jubilant Muesli Mix, 47
    Lemon Poppy Seed Muffins with Lemon
        Glaze, 239
    Maple Almond Strawberry Banana Rice
        Cake, 212
    Maple Cinnamon Coconut Chia Seed
        Pudding, 236
    Mixed Grains, Seeds, and Vegetable Bowl,
        179
    No-Bake Crispy Almond Pecan Bars, 227
    Nutty Fudge, 226
    Overnight Carrot Cake Oats and Walnuts,
        59
    Pumpkin Seed Dressing, 259
    Raspberry Lemon Chia Seed Jam, 246
    Roasted Pumpkin Seeds (with Cinnamon
        and Sugar option), 269
    salads with. See Salads
    smoothie bowls with. See Smoothies and
        smoothie bowls
    smoothies with. See Smoothies and
        smoothie bowls
    Strawberry Chia Seed Jam, 247
    SunButter and Jelly Crepes, 195
    Swiss Chard with Lentils, Pine Nuts, and
        Feta Cheese, 186
    Tahini Dressing, 259

Toasted Coconut Almond Millet, 112
Vanilla Maple Almond Butter, 286
Vegan Lemon Poppy Seed Muffins, 238
Vegan Parmesan Cheez, 287
Oats
    about: precautionary tip, 28, 38
    Autumn Breakfast Chia Bowl, 38
    Blueberry Granola Crisp, 237
    Chocolate Chip Energy Bites, 268
    Cinnamon Spice Granola, 38
    Cranberry Almond Granola, 57
    Cream of Muesli, 48
    Nut-Free Cranberry Granola Bars, 214
    Overnight Banana Chocolate Oats, 59
    Overnight Carrot Cake Oats and Walnuts,
        59
    Overnight Peanut Butter Pumpkin Spice
        Oats, 58
    Raspberry Lemon Oatmeal Bars, 51
oligosaccharides and fructans, 19–20
Onions, FODMAPs and, 20, 40
Onions, substitute for, 65
Open-Faced Shrimp Salad Sandwich with
    Cucumbers, 124
Orange, Red, and Green Buckwheat Salad, 89
Overnight Banana Chocolate Oats, 59
Overnight Carrot Cake Oats and Walnuts, 59
Overnight Peanut Butter Pumpkin Spice Oats,
    58
Pad Thai, vegan, 188
Paixão Smoothie, 276
Paleo Fudge, 225
Pancakes and crepes
    about: other pancake ingredients, 41
    Flourless Banana Cinnamon Pancakes, 41
    Flourless Vegan Banana Peanut Butter
        Pancakes, 41
    Ham and Cheese Crepes, 43
    Pumpkin Spice Crepes, 44
    SunButter and Jelly Crepes, 195
    Vegan Buckwheat Crepes, 42
Panko-Coconut Fish Sticks, 201
Pão de Queijo (Cheese Bread), 72
Papaya, 101
Parmesan-Crusted Chicken, 144
Parsnips
    Garlicky Parsnip and Carrot Fries, 110
    Roasted Parsnips with Rosemary, 109
    Root-a-Burgers, 113
Passionfruit, smoothies with, 46, 276
Pasta
    about: high-FODMAP to avoid, 305–6; low-
        FODMAP list of, 298; rice, making ahead
        and storing, 31
    Barbecue Pork Macaroni and Cheese, 148
    Greek Pasta Salad, 87
    Mac 'n' Cheese, 189
    Mac 'n' Cheese Taco Bake, 204
    Mediterranean Noodles, 185
    Rita's Linguine with Clam Sauce, 163
    Shrimp Puttanesca with Linguine, 168

Spaghetti and Meatballs, 202
squash alternatives. *See* Squash
Summer Vegetable Pasta, 177
Turkey Bolognese with Pasta, 142
Turkey Pasta with Kale, 154
Vegan Pad Thai, 188
Vegetable and Rice Noodle Bowl, 184
Peanuts and peanut butter
about: choosing natural peanut butter, 234
Flourless Vegan Banana Peanut Butter
Pancakes, 41
Overnight Peanut Butter Pumpkin Spice
Oats, 58
Paleo Fudge, 225
PB and J Kebabs, 211
Peanut Butter Banana Quesadilla, 202
Peanut Butter Chocolate Mug Cake, 243
Peanut Butter Cookies, 215
Peanut Butter Lover Smoothie, 277
Pumpkin Doughnuts, 234
Thai Peanut Dressing, 263
Vegan Pad Thai, 188
Peppers
Confetti Corn, 114
Latin Quinoa-Stuffed Peppers, 178
Mexican Risotto, 173
Red Pepper Soup, 83
sauces with. *See* Sauces, dressings, and
condiments
Stuffed Peppers with Ground Turkey, 133
Pesto Eggs Rice Bowl, 51
Pesto Sauce, 253
Pie Crust, 284
Pineapple
about: as digestive aid, 34
Carrot Pineapple Ginger Juice, 274
Pineapple Relish, 162
Pineapple Salsa, 157
Pineapple Sauce, 69
Pineapple Turmeric Smoothie, 279
Pizza
Barbecue Chicken Pizza, 205
Chicken Pizza Quesadilla, 207
Gluten-Free Pizza Dough, 285
Lemon and Mozzarella Polenta Pizza, 176
Mini Baked Eggplant Pizza Bites, 66
Mini Polenta Pizzas, 65
Quinoa Pizza Muffins, 210
Poached Salmon with Tarragon Sauce, 159
Polenta. *See* Corn and cornmeal
Polyols, 22
Pomegranate
Fennel Pomegranate Salad, 88
Pomegranate Salsa, 261
Zucchini Ribbon Salad with Goat Cheese,
Pine Nuts, and Pomegranate, 99
Popcorn, coconut cinnamon, 267
Pork. *See also* Ham
Bacon-Wrapped Maple Scallops, 167
Barbecue Pork Macaroni and Cheese, 148
Butter Lettuce Salad with Poached Egg

and Bacon, 103
Pork and Fennel Meatballs, 128
Pork Chops with Carrots and Toasted
Buckwheat, 136
Sourdough Meatballs, 149
Potatoes
about: precautionary tip, 28
Fish and Chips, 166
Goat Cheese and Potato Tacos with Red
Chili Cream Sauce, 182
Hasselback Potatoes, 117
Herbed Mashed Potatoes, 106
Potato and Kale Gratin, 111
Potato Soup, 82
Vegan Potato Salad, Cypriot-Style, 175
Warm Basil and Walnut Potato Salad, 98
Potpie, chicken, 206
Pretzels, dark chocolate–covered, 270
Pretzels, soft gluten-free cinnamon and sugar,
266
Probiotics, 34
Prosciutto. *See* Ham
Protein powders, 39
Pumpkin
about: canned, 147
Overnight Peanut Butter Pumpkin Spice
Oats, 58
Pumpkin Bread, 236
Pumpkin Doughnuts, 234
Pumpkin Maple Glaze, 257
Pumpkin Maple Roast Chicken, 147
Pumpkin Parfait, 194
Pumpkin Pie Mug Cake, 244
Pumpkin Seed Dressing, 259
Pumpkin Spice Crepes, 44
Pumpkin Spice Cupcakes, 235
Pumpkin Spice Pecan Cornbread, 244
Roasted Pumpkin Seeds (with Cinnamon
and Sugar option), 269
Quesadillas. *See* Snacks
Quinoa
about: make-ahead items, 31; storing, 31
Jubilant Muesli Mix, 47
Latin Quinoa-Stuffed Peppers, 178
Mixed Grains, Seeds, and Vegetable Bowl,
179
Quinoa, Corn, and Zucchini Fritters, 70
Quinoa, Egg, Ham, and Cheese Breakfast
Muffins, 52
Quinoa Cookies, 221
Quinoa Pizza Muffins, 210
Quinoa Tabbouleh, 119
Turkey Quinoa Meatballs with Mozzarella,
129
Raspberries. *See* Berries
Red Chili Cream Sauce, 182
Red pepper flakes, about, 184
Red Pepper Soup, 83
Relaxation and stress reduction, 35–36
Resources, additional, 311
Restaurants, low-FODMAP diet and, 31–33

Rice
about: make-ahead items, 31
Coconut Rice, 106
Crispy Baked Chicken with Gravy, 153
Maple Almond Strawberry Banana Rice
Cake, 212
Mexican Risotto, 173
Mixed Grains, Seeds, and Vegetable Bowl,
179
No-Bake Crispy Almond Pecan Bars, 227
Orange Tempeh and Rice Salad, 181
Pesto Eggs Rice Bowl, 51
Seafood Risotto, 156
Stuffed Peppers with Ground Turkey, 133
Turmeric Rice with Cranberries, 185
Vegetable and Rice Noodle Bowl, 184
Vegetable Fried Rice, 187
Rita's Linguine with Clam Sauce, 163
Roast Beef Tenderloin with Parmesan Crust,
130
Roasted Maple Dill Carrots, 116
Roasted Parsnips with Rosemary, 109
Roasted Pumpkin Seeds (with Cinnamon and
Sugar option), 269
Roasted Tomato Sauce, 251
Rolls, appetizer. *See* Appetizers
Roman Egg Drop Soup, 80
Root-a-Burgers, 113
Salad dressings. *See* Sauces, dressings, and
condiments
Salads, **77**
Abundantly Happy Kale Salad, 90
Baked Papaya and Chicken Salad with
Cilantro-Lime Dressing, 101
Butter Lettuce Salad with Poached Egg
and Bacon, 103
Citrus Fennel and Mint Salad, 89
Fennel Pomegranate Salad, 88
Filet Mignon Salad, 104
Glorious Strawberry Salad, 88
Greek Pasta Salad, 87
Kale Sesame Salad with Tamari-Ginger
Dressing, 97
Lemon Kale Salad, 99
Mediterranean Buckwheat Salad, 109
Mom's Chicken Salad, 102
Orange, Red, and Green Buckwheat Salad,
89
Orange Tempeh and Rice Salad, 181
Prosciutto di Parma Salad, 100
Vegan Potato Salad, Cypriot-Style, 175
Warm Basil and Walnut Potato Salad, 98
Zucchini Ribbon Salad with Goat Cheese,
Pine Nuts, and Pomegranate, 99
Salmon. *See* Fish and shellfish
Sandwiches and wraps, **121**–26. *See also* Tacos
Avocado, Goat Cheese, and Spinach Panini,
123
Baba Ghanoush Sandwich, 122
Barbecue Chicken Wrap, 126
Brie and Orange Marmalade Sandwich,

125
Chicken, Ham, and Blueberry Melt, 199
Chicken Burgers, 128
Collard Green Wraps with Thai Peanut
  Dressing, 191
Collard Green Eggs and Ham Breakfast
  Wrap, 209
condiments for. See Sauces, dressings, and
  condiments
Cornflake-Crusted Chicken Wraps, 197
Cucumber Goat Cheese Sandwich, 122
Curry Chickpea and Vegetable Spread
  Sandwich, 125
Greek Salad Wrap, 124
Open-Faced Shrimp Salad Sandwich with
  Cucumbers, 124
Turkey Pesto Wrap, 123
Turkey Sloppy Joes, 200
Vegetable and Cream Cheese Sandwich,
  199
Sauces, dressings, and condiments, 245–63
  about: choosing barbecue sauce, 205; high-
  FODMAP to avoid, 306; low-FODMAP list
  of, 301; make-ahead items, 30; vegan fish
  sauce, 187; wine for Bolognese sauce, 142
Aioli, 249
Artisanal Ketchup, 248
Basic Marinara Sauce, 252
Basic Mayonnaise, 247
Basil Sauce, 249
Basil Walnut Sauce, 168
Blueberry Chia Seed Jam, 246
Burger Sauce, 250
Caesar Salad Dressing, 260
Chermoula, 254
Chicken Gravy, 153
Cilantro-Lime Dressing, 101
Clam Sauce, 163
Clever Curry Mayonnaise, 255
Dill Dipping Sauce, 253
Fiesta Salsa, 262
Fresh Dill Sauce, 162
Garlic Turmeric Dressing, 260
Ginger Sesame Salad Dressing, 261
Maple Dressing, 258
Maple Mustard Dipping Sauce, 196
Maple Mustard Dressing, 258
Pesto Sauce, 253
Pineapple Relish, 162
Pineapple Salsa, 157
Pineapple Sauce, 69
Pomegranate Salsa, 261
Pumpkin Maple Glaze, 257
Pumpkin Seed Dressing, 259
Raspberry Lemon Chia Seed Jam, 246
Red Chili Cream Sauce, 182
Red Curry Paste, 255
Roasted Tomato Sauce, 251
Simple Brown Syrup, 263
Strawberry Chia Seed Jam, 247
Sweet Barbecue Sauce, 248

Sweet Chili Garlic Sauce, 256
Tahini Dressing, 259
Tamari-Ginger Dressing, 97
Tarragon Sauce, 159
Tartar Sauce, 254
Teriyaki Sauce, 184
Thai Peanut Dressing, 263
Tomato Paste, 251
Tomato Puree, 250
Tzatziki Dressing, 257
Sauerkraut, 34
Savory Baked Tofu, 186
Scallops, 164, 167
Scratch, ingredient recipes from, 281–87
Seafood. See Fish and shellfish
Seared Sesame Tuna, 158
Seeds. See Nuts and seeds
Serving amounts, 26–28
Sesame and Ginger Bok Choy, 118
Shakshuka for Two, 50
Shamrock Shake, 278
Shepherd, Dr. Sue, 12
Shrimp. See Fish and shellfish
Side dishes. See Vegetables and sides
Slow Cooker Chicken Tagine, 93
Smoked Salmon Hand Rolls, 68
Smoothies and smoothie bowls
  about: protein powders for, 39
  Banana-Nut Smoothie, 278
  Blue Moon Smoothie, 277
  Coconut Cacao Hazelnut Smoothie Bowl,
    45
  Green Dragon Smoothie Bowl, 39
  Gut-Friendly Smoothie, 275
  Jeremy's Revival Smoothie, 275
  Paixão Smoothie, 276
  Passionfruit Smoothie Bowl, 46
  Peanut Butter Lover Smoothie, 277
  Pineapple Turmeric Smoothie, 279
  Shamrock Shake, 278
  Strawberry Coconut Almond Smoothie, 274
  Strawberry Morning Smoothie, 279
Snacks, 265–70
  about: high-FODMAP to avoid, 304–5; low-
  FODMAP list of, 298–99; suggestions for
  menu plans and, 288–91; symptom diary
  for, 23
  Ants on a Trunk, 195
  Banana Nut Boat, 270
  Broccoli and Cheddar Quesadilla, 208
  Chicken Pizza Quesadilla, 207
  Chocolate Chip Energy Bites, 268
  Coconut Cinnamon Popcorn, 267
  Dark Chocolate–Covered Pretzels, 270
  Fiesta Nachos, 198
  Fruit and Cheese Kebabs, 211
  Gluten-Free Cinnamon and Sugar Soft
    Pretzels, 266
  Grilled S'mores Sandwich, 197
  Kale Chips, 267
  Maple Almond Strawberry Banana Rice

  Cake, 212
  PB and J Kebabs, 211
  Peanut Butter Banana Quesadilla, 202
  Pumpkin Parfait, 194
  Quinoa Pizza Muffins, 210
  Roasted Pumpkin Seeds (with Cinnamon
    and Sugar option), 269
  Strawberry Toast, 194
  SunButter and Jelly Crepes, 195
Sole Meunière, 163
Soups, 77
  about: make-ahead items, 31; storing, 31
  Beef with Buckwheat Soup, 92
  Carrot and Ginger Soup, 84
  Chicken and Dumplings Soup, 81
  Chicken Tortilla Soup, 96
  Coconut Curry Lemongrass Soup, 86
  Easy Onion- and Garlic-Free Chicken
    Stock, 78
  Fish Curry, 95
  Lentil Chili, 85
  Moroccan-Inspired Carrot Ginger Soup, 91
  Potato Soup, 82
  Red Pepper Soup, 83
  Roman Egg Drop Soup, 80
  Seafood Stock, 79
  Slow Cooker Chicken Tagine, 93
  Vegan Carrot, Leek, and Saffron Soup, 94
  Vegetable Stock, 82
Sourdough Meatballs, 149
Soy alternative, 101
Spaghetti and Meatballs, 202
Spaghetti Squash with Goat Cheese, 119
Spices, FODMAP levels, 302
Spinach
  Avocado, Goat Cheese, and Spinach Panini,
    123
  Beef with Spinach and Sweet Potatoes, 135
  Chicken, Sweet Potato, and Spinach Curry,
    151
  Eggs with Spinach and Chickpeas, 54
  Jeremy's Revival Smoothie, 275
  Mixed Grains, Seeds, and Vegetable Bowl,
    179
  Roman Egg Drop Soup, 80
  salads with. See Salads
  Savory Sourdough Strata, 61
  Shakshuka for Two, 50
  Spinach and Feta-Stuffed Chicken Breast,
    137
  Sweet and Savory Brazilian Meat and
    Cheese Tart, 145
  Tomato Spinach Frittata Muffins, 40
Squash
  about: mandolin for slicing zucchini, 146
  Herbed Yellow Squash, 108
  Mediterranean Flaky Fish with Vegetables,
    161
  Quinoa, Corn, and Zucchini Fritters, 70
  Spaghetti Squash with Goat Cheese, 119
  Summer Vegetable Pasta, 177

Zoodles with Pesto, 114
Zucchini Lasagna with Meat Sauce, 146
Zucchini Ribbon Salad with Goat Cheese,
    Pine Nuts, and Pomegranate, 99
Stocks. *See* Soups
Strawberries. *See* Berries
Stress, reducing, 35–36
Stuffed peppers, 133, 178
Sugar alcohols (polyols), 22
Sugar-free foods to avoid, 307
Sugars and sweeteners, 297, 306
Summer rolls, Vietnamese, 75
Summer Vegetable Pasta, 177
SunButter and Jelly Crepes, 195
Sweet and Savory Brazilian Meat and Cheese
    Tart, 145
Sweeteners, 297, 306
Sweet potatoes
    about: low-FODMAP amount, 115
    Beef with Spinach and Sweet Potatoes, 135
    Chicken, Sweet Potato, and Spinach Curry,
        151
    Collard Green Eggs and Ham Breakfast
        Wrap, 209
    Mixed Grains, Seeds, and Vegetable Bowl,
        179
    Sweet Potato with Maple Yogurt and
        Pumpkin Seeds, 115
Sweets. *See* Cookies and bars; Desserts; Snacks
Swiss chard
    Shakshuka for Two, 50
    Swiss Chard with Cranberries and Pine
        Nuts, 110
    Swiss Chard with Lentils, Pine Nuts, and
        Feta Cheese, 186
    Swiss Chard with Pine Nuts and Parmesan,
        107
Swordfish, 157, 167
Symptom diary, 23
Tabbouleh, quinoa, 119
Tacos
    Delicioso Breakfast Tacos, 55
    Goat Cheese and Potato Tacos with Red
        Chili Cream Sauce, 182
    Mac 'n' Cheese Taco Bake, 204
    Tempeh Tacos, 190
Tahini Dressing, 259
Tamari-Ginger Dressing, 97
Tarragon Sauce, 159
Tartar Sauce, 254
Teas, 272, 300, 307
Tempeh
    about: other uses, 181
    Orange Tempeh and Rice Salad, 181
    Tempeh Coconut Curry Bowls, 172
    Tempeh Tacos, 190
Teriyaki Sauce, 184
Tilapia, 165, 166, 201
Toasted Coconut Flake Butter, 286
Tofu
    Baked Tofu and Vegetables, 183

Savory Baked Tofu, 186
    Vietnamese Summer Rolls, 75
Tomatoes
    Artisanal Ketchup, 248
    Basic Marinara Sauce, 252
    eggs with. *See* Eggs
    Fiesta Salsa, 262
    Mediterranean Flaky Fish with Vegetables,
        161
    Roasted Tomato Sauce, 251
    Tomato Paste, 251
    Tomato Puree, 250
Tortilla soup, chicken, 96
Truffle oil, 113
Truffle salt. *See* Pizza
Turkey
    Cumin Turkey with Fennel, 138
    Meatloaf Muffins, 203
    Spaghetti and Meatballs, 202
    Stuffed Peppers with Ground Turkey, 133
    Turkey Bolognese with Pasta, 142
    Turkey Pasta with Kale, 154
    Turkey Pesto Wrap, 123
    Turkey Quinoa Meatballs with Mozzarella,
        129
    Turkey Sloppy Joes, 200
Turmeric Rice with Cranberries, 185
Tzatziki Dressing, 257
Vanilla extract, alcohol-free, 223
Vanilla Frosting, 237
Vanilla Maple Almond Butter, 286
Vegan and vegetarian main dishes, **171–91**
    about: vegan fish sauce, 187
    Baked Tofu and Vegetables, 183
    Broccoli Greenballs, 180
    Collard Green Wraps with Thai Peanut
        Dressing, 191
    Goat Cheese and Potato Tacos with Red
        Chili Cream Sauce, 182
    Latin Quinoa-Stuffed Peppers, 178
    Lemon and Mozzarella Polenta Pizza, 176
    Lentil Pie, 174
    Mac 'n' Cheese, 189
    Mediterranean Noodles, 185
    Mexican Risotto, 173
    Mixed Grains, Seeds, and Vegetable Bowl,
        179
    Orange Tempeh and Rice Salad, 181
    Savory Baked Tofu, 186
    Summer Vegetable Pasta, 177
    Swiss Chard with Lentils, Pine Nuts, and
        Feta Cheese, 186
    Tempeh Coconut Curry Bowls, 172
    Tempeh Tacos, 190
    Turmeric Rice with Cranberries, 185
    Vegan Pad Thai, 188
    Vegan Potato Salad, Cypriot-Style, 175
    Vegetable and Rice Noodle Bowl, 184
    Vegetable Fried Rice, 187
    Vegetable Nori Roll, 179
Vegan and vegetarian menu plans, 289–90

Vegan Buckwheat Crepes, 42
Vegan Lemon Poppy Seed Muffins, 238
Vegan Parmesan Cheez, 287
Vegetables and sides, **105**–19. *See also* Salads;
    specific vegetables
    about: high-FODMAP vegetables to avoid,
        303; low-FODMAP list of vegetables, 294–
        96; snack servings and suggestions, 292;
        starchy, precautionary tip, 28; storing, 31
    Coconut Rice, 106
    Confetti Corn, 114
    Garlicky Parsnip and Carrot Fries, 110
    Hasselback Potatoes, 117
    Herbed Mashed Potatoes, 106
    Herbed Yellow Squash, 108
    Lemon Pepper Green Beans, 118
    Potato and Kale Gratin, 111
    Quinoa Tabbouleh, 119
    Roasted Maple Dill Carrots, 116
    Roasted Parsnips with Rosemary, 109
    Root-a-Burgers, 113
    Sesame and Ginger Bok Choy, 118
    soups with. *See* Soups
    Spaghetti Squash with Goat Cheese, 119
    Sweet Potato with Maple Yogurt and
        Pumpkin Seeds, 115
    Swiss Chard with Cranberries and Pine
        Nuts, 110
    Swiss Chard with Pine Nuts and Parmesan,
        107
    Toasted Coconut Almond Millet, 112
    Vegetable and Cream Cheese Sandwich,
        199
    Vegetable Stock, 82
    Zoodles with Pesto, 114
Vegetarian main dishes. *See* Vegan and
    vegetarian main dishes
Vegetarian substitutes, FODMAP levels, 296,
    304
Victor's Chicken Parmesan, 139
Vietnamese Summer Rolls, 75
Wellness tips, 33–36
Wheat and gluten, 28–30
Whipped cream, coconut, 232
Wine, cooking with, 79
Wine, for Bolognese sauce, 142
Wraps. *See* Sandwiches and wraps
Yogurt
    about: smoothie bowls with, 39, 46; snack
        servings and suggestions, 291
    Pumpkin Parfait, 115
    Sweet Potato with Maple Yogurt and
        Pumpkin Seeds, 115
Zoodles with Pesto, 114
Zucchini. *See* Squash